THE
RESIDENT'S GUIDE
TO
AMBULATORY CARE

Frequently Encountered and *Commonly Confused* Clinical Conditions

FOURTH EDITION

2001-2002

Michael B. Weinstock, MD
Daniel M. Neides, MD

Anadem
Publishing

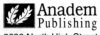
Anadem
Publishing
3620 North High Street
Columbus, OH   43214
Tel: 1 (800) 633-0055

THE RESIDENT'S GUIDE TO AMBULATORY CARE:
Frequently Encountered and *Commonly Confused* Clinical Conditions: Fourth Edition
Michael B. Weinstock
Daniel M. Neides

Second Printing

PRINTED IN THE UNITED STATES OF AMERICA

ISBN 1-890018-35-X

USING THIS BOOK
Publisher's Notes

The Guide is based upon information from sources believed to be reliable. In developing *The Guide* the publisher, authors, contributors, reviewers, and editors have made substantial efforts to make sure that the regimens, drugs, and treatments are correct and are in accordance with currently accepted standards. Readers are cautioned to use their own judgment in making clinical decisions and, when appropriate, consult and compare information from other resources since ongoing research and clinical experience yield new information and since there is the possibility of human error in developing such a comprehensive resource as this. Attention should be paid to checking the product information supplied by drug manufacturers when prescribing or administering drugs, particularly if the prescriber is not familiar with the drug or does not regularly use it.

Readers should be aware that there are legitimate differences of opinion among physicians on both clinical and ethical/moral issues in treating patients. With this in mind, readers are urged to use individual judgment in making treatment decisions, recognizing the best interests of the patient and his/her own knowledge and understanding of these issues. The publisher, authors, reviewers, contributors, and editors disclaim any liability, loss or damage as a result, directly or indirectly, from using or applying any of the contents of *The Guide*.

FOREWORD TO FIRST EDITION

Each year the scope of clinical problems encountered in Family Practice expands, especially as health care shifts to the ambulatory setting. Recognizing this, the authors have written *The Resident's Guide to Ambulatory Care*. An impressive list of outstanding physicians has also contributed to this book. It is a notable achievement, being written by residents for residents. *The Guide* is a collection of strategies, tips and practical information drawn from the authors' and contributors' observations and experience in the day-to-day management of outpatient problems. The authors are two highly committed, conscientious and hard working residents who have justifiably earned my support in their efforts. They have written this book in an easy to read and quick to reference style.

A manual of this type would be extremely valuable not only for any resident practicing ambulatory medicine, but for medical students and physicians alike. *The Resident's Guide to Ambulatory Care* belongs in the library of every person learning to provide ambulatory care.

Bill G. Gegas, M.D.
Associate Program Director
Family Practice Residency
Riverside Methodist Hospitals

Michael B. Weinstock, MD

Michael Weinstock finished his last year of Family Practice residency at Riverside Methodist Hospital in Columbus, Ohio in 1995. He is currently a Clinical Assistant Professor at The Ohio State University in the HIV clinic, a clinical instructor at Riverside Hospital's family practice program, and an emergency department attending at St. Ann's Hospital with Immediate Health Associates. Michael has practiced medicine on both a local and global scale, including volunteer medical work in Papua New Guinea, Nepal, and the West Indies. He plans to return to Nepal this fall. Michael obtained his bachelor's degree with a major in economics from Northwestern University and his medical degree from The Ohio State University College of Medicine. His medical interests include family medicine, HIV disease, tropical medicine, and emergency medicine. Other passions include skiing, backpacking, traveling and writing. He is a folk and blues acoustic singer-songwriter and recently completed a double compact disc. Michael and his wife Beth have a feisty one year old baby girl, Olivia. Daisy is the dog.

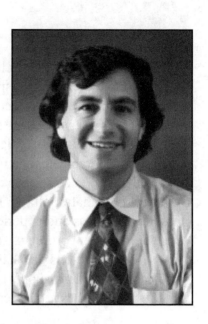

Daniel M. Neides, MD

Dr. Neides continues to practice Family Medicine in his hometown of Cleveland, Ohio. He is currently a staff physician with The Cleveland Clinic Foundation and an Assistant Professor of Family Medicine at The Ohio State University. Dr. Neides attended The Ohio State University earning both undergraduate and medical degrees. He completed his residency training at Riverside Methodist Hospitals in Columbus, Ohio. He has continued his involvement with medical education and was appointed to the admissions committee for the OSU College of Medicine. Dr. Neides was recently awarded the 1999-2000 Distinguished Educator of the Year from The Cleveland Clinic Foundation and The Ohio State University. His medical interests include pre-doctoral education and preventive medicine. When he is not practicing medicine, Dr. Neides enjoys spending time with his wife Karen, their children Melissa and David, and their golden retrievers Maggie and Bailey.

PREFACE TO FOURTH EDITION

The fourth edition of the Resident's Guide to Ambulatory Care completes an extensive review and updating of the existing chapters, and adds three new chapters; community acquired pneumonia, gout, and prevention and management of stroke. The references have been updated and some chapters have web links for continually updated information.

The Resident's Guide to Ambulatory Care was written by residents, for residents. While following a general format, each chapter is slightly different to reflect the unique insight of its resident author and the specific needs of the material presented. We have provided in-depth exploration of commonly encountered clinical situations, and left the "zebras" for other sources. We continue to provide "clinical pearls" at the end of each chapter, algorithms in selected chapters, and charts and tables for quickly finding information. Blank pages are provided for important pager and phone numbers.

Each chapter was reviewed by multiple primary care physicians, a specialist in the respective field, and a pharmacologist. There are contributions from the specialties of family medicine, internal medicine, pediatrics, cardiology, pulmonology, dermatology, ophthalmology, urology, surgery, infectious diseases, endocrinology, nephrology, gastroenterology, rheumatology, psychiatry, neurology, sports medicine, physical medicine and rehabilitation, and obstetrics and gynecology as well as physician assistants and nurses. Other contributors include medical students and medical educators.

Our mission has been to provide a reference that is tailored specifically to residents in the ambulatory care setting; this mission has expanded to include everyone working in the setting of ambulatory care. Each year has seen the book used by more physicians than ever —residents as well as attendings. This is a testament not only to the comprehensive and easy-to-understand nature of the book, but to each of its devoted authors and reviewers.

Michael B. Weinstock
Daniel M. Neides

PREFACE TO FIRST EDITION

Our goal in writing *The Resident's Guide to Ambulatory Care* is to provide a *framework* for the rapid diagnosis and management of ambulatory conditions commonly encountered by residents treating patients in the ambulatory setting. Whereas other ambulatory books attempt to incorporate everything that could possibly be encountered in the ambulatory setting, our goal is to provide more detailed chapters on some of the most *frequently seen* diagnoses. For example, this manual provides well organized, easily accessed, and detailed information on contraception, ambulatory management of HIV/AIDS, and hypertension, and leaves the management of less frequently encountered conditions (Waldenstrom's macroglobulinemia) to other references. It will neither provide a comprehensive didactic summary nor behave as a textbook for in-depth study.

This pocket manual incorporates essential topics covered by handbooks of internal medicine, family practice, pediatrics and obstetrics into one *easy to access* source. It is a "pocket companion / ancillary brain" for the resident who must be familiar with an extraordinary amount of medical knowledge, including:

1) *Office based care* (Diagnosis and management of frequently encountered clinical conditions)
2) *Preventive medicine* (Immunization schedules, cancer screening, cholesterol management)
3) *Surgery* (Pre-op evaluation, pain management, evaluation of abdominal pain, suturing)
4) *Geriatric medicine* (Drug-drug interactions, side effects more prevalent in the elderly, addressing code status, "pronouncing" a patient, incontinence, falls)
5) *Care of the pregnant woman* (Prenatal care, sample admission and delivery notes, answers to questions expecting parents commonly ask)
6) *Ambulatory management of HIV/AIDS* (Schedule of visits, prophylactic medications, algorithms for work-up of cough, diarrhea, headache, FUO, etc.)

The manual emphasizes the diagnostic importance of the history and physical exam, and the importance of preventive medicine in ambulatory care. We feel that these issues are important in an era of health care reform where cost effective ambulatory care is essential.

We have tried to enhance the readability of this reference by including "clinical pearls" at the end of each chapter, including algorithms in selected chapters, and providing charts and tables for quick comparisons. Blank pages are provided for important pager and phone numbers. Most chapters follow a consistent format, but some deviate due to the creative insight of the authors and in the interests of space.

Contributors include a broad spectrum of physicians from the specialties of family medicine, internal medicine, pediatrics, cardiology, dermatology, psychiatry, pulmonology, ophthalmology, urology, neurology, physical medicine and rehabilitation, and obstetrics and gynecology. Other contributors include medical students and medical educators. We hope *The Resident's Guide to Ambulatory Care* will serve as a helpful resource for residents, medical students, and clinicians in practice and that it will serve to improve ambulatory patient care and medical education. We welcome feedback for future editions.

Michael B. Weinstock
Daniel M. Neides

CONTRIBUTORS

Michael B. Weinstock, M.D.
Clinical Assistant Professor, HIV Clinic,
The Ohio State University College of Medicine
Clinical Instructor, Riverside Methodist Hospital Family Practice
Attending ED, St. Ann's Hospital with Immediate Health Associates
Columbus, Ohio

Daniel M. Neides, M.D.
Associate Staff Physician
Department of Family Medicine
The Cleveland Clinic Foundation
Cleveland, Ohio
Assistant Professor, Department of Family Medicine
The Ohio State University College of Medicine
Columbus, Ohio

Rugen Alda, M.D.
3rd year Family Practice Resident
Riverside Methodist Hospitals
Columbus, Ohio

Ann M. Aring, M.D.
Assistant Director, Riverside Family Practice
Riverside Methodist Hospitals
Columbus, Ohio

Thomas D. Armsey, Jr., M.D.
Assistant Professor
Director of Sports Medicine
Department of Family Practice
University of Kentucky Medical Center
Lexington, Kentucky

Kate Baltrushot, M.D.
3rd year Family Practice Resident
Riverside Methodist Hospitals
Columbus, Ohio

John G. Bartlett, M.D.
Chief, Division of Infectious Diseases
The Johns Hopkins University School of Medicine and
The Johns Hopkins Hospital
Baltimore, Maryland

Eric Bates, P.A.
St. Ann's Emergency Department
Immediate Health Associates
Columbus, Ohio

Julie Beard, M.D.
　　3rd year Family Practice Resident
　　Riverside Methodist Hospitals
　　Columbus, Ohio

Jonathan M. Bertman, M.D.
　　3rd year Family Practice Resident
　　Brown University Department of Family Medicine
　　Assistant Clinical Instructor, Brown University Medical School
　　Memorial Hospital of Rhode Island
　　Pawtucket, Rhode Island

Tom Boes, M.D.
　　Attending, Pulmonology
　　Riverside Pulmonary Associates, Inc.
　　Riverside Methodist Hospitals
　　Columbus, Ohio

Edward T. Bope, M.D.
　　Past President, American Board of Family Practice
　　Director, Riverside Methodist Hospital Family Practice
　　Clinical Instructor, The Ohio State University College of Medicine
　　Columbus, Ohio

Ed Boudreau, D.O.
　　Attending, St. Ann's Emergency Department
　　Immediate Health Associates
　　Columbus, Ohio

Pamela Jelly Boyers, Ph.D.
　　Director, Medical Education
　　Riverside Methodist Hospitals
　　Columbus, Ohio

Cari Brackett, Pharm. D., B.C.P.S.
　　Columbus, Ohio

Chad Braun, M.D.
　　2nd year Family Practice Resident
　　Riverside Methodist Hospitals
　　Columbus, Ohio

Darrin Bright, M.D.
　　3rd year Family Practice Resident
　　Riverside Methodist Hospitals
　　Columbus, Ohio

Steve Brook, M.D.
　　Chief Resident
　　Department of Family Practice
　　University of Kentucky Medical Center
　　Lexington, Kentucky

Brent Cale, M.D.
　　2nd year Family Practice Resident
　　Riverside Methodist Hospitals
　　Columbus, Ohio

John Carlin, PA-C
Department of Orthopedics
Southern California Permanente Medical Group
Bellflower, California

Miriam Chan, Pharm. D.
Riverside Family Practice Residency
Columbus, Ohio

Christine Costanza, M.D.
Attending, Psychiatry
Madison, Wisconson

Rob Crane, M.D.
Assistant Professor
Family Practice
The Ohio State University
Columbus, Ohio

Kathryn A. Crea, Pharm. D., B.C.P.S.
Westerville, Ohio

Laurie Dangler, M.D.
2nd year Family Practice Resident
Riverside Methodist Hospitals
Columbus, Ohio

Joseph DeRosa, M.D.
2nd year Family Practice Resident
Riverside Methodist Hospitals
Columbus, Ohio

Doug DiOrio, M.D.
3rd year Family Practice Resident
Riverside Methodist Hospitals
Columbus, Ohio

Mary DiOrio, M.D.
3rd year Family Practice Resident
Riverside Methodist Hospitals
Columbus, Ohio

Marc Duerden, M.D.
Clinical Assistant Professor
Department of Physical Medicine and Rehabilitation
Indiana University College of Medicine
Bloomington, Indiana

Geoffrey Eubank, M.D.
Attending, Neurology
Neurological Associates
Columbus, Ohio

Budd Ferrante, Ed.D., ABPP
Psychologist, Private Practice
Hilliard, Ohio

Deb Frankowski, M.D.
3rd year Family Practice Resident
Riverside Methodist Hospitals
Columbus, Ohio

Bill Gegas, M.D.
Associate Director, Riverside Methodist Hospitals Family Practice
Clinical Instructor, The Ohio State University College of Medicine
Columbus, Ohio

Joe Ginty, M.D.
Family Practice, private practice
Lancaster, Ohio

Carol Greco, M.D.
Attending, Obstetrics and Gynecology
Kingsdale Gynecologic Associates
Riverside Methodist Hospitals
Columbus, Ohio

Cathy Greiwe, M.D.
2nd year Family Practice Resident
Riverside Methodist Hospitals
Columbus, Ohio

Ken Griffiths, M.D.
2nd year Family Practice Resident
Riverside Methodist Hospitals
Columbus, Ohio

Eric Hansen, M.D.
2nd year Family Practice Resident
Riverside Methodist Hospitals
Columbus, Ohio

Ryan Hanson, M.D.
3rd year Family Practice Resident
Riverside Methodist Hospitals
Columbus, Ohio

Melissa Harris, M.D.
2nd year Family Practice Resident
Riverside Methodist Hospitals
Columbus, Ohio

Karen Hazelton, PA-C
Immediate Health Care Associates
Columbus, Ohio

Mike Hemsworth, M.D.
2nd year Family Practice Resident
Riverside Methodist Hospitals
Columbus, Ohio

Jonathan Jaffrey, M.D.
Internal Medicine Resident
University of Vermont
Burlington, Vermont

Susanne Johnson, M.D.
1st year Family Practice Resident
Riverside Methodist Hospitals
Columbus, Ohio

Wendy Johnson, M.D.
1st year Resident
Albuquerque Health Sciences
Albuquerque, New Mexico

Douglas Knutson, M.D.
3rd year Family Practice Resident
Riverside Methodist Hospitals
Clinical Instructor, The Ohio State University College of Medicine
Columbus, Ohio

Mary Kay Kuzma, M.D.
Associate Professor of Pediatrics
Columbus Children's Hospital
The Ohio State University College of Medicine
Columbus, Ohio

Loren Leidheiser, D.O.
Attending, St. Ann's Emergency Department
Immediate Health Associates
Columbus, Ohio

Charles E. Levy, M.D.
Clinical Assistant Professor
Department of Physical Medicine and Rehabilitation
The Ohio State University Hospitals
The Ohio State University College of Medicine
Columbus, Ohio

Steve Markovich, M.D.
Assistant Director, Riverside Family Practice
Riverside Methodist Hospitals
Columbus, Ohio

Kim Martin, P.A.
St. Ann's Emergency Department
Immediate Health Associates
Columbus, Ohio

Michael Martin, M.D.
3rd year Family Practice Resident
Riverside Methodist Hospitals
Columbus, Ohio

Susan May, M.D.
Attending, Pediatrics
Columbus Children's Hospital
The Ohio State University College of Medicine
Columbus, Ohio

Diane Minasian, M.D.
Assistant Clinical Professor
Department of Family Medicine
Brown University
Pawtucket, Rhode Island

Douglas L. Moore, M.D.
3rd year Family Practice Resident
Riverside Methodist Hospitals
Columbus, Ohio

Tina Nelson, M.D.
3rd year Family Practice Resident
Riverside Methodist Hospitals
Columbus, Ohio

Dana Nottingham, M.D.
Assistant Director, Riverside Family Practice
Riverside Methodist Hospitals
Columbus, Ohio

Michael Para, M.D.
Professor, Infectious Disease
The Ohio State University College of Medicine
Columbus, Ohio

Kathleen Provanzana, M.D.
3rd year Family Practice Resident
Riverside Methodist Hospitals
Columbus, Ohio

Mark Reeder, M.D.
Attending, Family Practice
Columbus, Ohio

Anita Schwandt, M.D.
2nd year Family Practice Resident
Riverside Methodist Hospitals
Columbus, Ohio

Tim Scanlon, P.A.
St. Ann's Emergency Department
Immediate Health Associates
Columbus, Ohio

Mrunal Shah, M.D.
3rd year Family Practice Resident
Riverside Methodist Hospitals
Columbus, Ohio

David Sharkis, M.D.
Chief Resident
Eastern Virginia School of Medicine
De Paul Hospital
Norfolk, VA

James Simon, M.D.
Attending, Urology
Columbus Urology, Inc.
Riverside Methodist Hospitals
Columbus, Ohio

Linda Stone, M.D.
Attending, Family Practice
U.S. Health Corporation
Riverside Methodist Hospitals
Columbus, Ohio

Lynn Stratton, R.N.C.
Perinatal nurse
Riverside Methodist Hospitals
Columbus, Ohio

Marti Y. Taba, M.D.
2nd year Family Practice Resident
Riverside Methodist Hospitals
Columbus, Ohio

Michael Taxier, M.D.
Attending, Gastroenterology
Mid-Ohio Gastroenterology Associates
Riverside Methodist Hospitals
Columbus, Ohio

Timothy Timko, M.D.
Attending, Cardiology
Clinical Cardiology Specialists, Inc.
Riverside Methodist Hospitals
Columbus, Ohio

John A. Vaughn, M.D.
3rd year Family Practice Resident
Riverside Methodist Hospitals
Columbus, Ohio

Elizabeth Walz, M.D.
Clinical Assistant Professor
Department of Neurology, The Ohio State University Hospitals
The Ohio State University College of Medicine
Columbus, Ohio

Beth Weinstock, M.D.
3rd year medical student
1st and 3rd year Family Practice Resident
Riverside Methodist Hospitals
Columbus, Ohio
Attending, Family Practice
Private practice
Columbus, Ohio

Frank J. Weinstock, M.D.
Professor, Department of Ophthalmology
Northeastern Ohio University College of Medicine
Canton, Ohio

Cindy Williams, M.D.
Attending, Endocrinologist
City of Hope
Los Angeles, California

Ivan Wolfson, M.D.
Director, Traveler's Aid Society of Rhode Island
Pawtucket, Rhode Island

Frank Wright, M.D.
Attending, Obstetrics and Gynecology
Wright, Goff, Krantz, Stockwell, Harmon, & Jones, M.D.s, Inc.
Riverside Methodist Hospitals
Columbus, Ohio

Steve Yakubov, M.D.
Attending, Cardiology
Mid-Ohio Cardiology Consultants, Inc.
Riverside Methodist Hospitals
Columbus, Ohio

Note: Contributors are listed by their academic/professional status at the time of their contribution.

Authors' Note: We would like to thank David C.F. Davisson, Nancy A. Eikenberry, Karla G. Gale, and Roman G. Shabashevich of Anadem Publishing, Inc. for all of their hard work and dedication in the preparation of this text. Thanks also to David R. Schumick of Cleveland, Ohio for the front cover art and many of the charts. Thanks to Miriam Chan, Pharm. D. for her support and hard work in reviewing all the medications in the book.

TABLE OF CONTENTS

IV. Preventive Medicine

V. Cardiology and Pulmonary Disorders

VI. Management of Common Ambulatory Conditions

XIII. Appendix

I. Care of Children

Related subjects:

Daniel M. Neides, MD
Julie Beard, MD

1. THE NEWBORN EXAM

I. HISTORY

Obtain perinatal, pregnancy, and family histories; inquire about feeding, stooling, and voiding

II. THE PHYSICAL EXAM

A. General: The neonate should be completely undressed prior to the exam. Observe for congenital anomalies, movement of all extremities, and respiratory pattern

B. Respiratory

1. Color: Central and peripheral (Peripheral cyanosis is normal for several hours after birth)
2. Breathing: Normal respiratory rate is 40–60/minute; *grunting* and *nasal flaring* are **not** normal—if detected, further work-up is necessary
3. Auscultation: Perform prior to any manipulation of the infant (holding the infant or providing a pacifier or a finger may quiet a crying infant). Listen for equal and bilateral breath sounds

C. Cardiovascular

1. Rate, rhythm, and detection of any murmurs
2. Heart rate is normally between 120–160/minute
3. Murmurs
    a. Not necessarily an important finding on the newborn exam; infants with major cardiac anomalies may not have a murmur while an infant with a closing ductus arteriosis may; it is important to take into account other factors: *color, perfusion, and blood pressure*
    b. If further work-up is warranted, start with a chest x-ray, ECG, and blood pressure in all 4 extremities
4. Pulses: Palpate femoral pulses (coarctation of the aorta)

D. Gastrointestinal: Because of relatively weak abdominal musculature, palpation of internal organs is possible

1. The liver should be palpable and often extends 2.5cm below the costal margin
2. The spleen usually is not palpable
3. Palpate for renal/abdominal masses (Wilms' tumor, neuroblastoma)

E. Genitourinary

1. Males
    a. Palpate testicles (run a finger from the internal ring down on either side of the shaft of the penis—this will trap the testes inside the scrotum). Hydroceles are common and will usually resolve within the first 6 months. Transilluminate to confirm a hydrocele
    b. Check the penis for hypospadias or epispadias—if present, consult a urologist and do *not* circumcise the infant
2. Females
    a. The labia majora may appear large because of maternal hormones
    b. Spread the labia, and observe for vaginal wall cysts or imperforate hymen
    c. A white discharge may be seen as well as pseudomenses (due to maternal hormones)
3. Rectal inspection: Check for position and patency (monitor for bowel movement). A fistula can be mistaken for a normal anus; however, position of a fistula is usually anterior or posterior to the location of a normal anus. Do *not* probe rectum with finger or instrument!

F. Extremities

1. Hip clicks: 2 maneuvers are performed
    a. **Barlow test:** Adduction and posterior pressure may produce a "clunk" of subluxation or dislocation
    b. **Ortolani test:** Abduct and lift hip back into place
2. Assess for club feet, polydactyly or syndactyly, and forefoot adduction
3. Examine for crepitus over the clavicles (most commonly fractured bones in infants)

4. Examine the back for pilonidal sinus tracts or sacral dimple. If a pilonidal sinus tract is detected and the base cannot be seen, spine films may be indicated (meningocele)

G. Head, eyes, and mouth
  1. Head:
     a. Examine the skull for cuts, bruises, or evidence of cephalohematomas
     b. Mobility of the suture lines is important to rule out craniosynostosis
     c. Fontanelles: If head circumference is normal (32–36cm) and suture lines are mobile, size of fontanelles are not important; anterior fontanelle should be palpated, but the posterior fontanelle may not be palpable
  2. Eyes: Examine for bilateral red reflex (congenital cataracts)—if there is difficulty opening neonate's eyes, try sitting infant up or holding upside down and rapidly bringing to an upright position (infant gets disoriented and instinctively opens eyes)
  3. Mouth: Palpate and visualize for cleft palate; small white cysts (Epstein's pearls) may be noted on the hard palate and are a normal finding

H. Neurologic: Most of the neurologic exam is done while performing the rest of the neonatal physical exam. Important aspects of the neurologic exam include watching the baby's movements, evaluating body tone when handled, and observing appropriate crying during the exam
  1. **Moro reflex:** Grasp the neonate's hands and carefully pull the baby up—as you bring the head back down toward the crib, let go and the Moro reflex should occur. (Abduction of arms and legs, extension of elbow and knees followed by flexion)
  2. **Sucking and rooting reflex:**
     a. Rooting occurs when the baby's lips are stroked laterally and the head turns toward the ipsilateral side
     b. Assess the suck reflex by placing a finger in the infant's mouth
  3. **Stepping reflex:** Hold the infant upright and lean him/her forward. This should cause the baby to instinctively produce a stepping action (this reflex does not always occur)
  4. **Head control:** Assess head control and head lag while holding the infant's hands and sitting him/her upright

I. Skin: Common normal findings include:
  1. **Milia:** Small cysts on the baby's nose
  2. **Nevi or Mongolian spots:** Brown/blue patches that typically disappear within months
  3. **Macular hemangiomas:** "Angel kiss" or "stork bites" on the face or neck

III. FOLLOW-UP INSTRUCTIONS
  1. Hepatitis B vaccine: See Chapter 3, Childhood Immunization Schedule
  2. If infant is discharged in less than 48hrs, a repeat PKU should be done at the initial exam at 2 weeks of age
  3. Follow-up at 2–4 weeks of age for routine exam (1–2 weeks if breast-feeding, See Chapter 4, Infant Formula and Breast-feeding)
  4. Discuss with the parents signs/symptoms of neonatal sepsis (*lethargy, poor feeding habits, crying and inconsolable, rectal temperature > 100.4° F*). Instruct parents to contact family physician if these problems arise

References

Shoen EJ, et al. The highly protective effect of newborn circumcision against invasive penile cancer. Pediatrics 2000;105(3):E36.

French LM, Dietz FR. Screening for developmental dysplasia of the hip. Am Fam Phys 1999;60:177–88.

Alexander M, Kuo KN. Musculoskeletal assesssment of the newborn. Orthop Nurs (United States), Jan–Feb 1997;16:21–31.

Pressler JL, Hepworth JT. Newborn neurologic screening using NBAS reflexes. Neonatal Netw (US), Sep 1997;16(6):33–46.

Cochran WD. History and physical examination of the newborn. In: Cloherty JP, et al., eds. Manual of neonatal care. 3rd ed. Boston: Little, Brown, 1993.

2. THE DEVELOPING CHILD

AGE of child	LANGUAGE	GROSS MOTOR	FINE MOTOR	SOCIAL
NEWBORN	crying	lacks control of muscle groups	no skill	fixes on objects; startles easily
1 MONTH	cooing; single vowel sounds	lifts chin briefly	no skill	indefinite stare at surroundings
2 MONTHS	cooing; single vowel sounds	lifts head up 45 degrees	hand to mouth	**social smile**
4 MONTHS	laughs; squeals	**rolls over**; head up 90 degrees (prone)	two hand reach and grasp	follows 180 degrees; recognizes bottle
6 MONTHS	monosyllable babbling	**sits alone without support**	reaches for dropped toy; palmar grasp	talks to mirror image and plays peek-a-boo
9 MONTHS	single syllables; responds to NO	crawls-pulls to stand; "cruises"	**thumb-finger (pincer) grasp**	stranger anxiety; shout for attention
12 MONTHS	**First word**; uses "mama", "dada" correctly	**walks alone**; pivots to pick up objects	fine pincer grasp; learns to use cup	takes toys off table to play on floor
15 MONTHS	4–6 words	stands without support	builds tower of two blocks	points to and vocalizes wants
18 MONTHS	**Two words together**; knows 6–10 words	walks up steps; kicks ball	turns pages two at a time; scribbles	performs simple tasks; hugs doll
2 YEARS	50 words; **2–3 word sentences**	walks down steps; overhand throw	copy vertical line; turns door knob	"MINE"; dry at night
3 YEARS	knows full name; 4 word sentences	jumps from bottom step; rides tricycle	zips and unzips; copy circle	**toilet trained; dresses with help**
4 YEARS	5 word sentences; sings songs	hops on one foot; running jump	laces shoes; buttons clothes	separates from parents; bathes self
5 YEARS	counts to 10; asks "why"	skips; balances on one foot	may tie shoe laces	dresses / undresses without help

NORMAL PEDIATRIC VITAL SIGNS

Age	Pulse	Resp	Blood Pressure*
NB	120–160	30–60	systolic = 60–70
< 1 yo	120–140	30–50	
1–2 yo	100–140	30–40	systolic = 70 + (2 × age)
3–5 yo	100–120	20–30	diastolic = 2/3 systolic
6–10 yo	80–100	16–20	

*Blood pressure is often an unreliable indication of hypovolemic shock. Assess peripheral perfusion

CLINICAL PEARLS
- It is reassuring to inform parents what they can expect developmentally before the next well-baby visit
- The chart items in **bold** are important milestones and easy ones to remember
- If a child falls significantly behind developmentally, complete developmental testing (e.g., Denver Development Screening Test) should be performed

Reference
Vaughn VC. Assessment of growth and development during infancy and early childhood. Pediatrics in Rev 1992;13:88–96.

3. CHILDHOOD IMMUNIZATION SCHEDULE

NOTE: On October 22, 1999, the Advisory Committee on Immunization Practices (ACIP) recommended that Rotashield® (RRV-TV), the only U.S.-licensed rotavirus vaccine, no longer be used in the United States (MMWR, Volume 48, Number 43, Nov. 5, 1999). Parents should be reassured that their children who received rotavirus vaccine before July are not at increased risk for intussusception now.

Recommended Childhood Immunization Schedule
United States, January–December 2000

Vaccines[1] are listed under the routinely recommended ages. Bars indicate range of acceptable ages for immunization. Catch-up immunization should be done during any visit when feasible. Shaded ovals indicate vaccines to be assessed and given if necessary during the early adolescent visit.

Age ▶ / Vaccine ▼	Birth	1 mo	2 mos	4 mos	6 mos	12 mos	15 mos	18 mos	24 mos	4–6 yrs	11–12 yrs	14–16 yrs
Hepatitis B[2]		Hep B										
			Hep B				Hep B				Hep B	
Diphtheria, Tetanus, Pertussis[3]				DTaP	DTaP	DTaP	DTaP[3]			DTaP	Td	
H,influenzae type b[4]			Hib	Hib	Hib	Hib						
Polio[6]			IPV	IPV		IPV[5]				IPV[5]		
Measles, Mumps, Rubella[7]						MMR				MMR[6]	MMR[6]	
Varicella[8]						Var					Var[7]	
Hepatitis A[8]										Hep A[8] - in selected areas		

Approved by the Advisory Committee on Immunization Practices (ACIP), the American Academy of Pediatrics (AAP), and the American Academy of Family Physicians (AAFP).

1 This schedule indicates the recommended ages for routine administration of currently licensed childhood vaccines as of 11/1/99. Additional vaccines may be licensed and recommended during the year. Licensed combination vaccines may be used whenever any components of the combination are indicated and its other components are not contraindicated. Providers should consult the manufacturers' package inserts for detailed recommendations.

2 **Infants born to HBsAg-negative mothers** should receive the 1st dose of hepatitis B (Hep B) vaccine by age 2 months. The 2nd dose should be at least one month after the 1st dose. The 3rd dose should be administered at least 4 months after the 1st dose and at least 2 months after the 2nd dose, but not before 6 months of age for infants.
Infants born to HBsAg-positive mothers should receive hepatitis B vaccine and 0.5 mL hepatitis B immune globulin (HBIG) within 12hrs of birth at separate sites. The 2nd dose is recommended at 1–2 months of age and the 3rd dose at 6 months of age.
Infants born to mothers whose HBsAg status is unknown should receive hepatitis B vaccine within 12hrs of birth. Maternal blood should be drawn at the time of delivery to determine the mother's HBsAg status; if the HBsAg test is positive, the infant should receive HBIG as soon as possible (no later than 1 week of age).
All children and adolescents (through 18 years of age) who have not been immunized against hepatitis B may begin the series during any visit. Special efforts should be made to immunize children who were born in or whose parents were born in areas of the world with moderate or high endemicity of hepatitis B virus infection.

3 The 4th dose of DTaP (diphtheria and tetanus toxoids and acellular pertussis vaccine) may be administered as early as 12 months of age, provided 6 months have elapsed since the 3rd dose and the child is unlikely to return at age 15–18 months. Td (tetanus and diphtheria toxoids) is recommended at 11–12 years of age if at least 5 years have elapsed since the last dose of DTP, DTaP or DT. Subsequent routine Td boosters are recommended every 10 years.

4 Three Haemophilus influenzae type b (Hib) conjugate vaccines are licensed for infant use. If PRP-OMP (PedvaxHIB® or ComVax® [Merck]) is administered at 2 and 4 months of age, a dose at 6 months is not required. Because clinical studies in infants have demonstrated that using some combination products may induce a lower immune response to the Hib vaccine component, DTaP/Hib combination products should not be used for primary immunization in infants at 2, 4 or 6 months of age, unless FDA-approved for these ages.

5 To eliminate the risk of vaccine-associated paralytic polio (VAPP), an all-IPV schedule is now recommended for routine childhood polio vaccination in the United States. All children should receive four doses of IPV at 2 months, 4 months, 6–18 months, and 4–6 years. OPV (if available) may be used only for the following special circumstances:
1. Mass vaccination campaigns to control outbreaks of paralytic polio.
2. Unvaccinated children who will be traveling in <4 weeks to areas where polio is endemic or epidemic.
3. Children of parents who do not accept the recommended number of vaccine injections. These children may receive OPV only for the third or fourth dose or both; in this situation, health-care providers should administer OPV only after discussing the risk for VAPP with parents or caregivers.
4. During the transition to an all-IPV schedule, recommendations for the use of remaining OPV supplies in physicians' offices and clinics have been issued by the American Academy of Pediatrics (see Pediatrics, December 1999).

6 The 2nd dose of measles, mumps, and rubella (MMR) vaccine is recommended routinely at 4–6 years of age but may be administered during any visit, provided at least 4 weeks have elapsed since receipt of the 1st dose and that both doses are administered beginning at or after 12 months of age. Those who have not previously received the second dose should complete the schedule by the 11–12 year old visit.

7 Varicella (Var) vaccine is recommended at any visit on or after the first birthday for susceptible children, i.e. those who lack a reliable history of chickenpox (as judged by a health care provider) and who have not been immunized. Susceptible persons 13 years of age or older should receive 2 doses, given at least 4 weeks apart.

8 Hepatitis A (Hep A) is shaded to indicate its recommended use in selected states and/or regions; consult your local public health authority. (Also see MMWR Oct. 01, 1999;48(RR12); 1–37).

NOTE: This schedule is provided by the American Academy of Family Physicians only as an assistance for physicians making clinical decisions regarding the care of their patients. As such, they cannot substitute for the individual judgment brought to each clinical situation by the patient's family physician. As with all clinical reference resources, they reflect the best understanding of the science of medicine at the time of publication, but they should be used with the clear understanding that continued research may result in new knowledge and recommendations.

CLINICAL PEARLS
- Recommendation for Pneumoccal Conjugated Vaccine from ACIP and AAFP (released 2/00):
  1. Heptavalent pneumococcal conjugate vaccine (**Prevnar**) should be given to all infants less than 2 years old and high risk children between 2–5 years of age (e.g., sickle cell, HIV, asplenia, chronic illness, immunocompromising conditions, Alaskan-Native, and American Indians)
  2. The dosing schedule of **Prevnar**
     a. For children < 6 months of age, 0.5mL given IM at 2 months, 4 months, 6 months, and 12–15 months
     b. For children > 7 months

Age of first dose	Total no. of doses	Dosing
7–11 months	3	2 doses at least 4 weeks apart 3rd dose after 12 months of age and at least 2 months after the 2nd dose
12–23 months	2	At least 4 weeks apart
>24 months–9 yr	1	

- A child with a minor illness (e.g., URI) but afebrile (<101°F) may still receive scheduled immunizations
- If the patient or a household contact is immunocompromised then Inactivated Polio Vaccine (IPV) should be used instead of the OPV
- Children with chronic diseases who are susceptible to pneumococcus (sickle cell, asplenia, renal disease, HIV and other immunodeficiency states) should receive the **Pneumovax** (given once) after age 2 years
- Children susceptible to influenza (severe asthma, cystic fibrosis (CF), bronchopulmonary dysplasia (BPD), cardiac disease, HIV and other immunodeficiency states) should receive the influenza vaccine yearly after age 6 months

Daniel M. Neides, MD
Mary DiOrio, MD

4. INFANT FORMULA AND BREAST-FEEDING

I. STANDARD MILK-BASED FORMULA: *First line formula*
Nutrient profile resembles human milk, heat-treated for easier digesting and to lower allergic potential. Begin with formula containing iron
*A. Carbohydrate: Lactose
*B. Protein: Whey, casein
*C. Fat: Soy, corn, coconut, safflower, or palm olein oils
Formula Available: Advance, Carnation, Gerber, Good Start, Enfamil, Similac, SMA

II. SOY FORMULAS: *Second line formula*
For infants with cow milk protein allergies or lactose intolerant. Begin with formula containing iron
*A. Carbohydrate: Sucrose or corn syrup
*B. Protein: Soy, L-methionine, L-carnitine, taurine
*C. Fat: Soy, corn, coconut, oleo, or safflower oils
Formula available: Isomil, Isomil SF (sucrose-free), Nursoy, Prosobee (sucrose-free)

III. SPECIAL NUTRITIONAL NEEDS
A. **Alimentum:** For infants with problems with digestion or absorption; hypoallergenic
B. **Nutramigen:** Lactose and sucrose free; hypoallergenic
C. **Portagen:** For infants who have difficulty digesting fats
D. **Progestimil:** For infants with malabsorption problems, allergies, intractable diarrhea, short-gut syndrome, or cystic fibrosis
* *Carbohydrate, protein, and fat content will vary with each formula; read the label for exact contents of each formula*

IV. FEEDING SCHEDULES
Formula-fed infants should eat 5–6 ounces of formula/kg/day (*See chart*). Solid foods (cereals) can safely be started at 4–6 months

Recommended Bottle Feedings for a Normal Infant by Age

AGE	Number	Volume per feeding
Birth – 1 week	6 – 10	1 – 3 oz
1 week – 1 month	7 – 8	2 – 4 oz
1 month – 3 months	5 – 7	4 – 6 oz
3 months – 6 months	4 – 5	6 – 7 oz
6 months – 9 months	3 – 4	7 – 8 oz
10 months – 12 months	3	7 – 8 oz

V. BREAST MILK: Gold standard of infant nutrition; can nurse up to 4–6 months without supplementing solids

A. Goals: Healthy People 2000 has a goal of having 75% of all mothers initiate breast-feeding and 50% continue breast-feeding at least 5 to 6 months. Roughly 50% of all mothers initiate breast-feeding. 25% quit within the first month and only 25% continue until 5 months or more

B. Benefits of breast-feeding
1. There is no better nutrition for the baby than breast milk. The caloric and nutritional content of the breast milk naturally changes as the baby ages, providing the optimal nutrition for the infant at any age. Also, the nutrients in breast milk are easier to assimilate than those in formula because breast milk is easier to digest
2. Mothers who breast-feed reduce their risks of getting ovarian and breast cancer
3. Breast-feeding utilizes calories (~200 kcal/day) and may help the mother regain her pre-pregnancy weight. Note: A higher caloric intake is required for lactation
4. Breast-feeding is convenient and saves money
5. Enhanced maternal-infant bonding
6. The early breast milk, colostrum, provides antibodies to the infant, decreasing the infant's incidence of upper respiratory infections, diarrheal illnesses, otitis media (etc.) in the first year of the child's life
7. Exclusively breast-feeding the infant for at least 3 months reduces the chance that the child will develop Type 1 Diabetes Mellitus—see reference 4
8. Breast-fed infants are less likely to develop food allergies, because the breast-milk antibodies prevent the absorption of allergy-provoking proteins
9. Colostrum has a laxative effect assisting with the early evacuation of meconium
10. Exclusive breast-feeding may be an effective birth control method for several months after delivery, although this should not be relied upon
11. The breast-fed baby's stools are relatively odor-free

C. Common breast-feeding problems
1. Breast engorgement
   a. Often occurs for the first time when the milk comes in, usually the second or third postpartum day. Can occur at any time when the mother has not breast-fed or pumped her breasts for awhile
   b. To decrease engorgement, the mother should pump or express her breasts to release some of the excess milk build-up. Warm compresses or a hot shower can help the milk let-down. Frequent nursing during this stage is important
2. Mastitis
   a. Initially women experience flu-like symptoms with myalgias, fevers, and chills. One of the breasts then becomes erythematous, tender, and edematous in a particular area
   b. Management
      i. Frequent breast-feedings (with both breasts being utilized), rest, plenty of fluids, acetaminophen
      ii. Warm compresses to the affected breast for pain relief
      iii. Antibiotics: The most commonly used antibiotics are the penicillins and cephalosporins which cover the most common mastitis-causing organisms, staphylococcus and streptococcus. Erythromycin can be used for penicillin-allergic patients. Duration of treatment is 10–14 days
   c. Bilateral mastitis: Rare and may be a sign of a Group B Streptococcal infection which has been transmitted to the mother from the infant. (This is a serious infection and would require immediate treatment of the infant and the mother)
3. Yeast infections: If the infant develops thrush, he can transmit the infection to the mother and she may develop "thrush nipples"
   a. The symptoms of "thrush nipples" are erythematous, edematous, cracked, painful nipples. Both the infant and the mother need to be treated
   b. The infant is given **Nystatin** 1mL PO QID for 2 weeks given after nursing
   c. The mother should apply an anti-fungal ointment after nursing
4. Breast abscess
   a. Rare complication of mastitis
   b. Treatment: Surgical drainage
5. Cracked or bleeding nipples

   a. Can occur at any time during the nursing process
   b. Prevention is important
      i. The infant needs to be properly positioned on the breast
      ii. The breasts need to be cared for properly
         a. A daily shower or bath with warm water is sufficient to keep the breasts clean. Soaps and detergents should not be used on the breasts since they are drying to the skin
         b. Breast creams are unnecessary and may actually cause sore nipples.
         c. Breast milk that is left on the breast after nursing may be gently rubbed on the nipples
         d. Plastic-lined breast pads and wet breast shields should be avoided.
         e. The mother should invest in several good cotton nursing bras that provide support but are not constricting. Bras that are too tight may lead to blocked ducts

D. Nursing frequency
   1. Initially, the infant should breast-feed frequently, usually 8–15 feedings in a 24hr period
   2. The infant can be kept on the first breast until interest lost in feeding (usually 10–20 minutes). Then remove from that breast, burp, and place on the second breast. May not feed as long on the second breast. Because of this, should start at this breast at the next breast-feeding session.
   3. Breast-feeding works on a supply-and-demand basis. The more an infant feeds, the more milk the breasts will produce. It is important the infant nurse frequently and for as long as desired so that an adequate milk supply will be produced
   4. Supplementation is not necessary and may hinder the establishment of a good breast-feeding relationship

E. Vitamin supplementation
   1. Vitamin D: If still exclusively breast fed, then consider supplementing with 400 IU of Vitamin D per day starting at 6 months of age, especially for those infants with darkly pigmented skin or those infants that do not receive enough sunlight exposure (i.e., those born in late fall or winter)
   2. Iron
      a. There is debate about when iron supplementation should be done
      b. The term newborn has about a 4 month store of iron accumulated during gestation. At 4 months of age the physician needs to decide if the infant needs iron supplementation or if the infant is eating enough iron-fortified cereal to meet iron needs
      c. The preterm infant should receive supplementation starting at birth
   3. Fluoride: If still exclusively breast fed, then consider supplementation with 0.25mg per day starting a 6 months
   F. Medications and Lactation: See Chapter 16, Medications during Pregnancy and Lactation

CLINICAL PEARLS
   • Infants should not receive cow's milk prior to 1 year of age secondary to increase risk of occult GI bleeding and subsequent anemia

References

Brent N, et al. Sore nipples in breast-feeding women. A clinical trial of wound dressings vs conventional care. Arch Pediatr Adolesc Med Nov 1998;152:1077–82.

Neifert MR. The optimization of breast-feeding in the perinatal period. Clin Perinatol (US), Jun 1998;25(2):303–26.

Sheard NF. Breast-feeding protects against otitis media. Nutrition Reviews 1993; 51(9):275–7.

Gerstein HC. Cow's milk exposure and type I diabetes mellitus. Diabetes Care 1994;17(1):13–9.

Pfluke. Breast-feeding and the active woman. Waco: WRS Publishing, 1995.

5. NEONATAL JAUNDICE

DEFINITION: An abnormality of bilirubin production, metabolism, or excretion which results in bilirubin levels high enough to discolor sclera or skin

I. HISTORY
Distinguish between physiologic and non-physiologic jaundice. The following cause/increase of non-physiologic jaundice:
   A. **Family history of jaundice or anemia:** Hereditary hemolytic anemia (spherocytosis), ABO incompatibility, breast milk jaundice, G6PD deficiency
   B. **Maternal illness during pregnancy:** Congenital infections (toxoplasmosis, rubella, cytomegalovirus, herpes simplex virus)
   C. **Maternal drugs:** Sulfonamides, Nitrofurantoin, or antimalarial drugs (in a G6PD deficient infant)
   D. **Labor and delivery history:** Trauma, asphyxia, delayed cord clamping or prematurity

II. CLINICAL SIGNS AND SYMPTOMS
Jaundice (apparent with bilirubin levels > 5mg/dL), lethargy, poor feeding, vomiting, poor Moro reflex, high-pitched cry, and constipation

III. PHYSIOLOGIC JAUNDICE
A transient increase of *unconjugated bilirubin* in the full-term infant apparent on the 3rd day of life that resolves by the 10th day of life
   A. **Laboratory:** Total bilirubin < 12mg/dL and direct bilirubin < 1.5mg/dL
   B. **Etiology**
      1. Increased bilirubin load secondary to polycythemia, birth trauma, decreased survival of fetal RBCs, increased enterohepatic circulation
      2. Decreased hepatic uptake of bilirubin
      3. Poor conjugation secondary to decreased glucuronyl transferase activity and decreased hepatic blood flow
      4. Decreased excretion of bilirubin

IV. NON-PHYSIOLOGIC JAUNDICE
   A. **Laboratory:** "The Rule of Toos"
      1. Bilirubin rises *too early*: Jaundice apparent in the first 24hrs of life
      2. Bilirubin rises *too fast*: Bilirubin increases more than 5mg/dL/day
      3. Bilirubin rises *too long*: Jaundice apparent > 10 days in a full-term infant—*or*— > 2 weeks in a pre-term infant
      4. Bilirubin rises *too high*: Total bilirubin > 12mg/dL in full-term infant—*or*— > 15mg/dL in a pre-term infant
      5. Bilirubin is *too direct*: Direct bilirubin > 1.5mg/dL
   B. **Etiology**
      1. Abnormal (excess) bilirubin production: ABO incompatibility, red cell membrane defects (spherocytosis), infection, drugs, hemoglobinopathies, disseminated intravascular coagulation (DIC), pyloric stenosis (increased enterohepatic circulation of bilirubin), dehydration, and polycythemia
      2. Abnormal bilirubin metabolism: Crigler-Najjar syndrome, Gilbert's disease, Dubin-Johnson syndrome, Rotor syndrome, galactosemia, hypothyroidism, and infants of diabetic mothers

V. BREAST MILK JAUNDICE
   A. Etiology: Inhibitor of conjugation present in breast milk and decreased excretion of bilirubin in stool
   B. Late-onset jaundice occurs in 1% of breast-fed infants
   C. Bilirubin increases after the 3rd day of life, can reach 30mg/dL by age 2 weeks, and

normalizes by 4–12 weeks
D. Cessation of breast-feeding is only recommended for diagnostic purposes, but is not necessary. Once stopped, bilirubin should decrease in 48hrs and rise only 2–4 mg/dL when breast-feeding is restarted
E. 70% recurrence rate in subsequent pregnancies

VI. LABORATORY EVALUATION OF JAUNDICE

The jaundiced infant with nonphysiologic characteristics should have the following labs:
A. Type and Coombs (infant and mother)
B. CBC and reticulocyte count and blood smear
C. Direct and indirect bilirubin
D. Consider: Liver function tests, thyroid function tests, TORCH titers, serum glucose, or a septic work-up depending on history and physical examination

VII. ALGORITHMIC APPROACH

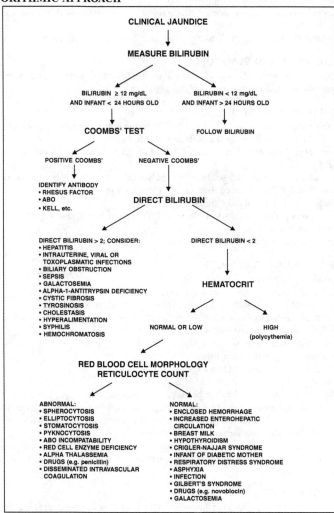

Source: Neonatal hyperbilirubinemia. Cloherty JP. In: Cloherty JP, et al., eds. Manual of neonatal care. 3rd ed. 1991:301. © Little, Brown and Company. Published by Little, Brown and Company. Boston. Used with permission.

VIII. TREATMENT

The goal is to prevent kernicterus which occurs when free, unconjugated bilirubin accumulates in the CNS

A. The level of bilirubin at which to start treatment remains unclear because there is not a specific level that is considered "safe" or "lethal" for all infants in every clinical situation

B. In otherwise healthy, full-term infants, kernicterus is unlikely with bilirubin < 20–25 mg/dL if the bilirubin is increasing slowly and the jaundice was not apparent before 24hrs of age

C. Infants who are preterm (< 37 weeks gestation), ill, or who have hemolytic disease have a higher risk of kernicterus with lower bilirubin levels

D. In all infants with hyperbilirubinemia:
1. Ensure adequate hydration with early Q2hrs feedings to help decrease enterohepatic circulation of bilirubin
   a. Monitor feeding behavior, stool output, and urine output
   b. Breast fed infants may need temporary supplements with formula—do not supplement with bottled water as it decreases hepatic function and stooling
2. Correct factors that decrease albumin's ability to bind bilirubin: hypoalbuminemia, sepsis, acidosis, hypoglycemia, increased free fatty acids, or sulfonamides
3. Correct factors that can disrupt the blood-brain barrier: Anoxia, ischemia, prematurity, hypothermia, and hypotension

E. Phototherapy: Alternating blue and white lights induces photoisomerization, which converts bilirubin to an isomer able to be excreted into stool and urine without conjugation in the liver
1. Begin phototherapy when an abnormal rise in bilirubin is detected, an early rise in bilirubin is detected, or when a level of bilirubin that could be toxic if increased further is detected
2. Start phototherapy at lower levels of bilirubin in those infants who are ill, preterm, or who have hemolytic disease
3. Discontinue when bilirubin level is no longer concerning and when the infant has matured enough to handle an increased bilirubin load (i.e., bilirubin <13mg/dL, at least 5 days old, and an otherwise healthy, full-term infant with physiologic jaundice)
4. Home phototherapy devices are available to decrease costs if parents can ensure adequate hydration
5. Placing jaundiced infants in direct sunlight is not advised, as severe hyperthermia may result

F. Exchange transfusion: Performed by a neonatologist in a neonatal ICU
1. Indications: Severe anemia, failure of phototherapy in an infant with a hemolytic disease, or hydrops
2. Double volume exchange will correct anemia, decrease bilirubin, and remove antibodies that can cause hemolysis

Recommendations for Management of Hyperbilirubinemia in the Healthy Term Newborn
(Total Serum Bilirubin Concentrations)

AGE (IN HRS)	CONSIDER PHOTOTHERAPY*	IMPLEMENT PHOTOTHERAPY	IMPLEMENT EXCHANGE TRANSFUSION IF PHOTOTHERAPY FAILS†	IMPLEMENT EXCHANGE TRANSFUSION
≤24 hours**	≥10 mg/dL (171µM/L)	≥15 mg/dL (257µM/L)	≥20 mg/dL (342 µM/L)	≥20 mg dL (342 µM/L)
25–48 hours	≥13 mg/dL (220 µM/L)	≥18 mg/dL (308 µM/L)	≥25mg/dL	≥30 mg/dL (513 µM/L)
49–72 hours	≥15 mg/dL (257 µM/L)	≥20 mg/dL (342 µM/L)	≥25 mg/dL (428 µM/L)	≥30 mg/dL (513 µM/L)
72 hours	≥17 mg/dL (291 µM/L)	≥22 mg/dL (376 µM/L)	≥25 mg/dL (428 µM/L)	≥30 mg/dL (513 µM/L)

* Phototherapy at these total serum bilirubin concentrations is a clinical option, meaning that the intervention is available and used on the basis of individual clinical judgment.

† Failure of phototherapy is defined as failure of the bilirubin level to stabilize or decline by at least 1 to 2 mg/dL within 4 to 6hrs in infants exposed to intensive phototherapy.

** It is recognized that the total serum bilirubin concentrations at 24hrs of age may not represent a healthy infant. Management of these infants requires investigation into the cause of hyperbilirubinemia, such as hemolytic disease.

Reproduced by permission of *Pediatrics*. Practice parameter: the management of hyperbilirubinemia in the healthy term newborn. *Pediatrics.* Vol 94 Page 560 Copyright 1994.

CLINICAL PEARLS

- Jaundice occurs in all infants as they transition from intra- to extra-uterine life
- Jaundice is usually a benign, self-limited condition that can be managed with close observation and reassurance
- Levels of bilirubin considered safe in healthy full-term infants may be pathologic in the sick or premature infant
- It is not necessary to stop breast-feeding in physiologic or breast milk jaundice
- Use the "Rule of Toos" to guide your investigation and treatment of the jaundiced infant

References
Gourley GR, et al. Neonatal jaundice and diet. Arch Pediatr Adolesc Med 1999;153:184–8.
Gartner LM. Neonatal jaundice. Pediatrics in Review 1994; 15:422–32.
Cloherty JP. Neonatal hyperbilirubinemia. In Cloherty JP, et al., eds. Manual of neonatal care. 3rd ed. Boston: Little, Brown, 1991:298–332.
Richardson DK, Alleyne CM. Management of the sick newborn. In: Graef JW, ed. Manual of pediatric therapeutics. 4th ed. Boston: Little, Brown, 1988: 148–53.

Daniel M. Neides, MD
Eric Hansen, MD

6. OTITIS MEDIA

I. INTRODUCTION
  A. Otitis media (OM) is the most common medical diagnosis made in children under age 15
  B. 85% of children have 1 episode of acute otitis media by age 3
  C. Environmental risk factors: Exposure to second-hand smoke, bottle feeding, and enrollment in day care

II. ETIOLOGY
  A. Bacterial: *S. pneumoniæ, H. influenzæ (nontypeable), M. catarrhalis, S. aureus,* Group A Strep
  B. Viral: Parainfluenza, RSV, Influenza, Adenovirus, Enterovirus

III. DIAGNOSIS
  A. Signs/Symptoms (Percentage of children affected in parentheses):
    1. Ear pain (47–83%)
    2. Fever (22–69%)
    3. Associated respiratory symptoms including cough and/or rhinitis (94%)
    4. Irritability (56%)
    5. Pulling at ear (12%)
    6. Drainage from ear (if tympanic membrane is ruptured)
  B. Physical Exam, predictive value in parentheses: (May need to remove cerumen prior to exam)
    1. Eyrthematous tympanic membrane (65%)
    2. Bulging tympanic membrane (89%)—occurs first in the postero-superior area
    3. Cloudy tympanic membrane (80%)
    4. Impaired mobility of tympanic membrane (78%)
    5. Note: Slightly impaired mobility of tympanic membrane (33%)
    6. Note: Slightly erythematous tympanic membrane (16%)

IV. TREATMENT: Since the causative agent of OM is usually unknown, initiate a 10 day course of empiric antibiotic therapy. See table below, Drugs Commonly Used with Otitis Media
  A. General
    1. Patients should be re-evaluated in 2 weeks to see if the treatment was successful. If there is presence of a middle ear effusion, consider:
      a. Re-evaluate in 6 weeks
      b. Re-treat with different antibiotic
    2. Antipyretics/Analgesics (oral)
      a. **Acetaminophen** 10–15mg/kg Q 4–6hrs (drops 0.8mL=80mg, susp. 160mL/5cc)
      b. **Ibuprofen** 5–10mg/kg Q 8hrs (drops 1.25mL=50mg, susp. 100mg/5cc)
    3. Analgesic (topical)
      a. **Auralgan otic suspension** 2–4 drops in affected ear QID (do not use with perforated TM)
  B. Acute Otitis Media (AOM): See table below, Drugs Commonly Used with Otitis Media
  C. Persistent OM: Occurs after initial course of antibiotics in up to 25% of patients
    1. Definition: Persistence of AOM within 6 days of beginning antibiotics or recurrence of AOM within a few days of completion of a 10 day course of antibiotics
    2. Consider other diagnosis
      a. Mastoiditis
      b. Meningitis
      c. Other infections
    3. Management: Change antibiotics to one that covers β-lactamase producing organisms
  D. Recurrent OM
    1. Definition: 3 episodes of OM in 6 months or 4 episodes in 12 months
    2. Consider other diagnosis
      a. Sinusitus

  b. Allergies
  c. Immune deficiencies (C3 and C5 deficiency)
  d. Submucous cleft palate
  e. Tumor of the nasopharynx
 3. Prevention
  a. Antibiotic prophylaxis
   i. **Amoxicillin** 20mg/kg PO QHS
   ii. **TMP/SMX** 4/20mg/kg PO QHS
   iii. **Erythromycin-Sulfisoxazole** 20mg/kg/day (if > 2 years old)
  b. Myringotomy with tympanostomy tube insertion
 E. Ruptured TM: Treat with **Cortisporin Otic Suspension** 2 drops QID for 3–5 days in addition to oral antibiotics per above recommendations
 F. Serous OM: Persistent middle ear effusion without infection; check hearing at 3 months. If decreased, then refer to ENT. There is no role for steroids or decongestants

DRUGS COMMONLY USED WITH OTITIS MEDIA

Drug	Dose	Availability	Common side effects
Amoxicillin	40-45mg/kg/day in 2 doses High risk patients 80-90mg/kg/day	Suspension: 125mg/5mL, 200mg/5mL, 250mg/5mL, 400mg/5mL Chewable: 125, 250mg Tabs: 250, 500mg	GI, urticaria, hyperactivity
TMP/SMX (Bactrim/Septra)	Children over 2 months: SMX 40mg/kg/day (TMP 8mg/kg/day) in 2 divided doses Adults: 1 DS tab BID	Suspension: SMX 200mg/5mL TMP 40mg/5mL Tabs: SS: SMX 400mg and TMP 80mg DS: SMX 800mg and TMP 160mg	GI, photosensitivity, neutropenia, thrombo- cytopenia. Use a different antibiotic if G6PD deficiency
Erythromycin Sulfisoxazole (Pediazole)	Children over 2 months: Erythro 50mg/kg/day (Sulf 150mg/kg/day) in 3 divided doses	Suspension: Erythro 200mg/Sulfisoxazole 600mg/5mL	GI, rash
Amoxicillin- Clavulanate (Augmentin)	30–40mg/kg/day in 3 divided doses In treatment failure: 80-90mg/kg/day of amoxicillin component (clavulanate dosing remains at 10mg/kg/day)	Suspension: 125mg/5mL 200mg/5mL, 250mg/5mL, 400mg/5mL Chewable: 125, 200, 250, 400mg Tabs: 250, 500, 875mg	Diarrhea, rash, urticaria
Loracarbef (Lorabid)	30mg/kg/day in 2 divided doses	Suspension: 100mg/5mL, 200mg/5mL Tabs: 200, 400mg * Empty stomach	GI, rash
Cefixime (Suprax)	8mg/kg/day in 1 dose per day (under 6 months — not recommended)	Suspension: 100mg/5mL Tabs: 200, 400mg	GI, rash, photosensitivity
Cefdinir (Omnicef)	7mg/kg/Q12hr or 14mg/kg/Q24hr	Suspension: 125mg/5mL Capsule: 300mg	GI, Drug interaction with antacids and iron supplements
Azithromycin (Zithromax)	Day 1: 10mg/kg 1 dose Days 2–5: 5mg/kg 1 dose	Suspension: 100mg/5mL, 200mg/5mL Caps: 250mg	GI
Clarithromycin (Biaxin)	15mg/kg divided BID	Suspension: 125mg/5mL, 250mg/5mL Tabs: 250, 500mg	GI, bad taste, HA
Ceftriaxone	50mg/kg x 1 IM max 1gm for severe infection can be given up to 3 shots	250mg, 500mg, 1000mg vials	Painful injection
Cefuroxime (Ceftin)	30mg/kg/day in 2 divided doses	125mg/5mL 250mg/5mL, 125, 250, 500mg tab	GI

CLINICAL PEARLS
- Decongestants, antihistamines, and glucocorticoids have not been shown to be helpful with AOM
- **Auralgan** drops (2 drops Q2hrs PRN) may decrease the symptom of ear pain. Do not use with perforated TM
- A crying child may have an erythematous TM because of crying—look for landmarks and light reflex
- Recurrent OM may result in hearing loss. Be alert for behavioral changes or learning difficulties
- Tympanostomy is not a benign procedure. Up to 10% of patients may develop tympanosclerosis with permanent hearing loss, and the child is exposed to the risk of general anesthesia

References

Cohen R, et al. One dose ceftriaxone vs. ten days of amoxicillin-clavulanate therapy for acute otitis media: clinical efficacy and change in nasopharyngeal flora. Pediatr Infect Dis J May 1999;18:403–9.

Hueston WJ, et al. Treatment of recurrent otitis media after a previous treatment failure. Which antibiotics work best? J Fam Pract 1999;48:43–6.

Weiss JC, et al. Acute otitis media: making an accurate diagnosis. Am Fam Phys 1996;53:1200–6.

Agency for Health Care Policy and Research. Managing otitis media with effusion in young children. Am Fam Phys 1994;50:1003–10.

Daniel M. Neides, MD

7. PHARYNGITIS

DEFINITION: An inflammatory process involving the mucous membranes and underlying structures of the oropharynx

I. PRESENTATION
A. History
   1. Chief complaint and associated symptoms (See below)
   2. Immunization history
   3. Sexual history (when indicated)
      a. Sexually active adolescents
      b. Abused children
      c. Inquire about current vaginal or penile discharge/dysuria
B. Signs and symptoms
   1. Sore throat
   2. Enlarged tonsils
   3. Fever, chills, headache, malaise, and anorexia
   4. Oropharyngeal erythema and/or exudate
   5. Rash
   6. Cervical adenopathy
   7. Rhinitis
C. Symptomatic triad of streptococcal pharyngitis
   1. Fever > 102.2° F (39° C)
   2. Cervical adenopathy
   3. Exudative tonsillitis

II. ETIOLOGY
A. Bacterial: Group A beta-hemolytic streptococcus, *Mycoplasma pneumoniæ, Hæmophilus influenzæ, Corynebacterium diphtheria, Neisseria gonorrhoeæ*
B. Viral: Adenovirus, Influenzæ viruses (A&B), Parainfluenza viruses, Epstein-Barr virus, Herpes simplex virus

III. EVALUATION
Laboratory
1. Rapid strep test—up to 96% sensitive
   a. Obtain specimen with 2 swabs
   b. If rapid test is positive, discard the 2nd swab
   c. If negative, perform blood agar throat culture with the second swab
2. Use appropriate culture medium if other bacteria (i.e., *Neisseria* or *Corynebacterium*) suspected

IV. TREATMENT
A. The goal of initiating therapy is to decrease the chance of secondary complications (including rheumatic fever). This therapy can safely be initiated up to 9 days after onset of symptoms and still be effective
B. The classic triad of fever, pharyngeal exudate and anterior cervical lymphadenopathy are present in only 15% of cases of strep pharyngitis
C. Medical personnel are correct in only 50–75% of cases where diagnosis is made based on clinical criteria alone
D. Compliance with antibiotics is a major problem with 71% of children discontinuing antibiotics by day 6
E. **Group A streptococcus**
   1. Oral penicillin
      a. Children: **Pen Vee K** 250mg PO BID–QID × 10 days
      b. Adolescents and adults: **Pen Vee K** 500mg PO BID–TID
   2. Intramuscular penicillin
      a. **Benzathine penicillin (Bicillin LA)**: Long acting PCN
         i. If greater than 1 month and < 27kg: 600,000 U
         ii. Children > 27kg and adults: 1.2 million U
      b. **Benzathine penicillin/Procaine penicillin (Bicillin C-R)**
         i. Injection may be less painful
         ii. There are different amounts of penicillin in the different preparations of Bicillin C-R. Use the above recommendations for the amount of Benzathine penicillin per injection
   3. Penicillin-Allergic
      a. **Erythromycin**
         Children: 30–50mg/kg/day divided TID–QID × 10 days
         Adults: 250mg PO QID × 10 days—*or* —
      b. **Cephalexin (Keflex)**
         Children: 25–50mg/kg/day divided BID–QID × 10 days
         Adults: 250mg PO QID × 10 days—*or* —
      c. **Azithromycin (Zithromax)** powder for oral suspension 12mg/kg once daily for 5 days, not to exceed 500mg/day. To be given at least 1hr before or 2hrs after a meal. Should **not** be taken with food. No refrigeration necessary
F. **Viral**
   1. Symptomatic relief:
      a. Gargle with warm salt water TID
      b. **Chloraseptic** spray or lozenges PRN sore throat
      c. **Acetaminophen** or **Ibuprofen** for pain, fever

V. COMPLICATIONS
A. Rheumatic fever (secondary to Group A Strep)
B. Post-strep glomerulonephritis (secondary to Group A Strep)
C. Peritonsillar abscess/Retropharyngeal abscess
D. Scarlet fever

CLINICAL PEARLS
- Untreated, streptococcal pharyngitis will resolve. Aggressive antibiotic therapy is necessary, however, to prevent complications including acute rheumatic fever and post-strep glomerulonephritis (PSGN)

- School-aged children who develop strep pharyngitis can return to school 24hrs after therapy is initiated
- Patients complaining of an associated rhinitis most likely have a viral etiology of their pharyngitis
- A Mono-spot test is a quick way to determine EBV (mononucleosis) infection; associated findings may include posterior cervical adenopathy, prolonged course of symptoms, or splenomegaly
- Once a peritonsillar abscess is suspected, immediate referral to ENT is indicated (for I & D)

References

Feder HM, et al. Once-daily therapy for streptococcal pharyngitis with amoxicillin. Pediatrics 1999;103:47–51.

Perkins A. An approach to diagnosing the acute sore throat. Am Fam Phys 1997; 55:131–8.

Emergency Medicine Reports. Inflammatory conditions of the head and neck. 1996;17:255–7.

Danjani AS, et al. Prevention of rheumatic fever. A statement for health professionals by the Committee on Rheumatic Fever, Endocarditis, and Kawasaki Disease of the Council on Cardiovascular Disease in the Young, the American Heart Association. Circulation 1988;78:1082–6.

Catanzaro FT, et al. The role of the streptococcus in the pathogenesis of rheumatic fever. Am J Med 1954;17:749–56.

Daniel M. Neides, MD

8. CROUP (Acute Laryngotracheitis)

DEFINITION: A viral illness characterized by a "barky" cough, inspiratory stridor, and fever

I. PRESENTATION
Affects children ages 3 months–3 years. Most frequently occurs in autumn
  A. Signs and symptoms: Gradual onset
    1. Barking, spasmodic cough, inspiratory stridor, hoarseness, and low-grade fever
    2. Upper respiratory infection (coryza) prodrome for 1–7 days
    3. Tachypnea, intercostal retractions, nasal flaring, dyspnea, and fatigue
    4. Cyanosis
  B. Differential diagnosis
    1. Epiglottitis
    2. Foreign body aspiration
    3. Bacterial tracheitis
    4. Subglottic stenosis

II. ETIOLOGY
  A. Viral
    1. Parainfluenza viruses (most common), Influenza viruses, RSV and Adenovirus
    2. Enteroviruses (coxsackievirus A & B and echovirus) are common causes of "summertime croup"
    3. Measles virus (endemic areas)
  B. Bacterial: *Mycoplasma pneumoniæ*

III. Evaluation: The diagnosis is usually a clinical diagnosis. More severe cases may warrant further work-up
  A. PA and lateral neck x-rays (obtain only if unsure of diagnosis)
    1. "Steeple Sign": Common x-ray finding secondary to subglottic narrowing
    2. Will help rule out epiglottitis ("thumb" sign on x-ray) as an etiology
  B. Laboratory
    1. WBC usually < 10,000/mm^3 with a predominately lymphocytic differential
    2. O$_2$ saturation

IV. MANAGEMENT: Mild cases can be effectively managed at home
   A. If symptoms improve with **saline aerosol treatments** patient may be sent home
   B. Dexamethasone 0.6mg/kg IM or PO as 1 time dose
   C. Place a **cool mist vaporizer** in the child's room
   D. Increase fluid intake, decrease agitation, observe carefully, follow-up closely
   E. Indications for admission:
      1. Stridor at rest
      2. Low oxygen saturation
      3. Tachypnea/retractions
      4. Ill appearance, poor color, decreased level of consciousness
      5. Questionable diagnosis (possible epiglottis, foreign body, etc.)

CLINICAL PEARLS
   • With the onset of symptoms, parents should place the child in a "steamy" bathroom or in the cool night air—symptoms will often improve
   • Spasmodic croup, a less severe form of croup, tends to occur at night and resolves quickly with mist therapy—the patient is usually afebrile and does not have x-ray changes
   • Antibiotic therapy is not indicated unless *Mycoplasma* is suspected

References
Johnson DW, et al. A comparison of nebulized budesonide, intramuscular dexamethasone, and placebo for moderately severe croup. N Engl J Med 1998;339:4989–503.
Custer JR. Croup and related disorders. Pediatr Rev 1993;14:19.
Kairys SW, et al. Steroid treatment of laryngotracheitis: a meta-analysis of the evidence from randomized trials. Pediatrics 1989;83:683.

Daniel M. Neides, MD

9. BRONCHIOLITIS

DEFINITION: An inflammatory process involving the bronchi and bronchioles

I. PRESENTATION
   Occurs mostly in winter and spring
   A. Criteria for diagnosis
      1. First episode of acute wheezing
      2. Age < 24 months
      3. Symptoms associated with viral infection (cough, fever, coryza)
      4. Pneumonia is ruled out as a cause of the wheezing
      5. No family history of atopy or asthma
   B. Signs and symptoms
      1. Expiratory wheezing and inspiratory rales
      2. Temperature usually < 101° F
      3. Grunting, intercostal retractions, dyspnea, tachypnea, prolonged expiratory phase
      4. Sore throat, cough, and coryza
      5. Associated otitis media
      6. Cyanosis
   C. Differential diagnosis
      1. Asthma
      2. Allergies (IgE-mediated hypersensitivity)
      3. Foreign body aspiration
      4. Pneumonia
      5. Gastroesophageal reflux disease (GERD)
      6. Congestive heart failure (CHF)
      7. Cystic fibrosis

II. ETIOLOGY

A. Viral: Respiratory syncytial virus (RSV), parainfluenza, adenovirus, rhinovirus, influenza virus

B. Bacterial: *Mycoplasma pneumoniæ, Chlamydia pneumoniæ*

III. EVALUATION

A. Chest x-ray (CXR)
1. Obtain on all "first-time wheezers" to rule out foreign body aspiration, pneumonia or CHF, and those patients requiring inpatient management
2. Common radiologic findings associated with bronchiolitis:
   a. Increased A-P diameter
   b. Atelectasis
   c. Flattening of the diaphragms

B. Laboratory: Only necessary for severe cases (See criteria for inpatient management below)
1. Arterial blood gas: monitor for hypoxemia, acidosis, and hypercarbia
2. Nasopharyngeal (viral) cultures: for detection of RSV
3. Continuous O_2 saturation monitoring

IV. MANAGEMENT

A. Home management
1. Most patients can and should be treated at home
2. Symptomatic relief
   a. Anti-pyretics (Tylenol, Pediaprofen)
   b. Anti-tussives (Dextromethorphan, Codeine-based syrup)
   c. Bronchodilator therapy (Ventolin syrup)
3. Adequate hydration
4. Avoid exposure to other children (incubation period of RSV is 4–6 days)
5. No smoking around child
6. Parents should be instructed to call the physician for worsening symptoms (respiratory distress)
7. Patients treated at home should have a follow-up appointment within 48hrs

B. Criteria for inpatient management of bronchiolitis
1. Tachypnea, marked intercostal retractions, increasing respiratory distress, cyanosis, or dehydration
2. Immunocompromised patients
3. Patients with a history of cardiopulmonary disease

Note: Steroids have *not* been shown to be beneficial in altering disease course

CLINICAL PEARLS

- 1 child in 50 will require hospitalization secondary to RSV bronchiolitis. Of these, 3–7% develop respiratory failure and 1% will die
- The mortality rate from nosocomial RSV in ill infants is as high as 20%
- Antibiotics should be withheld unless a bacterial etiology is suspected

References
DeBoeck K, et al. Respiratory syncytial virus bronchiolitis: a double blind dexamethasone efficacy study. J Pediatr 1997;131:919–21.
Horst PS. Brochiolitis. Am Fam Phys 1994;49:1449.

10. EVALUATION OF DIARRHEA IN CHILDREN

DEFINITION: An increase in the frequency, fluidity or volume of bowel movements as compared to the normal habit of the individual. Diarrhea may be acute (less than 2 weeks) or chronic

I. ETIOLOGY

A. Viral: Rotavirus (accounts for 35% of hospitalizations for acute diarrhea), adenovirus, Norwalk virus, enterovirus

B. Bacterial: *Aeromonas* species, *Vibrio cholerae, E. coli, Yersinia enterocolitica, Salmonella, Shigella, Clostridium difficile, Campylobacter jejuni*

C. Parasitic: *Cryptosporidium, Entamoeba histolytica, Giardia lamblia*

D. Formula intolerance, protein intolerance, carbohydrate intolerance, lactose intolerance

E. Post infectious diarrhea secondary to lactose intolerance

F. Overfeeding

G. Inflammatory bowel disease (IBD)

H. Chronic nonspecific diarrhea of infancy

I. Excessive fluid intake

J. Celiac disease, pancreatic disease

K. Constipation with overflow diarrhea

L. Functional tumors

M. Intestinal obstruction

N. Irritable bowel syndrome (IBS)

O. Laxative abuse

P. Non-GI causes: Otitis media, sepsis, toxic ingestion, immunodeficiency, hyperthyroidism

II. HISTORY

A. Chief complaint and associated symptoms (vomiting, tenesmus, malaise/lethargy, fever, weight loss, abdominal pain)

B. Medications

C. Onset and duration of illness

D. Dietary history (e.g., poorly cooked meats)

E. Frequency and character of stool (blood, pus, watery, foamy)

F. Hydration status
  1. Urine output
  2. Produces tears when crying
  3. Ability to take PO fluids/food

G. Family history (IBD, IBS, etc)

H. Past medical history

I. Travel history

J. Exposures and occupational history (day care center, sibling with diarrhea, etc.)

K. Well water vs. city water

L. Developmental history (monitor height & weight)

M. Ingestions

III. PHYSICAL EXAM

A. General: Fever, irritability, height, weight, head circumference

B. Hydration status: Tears when crying, capillary refill, dry mucous membranes

C. Cardiac: May detect murmur if dehydrated

D. Abdomen: Monitor for bowel sounds; tenderness including rebound; guarding

E. Skin: Rash, skin turgor

F. Rectum: Guaiac stool; look for mucus or pus in stool

DEGREE OF HYDRATION	
Percent dehydration	**Symptoms and signs**
Minimal: < 3% dehydration (10–20%ml/kg)	Increased thirst, mild oliguria
Mild: 3–5% dehydration (30–50ml/kg)	Increased thirst, oliguria, slightly dry lips, thick saliva
Moderate: 6–9% dehydration (60–90ml/kg)	Marked thirst, oliguria, irritable or listless, dry lips and oral mucosa, decreased or absent tears, depressed fontanelle, sunken eyes, delayed capillary refill, tenting of skin
Severe: > 10% dehydration (> 100ml/kg)	Clinical signs of moderate dehydration plus one or more of the following: Cyanosis, cold extremeties, rapid or thready pulse, grunting, tachypnea, lethargy, coma

IV. EVALUATION

   A. Stool studies: Based on presentation, history, and physical exam

     1. Reducing substances: Seen with lactose intolerance

     2. Occult blood

     3. Fecal leukocytes

     4. Stool cultures (e.g., *E. coli* 0157:H7): Consider if high likelihood of bacterial etiology:

       a. Abrupt onset of diarrhea

       b. Diarrhea which begins before vomiting

       c. Greater than 4 stools per day

       d. White cells on stool smear

       e. Blood in stool

     5. Ova and parasite exam (O&P): Diarrhea usually occurs > 10 days

     6. *Salmonella, Shigella, Campylobacter, Yersinia (S,S,C,Y)*

     7. Rotazyme

     8. pH

     9. *Clostridium difficile* toxin (C. diff): Especially if previous antibiotics given

     10. Stool volume while fasting

   B. Laboratory studies

     1. Electrolytes: Consider measuring with severe dehydration

     2. CBC with differential, consider peripheral smear

     3. ESR

     4. Total protein, albumin, liver function tests

     5. Stool trypsin

V. MANAGEMENT

   A. Fluid management

     1. Estimate degree of dehydration (see above table)

     2. Rehydration

       a. Severe dehydration: IV fluid replacement with normal saline (NS) or **Ringer's Lactate (LR)**—20–40mL/kg bolus every hour until circulatory status is restored, then oral rehydration solution (ORS)

       b. Moderate dehydration: May attempt to give PO replacement with ORS (above), and if unsuccessful, then proceed to IV fluid replacement

       c. Minimal or mild dehydration: Rehydration can usually be accomplished with oral rehydration solution (ORS), e.g., **WHO-ORS, Pedialyte**, etc. Calculate fluid deficit and replace

       d. If the patient is vomiting, then attempt to give small quantities frequently (5cc every 2–3 minutes) and, if unsuccessful, then consider antiemetics (phenergan or tigan rectal suppositories)

       e. If serum sodium is > 150, then replace the deficit over 12hrs to prevent seizures

       f. Correct any electrolyte abnormalities

B. Dietary management
1. Continue breast-feeding
2. Early re-feeding (within 4hrs of rehydration)

C. Symptomatic medications: Usually symptomatic medications are not indicated as rehydration is the most important therapy. If unsuccessful or with other circumstances, then consider **Bismuth Subsalicylate (Pepto-Bismol)**—20mg/kg 5 times/day in children 4–28 weeks

CALCULATION OF MAINTENANCE FLUID REQUIREMENTS	
Body weight (kilograms)	Milliliters water/kilogram
3–10	100
11–20	50
> 20	20

D. Medical therapy
1. Determine etiologic agent through focused laboratory evaluation
2. Commence appropriate pharmacologic therapy if indicated
3. Referral to specialist as necessary

E. Dietary therapy
1. When stool amount and frequency is markedly decreased, advance to half strength formula as tolerated
2. Advance to full strength feeds as tolerated
3. Solids as tolerated

F. Prevention: Good hygiene is the most effective intervention

CLINICAL PEARLS
- The leading worldwide cause of mortality in children under 5 years of age is dehydrating diarrhea (4.5 million deaths per year)
- In the United States, children under 5 years of age have 1.3–2.3 episodes of acute diarrhea per year
- In the United States, gastroenteritis is caused by viruses (30–40%), bacteria (20–30%) and unidentified agent (40%)
- Rotavirus has an incubation period of 1–3 days. Vomiting may occur for up to 3 days, and watery diarrhea for up to 8 days. May be accompanied by fever and URI signs
- Adenovirus causes more prolonged diarrhea than rotavirus. Norwalk virus usually occurs in epidemic outbreaks
- By the age of 4, most children will not become dehydrated from rotavirus infection

References
Duggan C, Nurko S. "Feeding the gut": the scientific basis for continued enteral nutrition during acute diarrhea. J Pediatr 1997;131:801–8.
Meyers A. Modern management of acute diarrhea and dehydration in children. Am Fam Phys 1995;51:1103.
Leung A, et al. Evaluating the child with chronic diarrhea. Am Fam Phys 1996;53:611.

Daniel M. Neides, MD
Julie Beard, MD

11. FEVER WITHOUT A SOURCE
(0–36 Months of Age)

DEFINITION: An acute febrile illness in which the etiology of the fever is not apparent after a careful history and physical exam
- Fever is defined as temperature ≥ 100.4° F (38.0° C)
- Concern for the possibility of occult bacteremia or underlying sepsis occurs in infants 0–90 days old with temperature > 100.4° F and in infants 3–36 months old with a temperature > 102.2° F (39.0° C)
- See Chapter 2, The Developing Child for a table of normal values for pulse, respiratory rate and blood pressure

I. DEFINITION OF HIGH RISK VS. LOW RISK PATIENTS
    A. High risk febrile infants: toxic appearing (lethargic, signs of poor perfusion, or marked hypoventilation, hyperventilation, or cyanosis)
    B. Low risk febrile infants: previously healthy with no focal bacterial infection on physical exam

II. FEVER WITHOUT A SOURCE < 28 DAYS OLD
Temperature > 100.4° F
    A. Risk factors: Prematurity, premature rupture of membranes(>18hrs), chorioamnionitis, maternal fever, maternal UTI, twin pregnancy, meconium aspiration
    B. Signs and symptoms: Temperature instability, respiratory distress, lethargy, feeding intolerance, jaundice, diarrhea, tachycardia, seizures, skin rash
    C. Diagnosis
        1. CBC with differential, electrolytes, serum glucose, CSF Gram stain and cell count
        2. Cultures from blood, CSF, and urine
        3. Group B strep antigen from urine and CSF
        4. Chest x-ray
        5. Other labs that may aid in the diagnosis: ABG, C-reactive protein, sed rate, serum calcium, haptoglobin, fibrinogen
    D. Management: Requires hospital admission and empiric parenteral antibiotics

III. FEVER WITHOUT A SOURCE 28–90 DAYS OLD
Temperature > 100.4° F: Obtain CBC with differential, urinalysis (send for culture)
    A. Low risk infants
        1. If WBC > 15,000/mm³:
            a. Obtain blood cultures and consider cerebrospinal fluid (CSF) for Gram stain and culture, cell count, glucose, and protein
            b. If positive CSF Gram stain (blood and CSF cultures will not be available for 24hrs) or abnormal CSF cell count, decreased CSF glucose or increased CSF protein, admit patient and begin parenteral antibiotics
            c. If negative CSF Gram stain (and CSF cell count, glucose, and protein are all normal), and negative urinalysis:
                i. **Ceftriaxone** 50mg/kg IM (Maximum dose is 1g) should be given
                ii. The patient should return for re-evaluation within 24hrs
        2. If positive urinalysis or urine culture:
            a. If patient is still febrile or unable to take PO, admit for parenteral antibiotics
            b. If afebrile and able to take PO, patient may receive oral antibiotics as an outpatient
            c. The patient should return for re-evaluation within 24hrs
            d. Follow-up with further studies. See Chapter 69, Urinary Tract Infections
        3. If the infant meets all low-risk clinical criteria and laboratory data are negative (WBC

< 15,000/mm³ and urinalysis and CSF Gram stain are negative) and the parents seem reliable and close follow-up is ensured, the infant can be managed as an outpatient. The patient should return for re-evaluation or call the physician's office with an update on the child's condition within 24hrs

B. High risk infants: Admit to hospital and begin parenteral antibiotics

IV. FEVER WITHOUT A SOURCE 3–36 MONTHS OLD

Temperature ≥ 102.2° and WBC ≥ 15,000/mm³ will be important factors in the treatment options for this age group

A. Low Risk Infants

1. If the child appears well and fever is < 102.2° F, no diagnostic tests or antibiotics are necessary; **Tylenol** (10–15mg/kg) may be given Q4hrs PRN fever; parents should be instructed to return if fever persists > 48hrs or patient's condition worsens

2. If temperature ≥ 102.2° F (39.0° C): Obtain **CBC with differential** and:
   a. **Urine culture** if the patient is male < 6 months or female < 2 years
   b. **Stool culture** if blood or mucus in stool or ≥ 5 WBCs/hpf in stool
   c. **Chest x-ray** only if dyspnea, tachypnea, rales, or decreased breath sounds are present
   d. **Blood cultures** if both fever ≥ 102.2° F and WBC ≥15,000/mm³
   e. **CSF cultures** are indicated when diagnosis of sepsis or meningitis is suspected based on history, observation, or physical exam

3. Empiric antibiotic therapy (parenteral **Ceftriaxone:** 50mg/kg (maximum dose of 1g) should be given if temperature ≥ 102.2° F (39.0° C) *and* WBC ≥ 15,000/mm³

4. Follow-up in 24–48hrs:
   a. If blood culture **positive**:
      i. Re-evaluate child within 24hrs and if child is still febrile or unable to take PO, admit for parenteral antibiotics
      ii. If child is afebrile and taking PO, patient may receive oral antibiotics as an outpatient (individualize therapy)
   b. If urine culture **positive**:
      i. If patient is toxic appearing or unable to take PO, admit for parenteral antibiotics
      ii. If afebrile and able to take PO, patient may receive oral antibiotics as an outpatient
      iii. Follow-up with further studies as outlined in Chapter 69, Urinary Tract Infections

B. High risk infants

1. Admit to hospital
2. Perform **sepsis** work-up including CBC with differential, blood, urine, and consider CSF analysis
3. Begin broad spectrum parenteral antibiotics

Remember: These are guidelines to help assist with managing a child who has a fever without a source. A careful history and physical exam are an essential part in determining treatment

CLINICAL PEARLS

- Children < 90 days old may not exhibit meningeal signs, despite having meningitis
- Impacted cerumen must be removed to completely visualize the tympanic membrane—the TM may be red from crying so obscured landmarks, a poor light reflex, or a bulging TM will confirm an otitis media
- Observation is a key component of the physical exam—a child who is smiling and/or playful is rarely septic

References

Finkelstein JA, et al. Fever in pediatric primary care: occurrence, management, and outcomes. Pediatrics 2000;105:260–6.

Shaw KN, et al. Prevalence of urinary tract infection in febrile young children in the emergency department. Pediatrics 1998;102:E16

Baraff LJ, et al. Commentary on practice guidelines. Pediatrics 1997;100:134–5.

Kramer MS, Shapiro ED. Management of the young febrile child: a commentary on recent practice guidelines. Pediatrics 1997;100:128–34.

Daaleman TP. Fever without a source in infants and young children. Am Fam Phys 1996;54: 2503–12.

Baraff LJ, et al. Practice guideline for the management of infants and children 0 to 36 months of age with fever without source. Pediatrics 1993;92(1):1–10.

Daniel M. Neides, MD
Marti Y. Taba, MD

12. CONSTIPATION IN CHILDREN

I. EPIDEMIOLOGY
   A. 1–3% children have chronic constipation
   B. In toddlers, incidence in male and female are equal, however, constipation is more prevalent in boys of school age

II. DEFINITION
   A. Normal stool pattern guidelines: (As long as the stool is soft, frequency doesn't matter. 5% of infants do not have a daily bowel movement)
     1. First 4 weeks of life: 4 stools a day
     2. Up to age 4 months: 2 stools a day
     3. Up to age 4 years: 1 stool a day
     4. Note: At age 3–4 the "Normal" stool patterns are 3 bowel movements a day to 3 bowel movements a week
   B. Constipation
     1. Hard, painful stool no matter what frequency
     2. Stool less than 3 times a week

III. ETIOLOGIES
The most common cause is functional constipation—neurologic and anatomic structures are normal but the child associates discomfort with defecation; other, less common causes include:
   A. Idiopathic: Due to low fiber diet, decreased water intake, painful stool passage causing retention, or insufficient opportunity to move bowels. Symptoms include pain, hard stool, soiling (incontinent liquid stool oozing past the impaction) abdominal pain relieved with a bowel movement, large stooling, anorexia
   B. Anatomic: Anal fissure, stenosis, or atresia; anterior displacement of the anus; rectal prolapse
   C. Metabolic and endocrine: Hypothyroidism, hypercalcemia, hypokalemia, diabetes insipidus, renal tubular acidosis
   D. Abnormal myenteric ganglion cells: Hirschsprung's (no passage meconium >48hrs, small-caliber stool, vomiting, failure to thrive, no stool in vault); Chagas' disease; von Recklinghausen's disease
   E. Neurologic: Myelomeningocele, spinal cord tumor, tethered cord (absent anal wink, decreased distal reflexes)
   F. Behavioral: Autism, ADHD, mental retardation
   G. Medications: Methylphenidate (Ritalin); Phenytoin (Dilantin); Imipramine (Tofranil); Phenothiazines; Codeine-containing cough syrups; iron supplements, lead toxicity

IV. PHYSICAL EXAMINATION
   A. General
     1. Height and weight
     2. Note any dysmorphic features
   B. Abdomen
     1. Abdominal distention seen in Hirschsprung's

2. A fecal mass may be palpable
C. Rectal Exam
Inspect for fissures, check for anal wink, rectal tone (tight with stenosis)

V. EVALUATION
Since most children have "functional" constipation, further work-up is not indicated unless suggested by information obtained from history and physical exam
A. Blood chemistry
Electrolytes, Ca^{++}, thyroid function tests
B. Barium enema
1. Bowel should be unprepped
2. Dilation of the rectum down to the anus is diagnostic of functional constipation
3. Hirschsprung's disease would reveal a narrow segment of colon above the narrow segment. Rectal manometry or rectal biopsy: Useful in diagnosing Hirschsprung's disease
C. Rectal manometry or rectal biopsy: Useful in diagnosing Hirschsprung's disease

VI. TREATMENT
A. If impacted on exam, need to disimpact if age > 1:
1. Mineral oil: 15–30mL/years PO QD–BID (max 8oz a day) for 3 days, watch for aspiration
2. Hypertonic phosphate enemas (3mL/kg) can be given up to twice daily up to 4.5 oz max QD no more than 3 days
   a. Contraindicated in CHF, renal impairment
   b. If not completely expelled, may lead to electrolyte imbalance and dehydration
   c. Due to side effects and potential problems, enemas are second line therapy
3. Golytely 90–120mL/kg over 1–2 days
B. Maintenance
1. Indications: Any child that needs disimpaction, child who defecates < 3 times/week, child who is passing firm, large stool or cries or strains excessively during defecation

Suggested Dosages of Commonly Used Laxatives

AGENT	PATIENT AGE	DOSAGE
Malt soup extract **(Maltsupex)**	Breast-fed infant Bottle-fed infant	1-2 tsp in 2-4 oz of water or juice BID 1-2 tsp with every other feeding X 3-4 days; then 1-2 tsp/day
Dioctyl sodium sulfosuccinate (Colace)	Infants	1/2 tsp PO BID
Lactulose	>6 Months	1/2 tps/kg/day
Milk of Magnesia	>6 Months	1/2 tps/kg/day in 2 doses
Mineral Oil	>6 Months	Same as Milk of Magnesia
Senna Syrup **(Senokot)**	1-5 Years 5-10 Years	1 tsp PO QHS (may increase to BID) 2 tsp PO QHS (may increase to BID)

2. Diet (in children > 1 year)
   a. Dietary fiber: Number of grams to be given per day = years old + 5
   b. Liquids > 1 quart a day
3. Toilet training:
   a. Discouraged during initial treatment of constipation
   b. Once the parent determines the onset of action of the laxative, the child should be placed on the toilet at that time (the same time every day) give 3–4, 5 to 10

minute opportunities a day after each meal
   c. Resume training 1 month after laxative treatment is begun
   d. Offer incentives for stooling/sitting, avoid embarrassment or punishment
   e. Keep stooling record
4. Follow-up care
   a. Goal: stooling >3 × a week with no soiling and no pain
   b. Follow-up 2 weeks after disimpaction then 1–2 months
   c. Many toddlers can discontinue laxative therapy within 3–6 months (rectal vault should return to normal size), while others may need them for up to 1 year or more

CLINICAL PEARLS
- Risk factors for developing chronic constipation: acute constipation, painful defecation, or harsh or too early toilet training
- Educate parents and provide them with support and encouragement

References

Felt B, et al. Guideline for the management of pediatric idiopathic constipation and soiling. Arch Ped Adolesc Med 1999;153:380–5.

Gold DM, et al. Frequency of digital rectal examination in children with chronic constipation. Arch Pediatr Adolesc Med April 1999;153:377–9.

Iacono G, et al. Intolerance of cow's milk and chronic constipation in children. N Engl J Med 1998;339:1100–4.

Worman S, Ganiats TG. Hirschsprung's disease: a cause of chronic constipation in children. Am Fam Phys 1995;51:487–94.

Leung AKC, et al. Constipation in children. Am Fam Phys 1996;54:611–8.

Michael Martin, MD

13. ENURESIS

I. DEFINITIONS
   A. Childhood enuresis is the involuntary loss of urine, classically after age 5
   B. Primary enuresis refers to a failure to ever achieve bladder control. Primary nocturnal enuresis accounts for 90% of all causes of enuresis
   C. Secondary enuresis refers to a return to incontinence after bladder control was previously achieved and is usually associated with psychological stressors (after birth of a sibling, significant loss or family discord)

II. ETIOLOGY: Probably multi-factorial; maturational delay of sleep and arousal mechanisms, delay in development of increased bladder capacity, and heredity (see clinical pearls)

III. HISTORY
   A. **Type and severity:** Determine if the episodes of enuresis are nocturnal (nighttime), diurnal (daytime), mixed (day and night) and primary or secondary. The severity of the enuresis should be evaluated by obtaining the number of enuretic nights per week, the number of episodes per night, and the amount voided with each episode
   B. **Voiding history:** Weak urinary stream, urgency, infrequent voiding, previous UTI, encopresis, constipation
   C. **Family history:** Enuresis or urinary tract abnormalities
   D. **Past medical history:** Diabetes mellitus or sickle cell anemia

IV. PHYSICAL
   A. Neurologic: Complete neurological exam is required, including perianal sensation, and anal sphincter tone, deep tendon reflexes, gait
   B. Spinal cord pathology: Patient's back should be inspected for evidence of sacral dimpling or cutaneous abnormalities suggesting spinal pathology
   C. Abdominal and genital exam

V. LABORATORY EVALUATION

A. Urinalysis and urine culture (all patients) to exclude renal, metabolic, and infectious pathology

B. If the history demonstrates a primary, nocturnal (or mild diurnal), normal stream enuresis, with no other accompanying symptoms, a normal physical exam, and a normal U/A and culture—then no further work-up is indicated

C. Any exception to V. B. (above) requires a renal sonogram, a voiding cystourethrogram, and spine films (if spinal pathology is suspected on history and physical)

VI. TREATMENT FOR PRIMARY NOCTURNAL ENURESIS

A. Reassurance: Family education and motivation are important to resolution. Inform the parents and child that enuresis is a developmental lag and not indicative of an emotional problem. Enuresis is no one's fault and the child should not be punished for bed wetting

B. Combinations of treatment options are most effective

C. Options include:

1. Alarm System: Often used as first line in combination with **Imipramine** or **Desmopressin**. Fairly inexpensive ($50–70) with a success rate of 70% and a relapse rate of 30%

2. **Imipramine:** 2.5mg/kg orally at bedtime. There is a high relapse rate, therefore, consider use when a short period of dryness is important (overnight visits or camp). ECG monitoring at baseline and during chronic therapy has been recommended

3. **Desmopressin (DDAVP):** 20–40 mcg (1–2 puffs) intranasally at bed time. Effective for short term control

4. **Oxybutynin (Ditropan):** Rarely beneficial

5. Bladder stretching: Child is instructed to withhold voiding for increasing amounts of time each day after an oral fluid load. Limited evidence to support use

6. Charting: Child keeps a chart of wet and dry nights and is given rewards for dry nights

7. Treat constipation

8. Hypnosis

9. Evening fluid restriction: Limited evidence to support use

CLINICAL PEARLS

- Primary nocturnal enuresis accounts for approximately 80% of all cases of enuresis
- Spontaneous remission occurs at about 15% per year
- 70% of children in whom both parents were enuretic will also be enuretic

References

Ullol-Minnich MR. Diagnosis and management of nocturnal enuresis. Am Fam Phys 1996;54:2259.

Robson WLM, Leung AKC. Advising parents on toilet training. Am Fam Phys 1991;44:1263.

14. ENCOPRESIS

DEFINITION: Fecal soiling occurring at least 1 time a month for 3 months after age 4

I. EPIDEMIOLOGY
A. Encopresis affects 2% of all children
B. 95% of encopresis is functional or idiopathic
C. Male: Female 3:1

II. TYPES
A. Retentive encopresis (psychogenic megacolon): Most common. Child withholds bowel movement leading to fecal impaction and then seepage of soft or liquid feces onto underclothing. Child is distressed that soiling occurs
B. Continuous encopresis: Child has never gained primary control of bowel function. Child and/or parents are prone to be socially or intellectually disadvantaged
C. Discontinuous encopresis: Encopresis after an extended period of bowel control. Loss occurs after a stressful event and child may put feces in "irritating places" as an expression of anger or as an attempt to be perceived as being younger than they are. Child is not distressed that soiling occurs
D. Toilet phobia: Child is afraid of the toilet (they are losing a part of themselves with each bowel movement)

III. HISTORY
A. Age when the symptoms first began
B. Stool size, consistency, and frequency
C. Constipation or diarrhea
D. Leg crossing to resist the urge to defecate
E. Abdominal pain
F. Urinary symptoms
G. Psych/social factors: Family stress, birth of sibling, recent death in family, marital disharmony

IV. PHYSICAL
A. Neurological exam
B. Rectal exam: Anal position, anal sphincter tone, scarring, anal wink, fecal mass, anal fissures, length of anal canal, presence of stool in rectal vault
C. Abdomen: Palpate for tenderness and mass
D. Back exam: Examine for palpable or cutaneous manifestations of spinal pathology
V. LABS AND OTHER TESTS: Obtain studies based on historical and physical findings and likely diagnosis
A. Abdominal flat plate to evaluate stool and gas pattern
B. Barium enema and/or rectal biopsy to evaluate possible anatomical or neurological (Hirshsprung's) pathology
C. Anorectal manometry may be beneficial

VI. MANAGEMENT
A. Functional constipation
   1. Definition: Less than 3 bowel movements per week or incomplete evacuation
   2. Most frequent cause of encopresis
   3. Usually accompanied with soiling in the underwear and not with large stool incontinence
   4. Often caused by reluctance to use the toilet
   5. Children complain of abdominal pain 50% of the time, daytime enuresis 27% of the time, and nocturnal enuresis 32% of the time

6. Regular visits to toilet. Have the child sit on the toilet for 5 minutes, 3–4 times per day, after each meal. The child should strain to have a bowel movement, and his or her feet should be able to touch the floor. See Chapter 12, Constipation in Children
7. Use positive reinforcements. Rewards for days without soiled underclothes

B. Organic Etiologies
1. Often have large bowel movements when incontinence occurs
2. Organic causes may have a constipation component
3. Etiologies
   a. Anterior anus: Most patients improve with medical treatment, but some need a posterior anoplasty or sphincterotomy
   b. Anal stenosis: Patients have stool of small diameter. This condition usually presents when solids are introduced into diet
   c. Spinal pathology: Patients most often are enuretic as well

CLINICAL PEARLS
- The management of encopresis involves the child and the parent. Parental distress needs to be addressed
- Encopresis is rare in adolescence

References
Kuhn B, et al. Treatment guidelines for primary nonretentive encopresis and stool toileting refusal. Am Fam Phys 1999;59:2171.
Howe AC, Walker CE. Behavioral management of toilet training, enuresis, and encopresis. Pediatr Clin North Am 1992;39:413.

II. Care of the Pregnant Patient

Related subjects:

Beth Weinstock, MD
Bill Gegas, MD
Sarah Alley, MD

15. PRENATAL CARE

OB

I. SCHEDULE OF PRENATAL VISITS: Schedules vary by patient population and practitioner. Ideally, first visit should be a pre-pregnancy counseling session. Patient should be given 400mcg **Folic Acid** supplement daily to reduce risk of neural tube defects, and rubella immunity should be checked prior to conception (consider MMR if patient is antibody negative)
  A. Every 4 weeks until 28–32 weeks
  B. Every 2 weeks from 32–36 weeks
  C. Every week from 32 weeks until delivery
  D. Bi-weekly non stress tests if post-term. Consider biophysical profile depending on risk factors
  E. Consider induction in uncomplicated patient between 41–42 weeks

II. INITIAL ASSESSMENT: Forms may vary by practice
  A. History
    1. Demographic data including current phone number, address
    2. Pregnancy: Date of first day of last menstrual period (LMP) and timing and flow (normal or light) of LMP
    3. Birth history: History of preterm labor, preeclampsia, gestational diabetes, incompetent cervix, Cesarean section (classical incision vs. low transverse), gestational age of previous births, birth weights, type of anesthesia used, use of vacuum or forceps, episiotomy
    4. Past medical history including history of depression, anxiety disorders, or post-partum depression, history of varicella, immunization history, sexually transmitted diseases (STDs)
    5. Past surgical history: Prior gynecologic surgery; in particular, cervical procedures
    6. Drug sensitivities/allergies
    7. Family history including history of genetic abnormalities
    8. Social history: Alcohol, tobacco and drug use, physical and/or emotional abuse
    9. Family support systems, involvement of "father of the baby"
    10. Diet and exercise, weight gain with past pregnancies
    11. Patient preferences: Anesthesia/analgesia, breast vs. bottle feeding, etc.
  B. Physical: Perform a full physical including thyroid, breast and pelvic exams
  C. Labs and other tests
    1. Routine
      a. Blood group type and Rh factor
      b. Indirect Coombs (antibodies to other blood group antigens)
      c. Hepatitis surface antigen (chronic hepatitis B)
      d. H/H
      e. Blood glucose
      f. Rubella antibody titer
      g. Syphilis serology
      h. HIV: If first test is negative and patient has significant risk factors, then repeat in 3–6 months
      i. Urinalysis and culture
      j. *Gonorrhea, Chlamydia* cultures (DNA probe)
      k. Pap smear
      l. If history of blood transfusions, check titers for Duffy and Kell antibodies. If increased, then patient is a candidate for amniocentesis
    2. Optional
      a. Sickle cell (at-risk populations)
      b. PPD (pregnancy mimics immunocompromised state): Consider in high-risk patients
      c. Ultrasound: Obtain if unsure of LMP or the LMP was abnormal. Not necessary if EDC by dates is reliable
      d. Toxo, CMV, varicella: Varicella zoster antibodies if patient has not been exposed

OB

D. Vaccines
  1. Influenza vaccine: OK to administer in pregnancy
  2. **Varicella (Varivax):** Should *not* be given to pregnant women. Women should avoid pregnancy within 1 month of receiving the vaccine

III. INITIAL VISIT—28 WEEKS

A. History
  1. Contractions: Frequency, intensity
  2. Fetal movements (First felt at 18–20 weeks in primip, 16–18 weeks in multip)
  3. Vaginal discharge or bleeding
  4. Symptoms of preeclampsia
      a. Edema (distinguish ankle edema vs. hand/face edema—latter is more significant for preeclampsia, particularly in third trimester)
      b. Headache
      c. Blurred vision
      d. Abdominal pain (round ligament pain begins at approx. 20 weeks)
  5. Alcohol or drug use
  6. Compliance with prenatal vitamins

B. Physical
  1. Blood pressure (should be below 140/90)
  2. Weight gain: Based on body mass index
      a. Underweight women: 28–40 pounds desired weight gain
      b. Normal weight women: 25–40 pounds (approx. 1 lb per month for the first 3 months and then 1 lb per week to term)
      c. Overweight women: 15–25 pounds (need supervision and good diet)
  3. Fetal heart tones: Heard by doppler at 10–12 weeks
  4. Fundal height (FH): Measure with bladder empty and legs extended, from the pubic symphysis to top of uterine mass (full bladder can increase FH 3 cm)
  5. Urine dip (done in office at every visit) : Check for protein, glucose, ketones and leukocytes
      a. Protein: "Trace" or 1+ is WNL. If 2+ or more, then check 24hr urine for protein
      b. Glucose: "Trace" is normal with pregnancy due to increased GFR. If risk factors or more than "trace," then consider one 1hr glucola screen
      c. Asymptomatic bacteriuria (incidence during pregnancy is 2–7%): Major cause of maternal and fetal morbidity. If untreated, 25–30% may develop acute pyelonephritis
          i. Diagnosis based upon isolation of $> 10^5$ organisms per mL of urine in 2 consecutive clean-catch specimens. *E Coli* is most common offending organism
          ii. Give 3 day course of Nitrofurantoin (Macrobid) or Amoxicillin and screen with Q month cultures
          iii. If greater than 1 UTI or more than 1 incidence of asymptomatic bacteriuria: Need prophylaxis for duration of pregnancy
          iv. Symptomatic bacteriuria (hematuria, dysuria, urgency, fever, flank pain, etc): Give a 7 day course of Amoxicillin or Nitrofurantoin (Fluoroquinolones are contraindicated in pregnancy)

C. Labs: *Optional testing*
  1. **Maternal serum alpha fetal protein (MSAFP)**
      a. Indication: To screen pregnancies for neural tube defects or trisomies (including Down's syndrome)
      b. When AFP is combined with HCG and unconjugated estriol (the "triple test" or "AFP³"), the sensitivity for Down's syndrome increases from 20% to 60–65%. Some clinicians use the "triple test" for women > age 35, and others use it for all women. The classic laboratory results of the "triple test" will be a low AFP, low unconjugated estriol, and high HCG
      c. Perform at 16–18 weeks
      d. If abnormal, then obtain ultrasound to ensure dates are correct (if not already done)
      e. *If AFP is low* then fetus has increased incidence of Down's syndrome. Perform level II ultrasound and amniocentesis (See below)
          i. Statistically 4–5% of all AFPs will be low
          ii. Down's syndrome occurs in 1.3 of 1000 live births

    f. *If AFP is high* then AFP needs to be repeated. If still high, then fetus has increased incidence of neural tube defects. Other causes of elevated AFP include threatened abortion, twins, fetus misdated, and abdominal wall defects. Perform amniocentesis (See below)

        i. Statistically 3–5% of all AFPs will be high. Of 100 high AFPs, 95 will be "unexplained high" AFPs. These patients do not have neural tube defects, but will be at increased risk for problems in pregnancy. These women should have NSTs Q week after 32 weeks

        ii. Neural tube defects occur in 1–2 of 1000 pregnancies. If there is a positive family history, the risk rises to 2%

2. Chorionic Villus Sampling

    a. Indication: To determine karyotype and genetic disorders in women with advanced maternal age (> 35) or high risk for genetic abnormalities. Does *not* evaluate for spina bifida

    b. Perform at 10–12 weeks

    c. Risk of fetal loss is 3–5%

3. Amniocentesis: *Optional, but strongly suggested if > age 35*

    a. To test for chromosomal abnormalities including Down's, Tay-Sachs, Sickle cell disease

    b. Indications

        i. Advanced maternal age (> 35) or women at high risk for genetic abnormalities

        ii. Follow up abnormal AFP values

    c. Perform at 15–20 weeks

    d. The chance of fetal trisomies at age 35 is 1 in 200; at age 45 it is 1 in 20

    e. There is a <1% risk of fetal loss from the procedure if used with ultrasound guidance

IV. WEEKS 28—36

A. History: Same as above. If patient reports > 4 contractions/hr, she should be evaluated immediately. This holds true for symptoms of leaking fluid or vaginal bleeding, as well as UTI symptoms

B. Physical: Same as above

C. Other

    1. **1 hour post glucola (1 hour PG):** Done at 26–30 weeks

      a. Consists of 50g glucose load

      b. 15% of population will be abnormal. 1–2% of pregnant mothers are diabetic

      c. Normal is < 140. If > 140 then obtain 3hr GTT

      d. 3hr GTT is abnormal if 2 or more values are abnormal:

        i. Fasting < 105

        ii. 1hr < 190

        iii. 2hrs < 165

        iv. 3hrs < 145

    2. H/H: 28 weeks (get with 1 hour PG)

    3. Repeat *GC/chlamydia* and syphilis serology in high risk population. Bacterial vaginosis screen if higher risk of premature labor

    4. If mother is Rh negative: **RhoGAM 300mcg IM** at 28–32 weeks. If "father of baby" is Rh+, check indirect Coombs prior to giving RhoGAM

    5. If desired, sign consent for tubal ligation/tubal referral

    6. Discuss premature labor: Assess Group B β-Hemolytic *strep* infection risk (see section below). Guidelines for treating contractions in pregnancy vary. Prophylaxis in labor if positive risk including: prior affected infant, preterm, PROM

    7. Counsel patient on fetal movements/give kick graph. (She should feel 10 fetal movements by 6 PM. If not, then she must call and may need to be scheduled for a NST)

    8. Discuss birthing classes (Lamaze or patient's preference)

V. WEEK 36—DELIVERY

A. History: Same as above

B. Physical: Same as above—*plus*—

    1. Weekly cervical exams beginning at 37 weeks

    2. Palpate abdomen for fetal lie and position

C. Labs: Group B strep screening per recommendations below

OB

D. **Discuss** anesthesia during labor (Epidural, Nubain), episiotomy, and labor and delivery procedures. Offer patient opportunity to watch labor and delivery videotape if available

E. **Advise** patient to call physician or report to Labor and Delivery if:
1. She suspects ROM
2. If contractions are Q 5–6 minutes for 1hr for primip, Q 8–10 minutes for 1hr if multip
3. Vaginal bleeding
4. Reduced or absent fetal movement (<10 kicks/hr)

VI. **RECOMMENDATIONS FOR PROPHYLAXIS OF GROUP B *STREPTOCOCCUS*** (Centers for Disease Control guidelines)

A. Intrapartum treatment based on risk factors (see table below) vs. universal screening. Vaginal and perirectal culture at 35–37 weeks gestation. All positive cultures should be treated with intrapartum prophylaxis (see below)

B. Summary of Recommendations for Prevention of Neonatal Group B Streptococcus Disease

---

STRATEGY 1

Give intrapartum chemoprophylaxis to all women who previously had an infant with invasive group B streptococcal disease, who have group B streptococcal bacteriuria in the present pregnancy or who go into labor or have rupture of the membranes before the fetus has reached an estimated gestational age of 37 weeks

Perform prenatal screening when the fetus is at an estimated gestational age of 35 to 37 weeks and offer intrapartum chemoprophylaxis to all maternal carriers of group B streptococci

Give intrapartum chemoprophylaxis to all maternal carriers of group B streptococci who have intrapartum risk factors and to pregnant women without group B streptococcal culture results who have risk factors†

STRATEGY 2

Give intrapartum chemoprophylaxis to all women with intrapartum risk factors‡

---

* Source of recommendations: Centers for Disease Control and Prevention (1996), American College of Obstetrics and Gynecology (1996) and American Academy of Pediatrics (1997)

† These risk factors include rupture of the membranes for 18 hours or more or an intrapartum fever (temperature: 38°C [100.4°F]) or higher)

‡ These risk factors are a previous infant with invasive group B streptococcal disease, group B streptococcal bacteriuria during this pregnancy, labor or rupture of the membranes when the fetus has an estimated gestational age of less then 37 weeks, rupture of the membranes for 18 hours or more or an intrapartum fever (temperature: 38°C [100.4°F] or higher)

Source: Keenan C. Prevention of neonatal Group B streptococcal infection. Am Fam Phys 1998;57:2713, table 3. Used with permission.

C. **Antibiotics**
1. **Penicillin G** IV 5 million units initially then 2.5 million units Q 4hrs until delivery—*or*—
2. **Ampicillin** IV 2g, then 1g Q 4hrs until delivery
3. PCN allergic:
   a. **Clindamycin** 900mg IV Q 8hrs until delivery
   b. **Erythromycin** 500mg IV every 6hrs until delivery

CLINICAL PEARLS
• 5–10% of patients will deliver on their due date
• All patients should be given a prescription for prenatal vitamins on their first visit
• Women should ideally receive folate at 28 days prior to conception through the first 8 weeks of pregnancy to decrease the risk of neural tube defects. If patient has had a previous pregnancy affected by a neural tube defect, then a daily 4mg dose of folate is recommended

- A 20 week uterus will be palpated at the umbilicus
- If patient experiences vaginal bleeding associated with a closed cervix, and a fetus is seen on ultrasound, then miscarriage rate is < 3%
- Antiretroviral use during pregnancy decreases risk of transmission of HIV by at least ⅔ and should be *strongly* recommended (in consultation with an HIV specialist) to every HIV positive woman

OB

References

Werler MM, et al. Achieving a public health recommendation for preventing neural tube defects with folic acid. Am J Public Health Nov 1999; 89:1637–40.

Keenan C. Prevention of neonatal Group B streptococcal infection. Am Fam Phys 1998;57:2713.

Haddow JE, et al. Screening of maternal serum for fetal Down's Syndrome in the first trimester. N Engl J Med 1998;338:955–61.

Cnattingius S, et al. Prepregnancy weight and the risk of adverse pregnancy outcomes. New Engl J Med 1998;338:147–52.

Cheng EY, et al. A prospective evaluation of a second-trimester screening test for fetal Down syndrome using maternal serum α-fetoprotein, hCG, and unconjugated estriol. Obstet Gynecol 1993;81(1):72–7.

American College of Obstetricians and Gynecologists. Ultrasonography in pregnancy. ACOG technical bulletin No. 187. Washington, D.C., Dec. 1993.

Fargason CA, et al. The pediatric costs of strategies for minimizing the risk of early-onset group B streptococcal disease. Obstet Gynecol 1997;90:347–52.

Centers for Disease Control and Prevention. Prevention of perinatal group B streptococcal disease: a public health perspective. MMWR 1996;45(RR–7):1–24 [Published erratum appears in MMWR 1996;45(31):679].

Mary DiOrio, MD
Douglas Knutson, MD
Michael B. Weinstock, MD

16. MEDICATIONS DURING PREGNANCY AND LACTATION

I. INTRODUCTION: Although most medications with systemic effects in the mother will cross the placenta, many of these medications do not seem to adversely affect the fetus. Still, many effects of medications are not known, and it is important to not prescribe medications during pregnancy unless the benefit will outweigh the risk

II. FDA CLASSIFICATIONS

Schedule A: Controlled studies *in humans* have demonstrated no fetal risks

Schedule B: *Animal studies* have indicated no fetal risk, but there are no human studies to support the data, *OR*, fetal risks have been demonstrated in animals, but *not* in well-controlled human studies

Schedule C: *No adequate studies* in either humans or animals have been done—*or*—adverse effects have been seen in animal studies, but there is no human data available

Schedule D: There is *evidence of fetal risk*, but the benefits of the medication may outweigh the risks to the fetus

Schedule X: There are *proven fetal risks* which clearly outweigh the benefits of using the medication

III. OTC DRUGS GENERALLY CONSIDERED SAFE TO USE IN PREGNANCY

A. Pain relief: Acetaminophen (Tylenol): 650mg PO Q4–6hrs

B. Cough: Robitussin DM (Dextromethorphan 10mg and Guaifenesin 100mg per 5mL): 10mL PO Q4hrs

C. Constipation: Psyllium (Metamucil): 1 tsp in 8 oz water or 1 wafer QD–TID. **Perdiem (Senna-fiber):** Start with 1 tsp PO QD, may increase to 2 tsp PO QID

D. Indigestion: Maalox, Mylanta, Rolaids, Tums

E. Diarrhea: Kaopectate, Imodium AD

F. Sinus congestion: Sudafed, Actifed, or **Afrin** nasal spray (short-term use)

G. Nausea/vomiting: Emetrol: 15–30mL PO Q1–2hrs as tolerated

OB

IV. DRUGS USED DURING PREGNANCY FOR VARIOUS CONDITIONS

Schedule A and B medications are generally considered to have minimal effects on the fetus. Use only if benefits outweigh risks

Classification by indication of some drugs and medications used during pregnancy*

Asthma	Infections	Nausea and Vomiting
Albuterol C	Acyclovir C	Chlorpromazine C
Corticosteroids B, C, D	Amoxicillin B	Cyclizine B
Cromolyn B	Amphotericin B	Meclizine B
Ephedrine C	Azithromycin B	Prochlorperazine C
Epinephrine C	Aztreonam C	Promethazine C
Metaproterenol C	Cephalosporins B	Trimethobenzamide C
Terbutaline B	Chloroquine C	**OTC Meds**
Theophylline C	Clarithromycin C	Antihistamines B, C
Cardiovascular	Erythromycin B	Diphenhydramine C
β-blockers C	Famciclovir B	Guaifenesin C
Captopril D	Lindane B	Phenylpropanolamine C
Coumadins D	Metronidazole B	Pseudoephedrine C
Digoxin C	Mebendazole C	**Pain and Inflammation**
Enalapril D	Miconazole B	Acetaminophen B
Furosemide C	Nitrofurantoin B	Aspirin C
Heparin C	Nystatin B	Codeine C
Methyldopa C	Penicillins B	Ibuprofen B/D
Procainamide C	Pyrantel C	Indomethacin B/D
Quinidine C	Quinine D	Meperidine B
Thiazides D	Sulfonamides B	Morphine B
Verapamil C	Tetracyclines D	**Psychiatric Disorders**
Convulsive Disorders	Trimethoprim C	Amitriptyline D
Carbamazepime C	Valacyclovir B	Chlordiazepoxide D
Phenobarbital D	Vancomycin C	Diazepam D
Phenytoin D	Zidovudine C	Imipramine D
Trimethadione D	**Miscellaneous**	Lithium D
Valproic acid D	Barbiturates C	Nortriptyline D
GI Meds	Caffeine B	Phenothiazines C
Cimetidine B	Cyclosporins C	**Rheumatic Diseases**
Cisapride C	Dextroamphetamine C	Azathioprine D
Famotidine B	Heroin B/D	Betamethasone C
Lansoprazole B	Insulin B	Chlorambucil D
Metoclopramide B	Isotretinoin X	Cyclophosphamide D
Nizatidine B	Thyroid A	Cyclosporin A, C
Omeprazole C	Vaccines C, X	Dexamethasone C
Ranitidine B		6–Mercaptopurine D
Sucralfate B		Methotrexate X
Hormones		Methylprednisolone B
Clomiphene X		Prednisone B
Contraceptives X		
Estrogens X		
Progestins D		

* Categories according to Food and Drug Administration guidelines, whether by manufacturer or according to Briggs and colleagues (1990)

V. MEDICATIONS USED DURING LACTATION

Contraindicated	Avoid or Give with Great Caution	Probably Safe but Give with Caution
Antineoplastic agents	Anthraquinones (laxatives)	Anesthetics
Amphetamines	Aspirin (salicylates)	Acetaminophen
Azathioprine	Atropine	Aldomet
Bromocriptine	Bromides	Antibiotics (not Tetracycline,
Clemastine	Calciferol	Quinolones)
Chlorambucil	Cascara	Antithyroid (not Methimazole)
Chloramphenicol	Clindamycin	Antiepileptics
Cocaine	Danthron	Antihypertensive/cardiovascular
Cyclophosphamide	Dihydrotachysterol	Bishydroxycoumarin
Cyclosporin A	Diphenhydramine	Chlorpheniramine*
Cyclosporine	Estrogens	Chlorpromazine*
Diazepam	Estrogen/progesterone	Codeine*
Diethylstilbestrol	combination contraceptives	Digoxin
Doxorubicin	Ethanol	Dilantin
Ergots	Imipramine	Diuretics
Gold salts	Metoclopramide	Furosemide
Heroin	Metronidazole	Haloperidol*
Immunosuppressants	Narcotics	Hydralazine
Iodides	Nitrofurantoin	Indomethacin
Isoniazid	Phenobarbital *	Methadone*
Lithium	Primidone	Muscle relaxants
Meprobamate	Psychotropic drugs	Prednisone
6–Mercaptopurine	Reserpine	Progestin-only contraceptives
Methimazole	Salicylazosulfapyridine (Sulfasalazine)	Propranolol
Methotrexate	Sulfonamides	Propylthiouracil
Methylamphetamine	Tetracycline	Sedatives*
Nicotine (smoking)		SSRIs
Phencyclidine (PCP)		Theophylline
Phenindione		Vitamins
Radiopharmaceuticals		Warfarin
Tetracycline		
Thiouracil		

* Watch for sedation

Source: Behrman RE. Nelson's textbook of pediatrics. Philadelphia: W.B. Saunders, 1996:439. Used with permission.

References

Koren G, et al. Drugs in pregnancy. N Engl J Med 1998;338:1128–37.

Briggs GG, et al. Drugs in pregnancy and lactation. 4th ed. Baltimore: Williams & Wilkins, 1994.

Smith J, Taddio A, Koren G. Drugs of choice for pregnant women. In: Koren G, ed. Maternal-fetal toxicology: a clinician's guide. 2nd rev. ed. New York: Marcel Dekker, 1994:115–28.

Broussard CN, et al. Treating GERD during pregnancy and lactation: what are the safest therapy options? Drug Safety 1998 Oct;19(4):325–37.

Ramsey-Goldman R, et al. Immunosuppressive drug use during pregnancy. Rheum Dis Clin North America Feb 1997; 23(1):149–67.

Reed BR. Dermatologic drugs, pregnancy, and lactation. a conservative guide. Arch Dermatology 1997; 133(7):894–8.

Lynn Stratton, RN
Michael B. Weinstock, MD

OB

17. QUESTIONS EXPECTING PARENTS COMMONLY ASK

Many of these issues should be discussed with your patients before they ask

I. WHAT ACTIVITIES ARE SAFE TO PARTICIPATE IN?

Pregnancy is not an illness and expecting mothers should not be treated as if they were sick. Pregnant women may have sexual intercourse, drive a car, fly in an airplane, go swimming, take tub baths and paint the nursery. Adequate rest, exercise and nutrition are advisable for the best pregnancy outcomes

II. WHAT ACTIVITIES SHOULD BE AVOIDED?

Douching, cleaning the litter-box, dieting to lose weight, high risk activities (skiing, sky diving), new vigorous exercise programs, high impact aerobics, vibrating machines, tanning booths, saunas

III. WHICH DANGER SIGNS SHOULD NOT BE IGNORED?

A. Bleeding (more than a few spots) from the vagina
B. A sudden gush of fluid or a slow leak of fluid
C. Severe abdominal pain
D. Chills and fever
E. Fainting
F. Pain or burning with urination

IV. WHAT CAN BE DONE TO HELP WITH MORNING SICKNESS?

Eat crackers or toast before getting out of bed. Sit on the edge of the bed for several minutes before getting up in the morning. Eat more frequently, but smaller meals (5–6 times per day). Avoid greasy and spicy foods. Drink water freely between meals. Take the prenatal vitamin after eating. Participate in stress relieving activities like walking outside 20–30 minutes 5 times per week or practicing deep breathing, asking others to help with stressful activities, and participating in organized stress relief groups. **Vitamin B$_6$** 50mg PO TID; **Emetrol** 15–30mL PO Q1–2hrs as tolerated

V. TENDER BREASTS

Wearing a good support bra may help. If not effective, consider wearing it at night. Leaking breasts may be managed with nursing pads or tissues placed in the bra

VI. CONSTIPATION

Increase intake of fresh fruits and vegetables, grains and bran. Increase fluid intake and consider a cup of hot water 3 times per day. Continue to exercise including walking 20–30 minutes 5 times per week. **Psyllium (Metamucil):** 1 tsp in 8 oz water or 1 wafer QD–TID. **Perdiem (Senna-fiber):** Start with 1 tsp PO QD, may increase to 2 tsp PO QID

VII. LOW BACK PAIN

Reassure that this is to be expected. Rest frequently during the day. Maintain good posture. Use a footstool while sitting. Wear low heeled shoes and avoid overly soft beds and chairs

VIII. PELVIC PAIN (ROUND LIGAMENT PAIN)

As the uterus enlarges the ligaments supporting it will stretch, causing pelvic pain. May use **Tylenol** as needed. Do not make sudden movements. Get out of bed slowly. Massage may be helpful

IX. ARE DENTAL PROCEDURES SAFE DURING PREGNANCY?

Use of local anesthetic agents are generally considered safe in pregnancy. Teeth cleaning/plaque control is considered safe. Dental radiographs are probably safe with use of a lead apron, but should be obtained only when absolutely necessary

X. IS CAFFEINE SAFE DURING PREGNANCY?

Drinking *large amounts* of caffeine has been associated with increased fetal loss, and women should be counseled on decreasing the amount of caffeine from coffee as well as other sources (tea, colas, chocolate, OTC drugs). In addition, *heavy* caffeine use may cause caffeine withdrawal in newborns. Most physicians consider drinking low to moderate amounts of caffeine acceptable during pregnancy

XI. IS ASPARTAME (NUTRASWEET) SAFE DURING PREGNANCY?

Studies have not shown adverse fetal or maternal effects from aspartame during pregnancy

XII. IS THERE A PROBLEM WITH VIDEO DISPLAY TERMINALS?

No. They are considered safe during pregnancy

XIII. ARE INSECTICIDES SAFE?

Pregnant women should avoid use of insecticides and fumigants in the home or in the yard

XIV. WHAT OTC MEDICATIONS ARE SAFE TO USE?

See Chapter 16, Medications during Pregnancy and Lactation

XV. SHOULD SEAT BELTS BE WORN DURING PREGNANCY?

The leading nonobstetric cause of fetal death is maternal trauma. The use of a diagonal shoulder strap and a lap belt is strongly recommended during pregnancy

References

Hueston WJ, et al. Common questions patients ask during pregnancy. Am Fam Phys 1995;52:1465–72.

American College of Obstetricians and Gynecologists. Exercise during pregnancy and the postpartum period. ACOG technical bulletin No. 189. Washington D.C., Feb 1994.

Michael B. Weinstock, MD

OB

18. OB ADMISSION NOTE

HISTORY: Patient is a __ y/o woman G__P__Ab__ with a __ week intra-uterine pregnancy and EDC of __/__/__ by LMP (and/or) __ week ultrasound who presents to labor and delivery with complaint of ******. She ___(denies/reports) vaginal bleeding or ROM. She reports ___(frequent) fetal movements. Her pregnancy has been complicated by _____ (smoking/alcohol/drugs, multiple gestation, infections, abnormal Pap, PIH, gestational diabetes, etc.)
   **Examples:
     1. Contractions occurring every__minutes which last__seconds each and have been occurring for __hours
     2. "My water broke" __hours ago with ___(clear, green, malodorous) fluid
     3. Post-dates for induction of labor

PRENATAL LABS: Blood type and Rh status, antibody screen, HBsAg, HIV, *gonorrhea* and *chlamydia* cultures, rubella, Pap results, H/H, UA, sickle prep if increased risk group. Note if RhoGAM was given, and if so, when. Results of 1 hour PG

PAST MEDICAL HISTORY:
   Past illness
   Medications (Prenatal vitamins/iron)
   Past surgical history
   Allergies
   Birth History: List each birth by year, length of gestation, weight and sex, route of delivery, and complications

PHYSICAL EXAM:
    1. Cervix: dilation/effacement/station
    2. Fetal lie, presentation, and position (if possible)
    3. Fetal monitor shows _____ (good short- and long-term variability) with a rate of _____
    4. Status of amniotic fluid is _____ (clear, cloudy, green, thick, foul smelling)

ASSESSMENT: __y/o woman with __week IUP in ___(active) labor with ___(frequency Q___ minutes) contractions and prenatal course complicated by ___

PLAN: Admit to L & D. Monitor. CBC, Type and screen, UA. Anticipate spontaneous vaginal delivery (SVD) or will augment labor with ___(Pitocin)

Michael B. Weinstock, MD

19. OB DELIVERY NOTE

1. Type of birth _____(e.g., NSVD, suction, forceps)
2. Surgeon (name of person delivering plus attending/assistant)
3. Birth of viable ___(male/female) with Apgar score of __/__
4. Anesthesia (epidural/spinal/pudendal block/local)
5. Estimated blood loss (EBL)—average for vaginal delivery is 300–500cc and for C-section is 800–1000cc
6. The placenta was delivered ____ (spontaneously, manually), was ___ (intact) and had a __ (e.g., 3) vessel cord
7. Uterus (was) explored without retained material
8. Episiotomy was ___(e.g., midline) ___(with, without) extension and was repaired with ____(e.g., suture). There were lacerations at _____ (periurethral, left vaginal wall, cervical)
9. Complications (meconium, nuchal cord, retained placenta, bleeding, etc.)
10. Time of first, second and third stages of labor

OB

20. POSTPARTUM DISCHARGE INSTRUCTIONS

These issues should be discussed with all home going mothers by the physician

A. No heavy lifting (anything heavier than the baby) or driving for 1–2 weeks. This needs to be individualized as the reason not to drive is that episiotomy pain may cause hesitancy while driving

B. No vaginal intercourse, tampons or douching for 6 weeks. This allows the vaginal musculature to tighten and the episiotomy to heal

C. Sitz baths (sitting in a warm bath) may help episiotomy pain

D. Contraception: Ask all mothers what type of birth control they will be using. Breast-feeding alone is a poor contraceptive. **Norplant** and **Depo-Provera** can be started on postpartum day 1. Progesterone-only oral contraceptives can be started on day 1 even for mothers who are breast-feeding. An estrogen-containing contraceptive may decrease milk production and contribute to the normal hypercoagulable state of postpartum patients. An estrogen-containing oral contraceptive may safely be started after 3 to 4 weeks. For undecided patients, encourage using a condom with or without contraceptive foam until first postpartum visit

E. Pain medications: **Tylenol** will usually be all that is needed for vaginal deliveries. Sitz baths may help episiotomy pain. A narcotic after C-section is reasonable. **Vicodin** or **Percocet** are good choices

F. Postpartum depression: If lasts longer than 72hrs or is accompanied by lack of interest in the infant, suicidal or homicidal thoughts, or hallucinations, patient should seek treatment

G. Call office if temperature > 100.5°F or with increased pain

H. Consider a stool softener (**Colace** 100mg PO BID)

I. Vaginal bleeding: Patients can expect some lochia for 3–4 weeks postpartum. Anything heavier than a normal menstrual period should be evaluated

J. Breast-feeding. See Chapter 4, Infant Formula and Breast-feeding

III. Women's Health

Michael B. Weinstock, MD
Beth Weinstock, MD
Kate Baltrushot, MD

21. CONTRACEPTION

GYN

I. ORAL CONTRACEPTIVES (OCs)

OCs act by suppression of ovulation and thickening of cervical mucus

A. Advantages

1. Very effective contraception: Theoretical and actual failure rates of 0.5% and 3% respectively (failure rate of inner city teens as high as 15%)
2. Decreased risk of ovarian and endometrial cancer by 40% and 50%, respectively
3. Decreased risk of ectopic pregnancy (occur 500 times less often in OC users) and pelvic inflammatory disease (PID)
4. Lighter menstrual flow, relief of dysmenorrhea, decreased ovarian cysts
5. Decreases endometriosis, PMS symptoms and acne
6. Decreased incidence of fibrocystic breast disease and fibroadenoma
7. Fertility returns within 3 months of discontinuing OCs in most patients

B. Indications:
Women seeking a reliable form of birth control. Patients must be cautioned that OCs do not protect against sexually transmitted diseases and a condom should be used. Women can use OCs until menopause (See section G) unless they are smokers, in which case they should stop use at age 35. In many states minors may be prescribed OCs without parental consent

C. Contraindications

1. Absolute (applies to *Estrogen-containing OCs* only)
   a. Pregnancy
   b. Thrombophlebitis or thromboembolic disorders past or present
   c. CVA or CAD
   d. Undiagnosed vaginal bleeding
   e. Breast cancer or Estrogen dependent cancer (Some feel this is a relative contraindication)
   f. Benign or malignant tumor of the liver (past or present)
2. Relative
   a. Age >35 and smoker
   b. Cervical dysplasia
   c. Hypertension
   d. Cardiac, renal, gallbladder, sickle cell disease
   e. Migraines, history of severe depression, history of toxemia
   f. Active hepatitis or infectious mononucleosis
   g. Diabetes, surgery, fracture, severe injury (prolonged bedrest with increased risk of DVT), lactation, significant depression

D. Drug interactions:
Patients taking the following drugs will need to use another form of contraception: Rifampin, Phenobarbital, Phenytoin (Dilantin), Griseofulvin, Primidone (Mysoline), Carbamazepine (Tegretol), and antibiotics. OCs can also decrease the hepatic metabolism of certain drugs, resulting in increased toxicity (some Benzodiazepines, β-blockers, Theophylline, TCAs). Pioglitazone (Actos) and Ethosuximide can decrease effectiveness

E. Follow-up:
Return 3 months after beginning OCs to have blood pressure checked. Inquire about side effects, spotting, failure to withdrawal bleed (See following tables.) Then follow-up every year. Check blood lipids in same fashion as for non-pill users—check baseline *non-fasting* total cholesterol and HDL, then every 5 years unless high risk (See Chapter 37, Hyperlipidemia)

GYN

F. Beginning OCs: *It is safe to begin all contraceptives on the first Sunday after the onset of menses or on the first day of menses.* If menses begins on a Sunday, start that night and no other form of contraception is required. If OC is not started within 5 days of onset of menses, then some clinicians advise using an alternate form of birth control for the first week (e.g., condoms and spermicidal foam). When starting OCs, pick one with 30–35mcg of Estrogen. Most physicians will start with any of the OCs except a Progestin-only pill (failure rates ~3%). Modify according to side effects

G. Age greater than 35
  1. Smokers: Discontinue OC's or change to progesterone only pill
  2. If patient is a non-smoker and blood pressure and lipids are within normal limits, then OCs may be continued until menopause. Use a low dose (20mcg **Ethinyl Estradiol**) OC if patient > age 40, e.g., **Loestrin 1/20**
  3. Women > age 45 on OCs should have FSH checked every year (at the end of pill pack) and be changed to Estrogen replacement therapy (ERT) when FSH > 30
  4. Loestrin 1/20 is 4 times as potent as Premarin 0.625mg

H. Missed pills
  1. 1 missed pill: Take as soon as patient remembers, take next pill on schedule, no back-up required
  2. 2 missed pills: Take 2 pills on each of next 2 days and use a back-up for 7 days
  3. 3 missed pills: Continue to take pills and use back-up until menstruation

I. Amenorrhea while taking OCs:
  1. For 1–2 cycles: Check β-hCG
  2. For 3 cycles: Increase estrogen or decrease progestin

J. Lactation: Use a Progestin-only pill or Depo-Provera because Estrogen may cause a decrease in production of milk. The failure rate of Progestin-only minipill is extremely low when combined with the contraceptive action of prolactin due to lactation. Estrogen containing pills *are safe* for lactating mothers

K. Postpartum: Use a Progestin-only pill or wait until the first postpartum (2–4 weeks) visit due to increased coagulable state with Estrogen-containing OCs

L. Postponing menstruation: Often desired for wedding, vacation. Patient should omit the 7 day hormone-free interval. She should start a new pack the next day after finishing the 21 active pills

M. Pregnancy occurring while on OCs: Using OCs during early pregnancy does not appear to increase the risk of fetal deformities. The OC should be stopped after pregnancy is diagnosed

N. Types of oral contraceptives
  1. Estrogen-Progestin Combinations:
      a. Two most commonly used Estrogen compounds are Ethanyl Estradiol (EE) or Mestranol. Mestranol is estimated to be 50% less potent than EE
      b. Progestational component in OCs varies in both dose and type of Progestin—leads to differences in pharmacologic effect, see chart:

Type of Progestins	Progestin	Estrogen	Antiestrogen	Androgen
Norgestrel	+++	0	++	+++
Desogestrel	+++	0/+	+++	0/+
Norgestimate	+++	0	+++	0
Ethynodiol diacetate	++	+	+	++
Norethindrone acetate	+	+	+++	++
Norethindrone	+	+	+	++
Norethynodrel	+	+++	0	0

    c. Biphasic and triphasic OCs vary dose of Progestin (and often Estrogen) in 2 or 3 phases. These attempt to duplicate the pattern of a normal menstrual cycle. Clinically, very little difference is observed between monophasic and multiphasic OCs
    d. OCs most frequently prescribed contain 30–35mcgs of EE and a Progestin that is less androgenic (Norgestimate or Desogestrel)
    e. Low Estrogen-Progestin combinations are now available. Alesse is a monophasic OC containing 20 mcg EE/0.1mg Levonorgestrel, Mircette is a biphasic OC containing 20/10mg EE/0.15mg desogestrel

2. Progestin-only products ("mini-pills")
    a. Contain decreased dose of Progestin relative to combination OCs
    b. Preferred for use during breastfeeding (Estrogen may decrease milk production), and for women who have contraindication to estrogens (especially smokers > age 35)
    c. Have a slightly higher failure rate (1–4%) and may lead to more irregular bleeding

ORAL CONTRACEPTIVE SIDE EFFECT ADJUSTMENTS

SYMPTOM	PROBABLE ETIOLOGY	CHANGE REQUIRED
Break through bleeding (BTB) spotting first 10 days	Estrogen deficiency	Increase estrogen*
BTB or spotting second 10 days	Estrogen and/or progesterone deficiency	Increase estrogen* or progesterone
Prolonged or heavy menses	Progestin deficiency	Increase progestin
Delayed onset of menses	Progestin deficiency	Increase progestin
Shortened menses	Progestin excess	Decrease progestin
No menses	Progestin excess or estrogen deficiency	Continue one cycle then increase estrogen
Weight gain	Progestin excess	Decrease progestin
Hirsutism, loss of scalp hair, acne	Progestin excess	Decrease progestin or change to progestin with low androgenicity
Cervicitis, candidal vaginitis	Progestin excess	Decrease progestin
Depression, decreased libido, fatigue	Progestin excess	Decrease progestin
Nausea, vomiting	Estrogen excess	Decrease estrogen
Chloasma (skin discoloration)	Estrogen excess	Decrease estrogen
Uterine cramps	Estrogen excess	Decrease estrogen
Edema, bloating, breast tenderness and enlargement, headaches	On pills — Estrogen excess On placebo week — Progestin excess	Decrease offending steroid, diuretics
Migraine, blurring of vision	Estrogen excess	Needs further evaluation, consider stopping pills
Androgenic symptoms		Change to 3rd generation progestin
Dyslipidemia	Progestin excess	Change to 3rd generation progestin

* An easy way to increase the Estrogen without decreasing the Progesterone is to administer Conjugated Estrogen (Premarin) 1.25mg QD × 7 days. This may be attempted no matter where patient is in her cycle

Composition of Combination OCs					
Type	Name	Estrogen	mcg	Progestin	mg
Low Androgenic Activity of Progestin Component					
Monophasic	Modicon Brevicon Nelova 0.5/35 NEE 0.5/35	EE	35	norethindrone	0.5
	Ovcon 35	EE	35	norethindrone	0.4
	Ortho-Cyclen	EE	35	norgestimate	0.25
	Ortho-Cept Desogen	EE	30	desogestrel	0.15
Triphasic	Ortho Tri-Cyclen	EE	35/35/35	norgestimate	0.18/0.215/0.25
Medium Androgenic Activity of Progestin Component					
Monophasic	Norlestrin 1/50	EE	50	norethindrone acetate	1.0
	Ovcon 50 Genora 1/50 Norethin 1/50M	EE	50	norethindrone	1.0
	Ortho-Novum 1/50 Norinyl 1 + 50	mestranol	50	norethindrone	1.0
	Demulen	EE	50	ethynodiol diacetate	1.0
	Demulen 1/35	EE	35	ethynodiol diacetate	1.0
	Ortho-Novum 1/35 Norinyl 1 + 35 Genora 1/35 Norethin 1/35E Norcept-E 1/35 Nelova 1/35 NEE 1/35	EE	35	norethindrone	1.0
	Loestrin 1/20	EE	20	norethindrone acetate	1.0
Biphasic	Ortho-Novum 10/11 NEE 10/11 Jenest-28	EE	35/35	norethindrone	0.5/1.0
Triphasic	Ortho-Novum 7/7/7	EE	35/35/35	norethindrone	0.5/0.75/1.0
	Tri-Norinyl	EE	35/35/35	norethindrone	0.5/1.0/0.5
	Triphasil Tri-Levlen	EE	30/40/30	levonorgestrel	0.05/0.075/0.125
High Androgenic Activity of Progestin Component					
Monophasic	Ovral	EE	50	norgestrel	0.5
	Norlestrin 2.5/50	EE	50	norethindrone acetate	2.5
	Loestrin 1.5/30	EE	30	norethindrone acetate	1.5
	Lo-Ovral	EE	30	norgestrel	0.3
	Nordette	EE	30	levonorgestrel	0.15
	Levlen	EE	30	levonorgestrel	0.15
Composition of Progestin-Only OCs					
Type	Name	Estrogen	mcg	Progestin	mg
Monophasic	Micronor	None	N/A	norethindrone	0.35
	Nor-QD	None	N/A	norethindrone	0.35
	Ovrette	None	N/A	norgestrel	0.075

- Failure rates with the progestin-only minipill are higher than other OCs (1–4%). They also do not offer protection against functional ovarian cysts
- Ethynodiol, Desogestrel and Norgestimate have a low amount of androgenicity and may be good first line agents for women with acne and hirsutism
- Some clinicians feel that assessing the relative progesterone potency is not clinically useful

II. PROGESTERONE IMPLANTS AND INJECTIONS

A. Depo-Provera (Medroxyprogesterone Acetate) 150mg IM Q3 months
1. Failure rate of 0.3%
2. Check urine pregnancy test before administering first dose. Should also check urine pregnancy before re-administering Depo-Provera if patient > 1 week late for injection
3. If first dose is given during menstruation, contraception begins immediately. If not, then use alternate form of contraception until next menses
4. May give postpartum even if mothers are lactating
5. Side effects: Irregular bleeding, amenorrhea, weight gain (5–10 lbs), headache, may increase risk of bone loss with long-term use. Inform patient to anticipate these effects when medication is begun!
6. If spotting occurs, patient should be informed that irregular bleeding usually disappears after 1 year. Consider giving **Premarin** 1.25mg QD × 7 days which may be increased to 2.5mg QD × 7 days or 2.5mg QD × 21 days. This therapy should not be continued longer than 1–2 months. If unsuccessful then consider another form of contraception

B. Norplant (Medroxyprogesterone): Same basic description as Depo-Provera. Good for 5 years of contraception. Often difficult to remove

III. MALE CONDOM

A. Theoretical and actual failure rates: 2% and 10%, respectively. Patients should be instructed in use as the actual failure rate can fall dramatically with correct use
B. Better protection against STDs (including HIV if condoms with nonoxynol-9 are used)
C. Patients should be instructed not to use with oil-based lubricants, such as Vaseline
D. If used with a spermicidal vaginal foam, contraception failure rates approach OCs

IV. FEMALE CONDOM

A. Failure rate 5–20%
B. Difficult to use
C. Protects against STDs
D. Can use any lubricant

V. DIAPHRAGM

A. Theoretical and actual failure rates: 2% and 20% when used with spermicide
B. Provides protection against pelvic infection and cervical dysplasia. Increased risk of UTIs
C. Must be inserted prior to intercourse, but does not need to be removed and reinserted for subsequent intercourse for next 12hrs (do need to use extra spermicide after 6hrs). Cannot be left in longer than 12–18hrs (increased risk of UTIs)

VI. CONTRACEPTIVE SPONGE, FOAM, CREAM AND JELLY

A. Failure rates from 3–20% per year
B. Inserted before intercourse and may be used without replacement for repeated acts of intercourse for 12–18hrs. Cannot be left in longer than 12–18hrs

VII. INTRAUTERINE DEVICES (IUDs)

A. Failure rates 1–2%
B. There are 2 brands: Progestasert (secretes progesterone) and Copper T380A
C. Implant during menses, mid-cycle to prevent implantation, or 12 weeks postpartum. Progestasert should be changed annually, and Copper T380A, every 10 years
D. Especially useful in women who have completed child bearing and have only 1 sexual partner. Risk of PID are increased, therefore only use with caution in women in child bearing years. Increased risk of ectopic pregnancy

GYN

VIII. COITUS INTERRUPTUS
Failure rates 20–25% per year

IX. FERTILITY BASED AWARENESS (Basal body temperature, calendar)
Failure rates from 2–20% depending on expertise of user

X. STERILIZATION:
A. Male
1. Failure rate of only 0.1%
2. Couple needs to be sure that no more children are desired
3. In office procedure with 'scalpel-less' procedure
4. Easy to perform, local anesthesia

B. Female
1. Failure rates depend on procedure used—most effective post partum
2. Failure rates increase over 10 years from 0.8% to 4%. Counsel the couple on their certainty of sterilization. Can possibly be reversed, but at a cost of ~$10,000
3. Salpingectomy (part of tube removed and ends tied) is most effective

XI. NO METHOD
Pregnancy rate of 85–90% per year

XII. POSTCOITAL CONTRACEPTION
A. May be used for unprotected sex, broken condom (mid-cycle), rape
B. First dose must be given within 72hrs with the second dose administered 12hrs later
C. Perform pregnancy test first!
D. Failure rates of ~1.5%. If pregnancy occurs then elective abortion is an option
E. Available kits are: **Ovral**–2 pills/dose
Nordette–4 pills/dose
Triphasil–4 pills/dose
Plan B–1 pill/dose
Preven kit–2 pills/dose
F. Important to include Rx. for antiemetic—e.g., **Phenergan** 25mg PO or PR Q 4–6hrs PRN
G. Should experience bleeding in 3–4 weeks. If not, the patient needs a pregnancy test

CLINICAL PEARLS
• Most cases of condom failure result from inappropriate usage. The number of condoms that break is less than 2 per 100
• The number of women with *chlamydia* and *gonorrhea* who later develop infertility ranges from 10–40%. Correct use of a male (or female) condom can drastically reduce the chance of contracting a sexually transmitted disease

References
Abma JC, et al. Fertility, family planning and woman's health: new data from the 1995 national survey of family growth. Vital Health Stat 1997;23(19):1–114.
Beral V, et al. Mortality associated with oral contraceptive use: 25 year follow up of cohort of 46,000 women from Royal College of General Practitioners' oral contraception study. BMJ Jan 9, 1999;318: 96–100.
Cerel-Suhl SL, Yeager BF. Update on oral contraceptive pills. Am Fam Phys 1999;60:2073–84.
International Federation of Fertility Societies. Consensus conference on combination oral contraceptives and cardiovascular disease. Fertil Steril 1999;71(suppl 3):1s–6s.
Scholes D. et al. Bone mineral density in women using depot medroxprogesterone acetate for contraception. Obstet Gynecol Feb 1999; 93:233–8.
Hatcher RA, et al. Contraceptive technology. 17th rev. ed. New York:Ardent Media, 1998.
American College of Obstetricians and Gynecologists. Hormonal contraception. ACOG technical bulletin No. 198. Washington, D.C., Oct. 1994.

Michael B. Weinstock, MD
Kate Baltrushot, MD

22. PAP SMEARS:
INDICATIONS AND INTERPRETATION

GYN

I. INDICATIONS AND SCHEDULE

A. To begin with onset of sexual activity, age 18, or with first pelvic exam, whichever comes first

B. Perform Pap smears, pelvic and breast exam yearly. If a patient has no risk factors (See below) and 3 normal Paps, then consider performing Paps Q2–3 years. Patient should continue with yearly pelvic and breast exams

C. Risk factors for cervical cancer

1. Early first intercourse
2. Large number of lifetime sexual partners
3. History of STDs, especially human papilloma virus (HPV)
4. High risk sexual partners
5. Cigarette smoking
6. Lack of normal immune response (HIV increases chances of cervical cancer 8–11 times)

II. TECHNIQUE FOR USING ARYST SPATULA AND CYTOBRUSH (Note: May use "broom" to get both cervical and endocervical components)

A. Perform mid-cycle. Patient should not douche or have sexual intercourse for 24hrs before Pap

B. Visually inspect cervix

C. Rotate wooden spatula (aryst spatula) 720° to sample squamocolumnar junction

D. Slowly rotate cytobrush 720° in endocervix

E. Use fixative as quickly as possible (within seconds)

F. Perform pelvic examination

III. NEW TECHNIQUES FOR SCREENING:

A. Autopap or Papnet: Computerized rescreening of all manually screened slides. Attempt to decrease number of false negative slides. Computerized to decrease human error from fatigue, time limits, etc.

B. Fluid based technology: Thinprep, Cytorich (not currently approved by FDA). Uses the same technique for getting sample. The brush is then washed in preservative solution. This increases the yield of cells while maintaining the integrity of the sample better than traditional methods. The preservative solution also lyses fresh RBC's, kills bacteria and dispenses mucus all of which can affect the sample. This is a new technique and requires different training to interpret the slides. It also costs more and will require a higher cost to the patient

IV. PATHOLOGY REPORT AND ACTION TO TAKE

Letters A–G (below) describe the possible descriptive diagnosis a Pap can be. A **low grade squamous intraepithelial lesion (LGSIL)** Pap is further broken down into dysplasia (CIN I) and HPV. A **high grade squamous intraepithelial lesion (HGSIL)** Pap is further broken down into moderate dysplasia (CIN II), severe dysplasia (CIN III) and carcinoma in situ (CIN III). The Bethesda system combines these 3 entities into one (HGSIL) because they are managed the same, and because the differentiation has not been shown to be reproducible

A. Within normal limits

Action: Repeat in 1 year. (Pap smears have a 15–40% false negative rate)

B. Benign cellular changes: Inflammation, infection, atrophy

Action:

1. **Clindamycin Phosphate** vaginal cream (**Cleocin**): Apply intravaginally QHS × 7 days. Repeat Pap in 2–3 months—*or* —
2. **Betadine** douche and gel: Use gel QHS × 5–7 days or douche QD × 5–7 days. Repeat Pap in 2–3 months

GYN

3. Treat infection if culture positive for *chlamydia* or *N. gonorrhea*. See Chapter 28, Vaginitis and Sexually Transmitted Diseases

4. **Conjugated Estrogens (Premarin)** vaginal cream for atrophic vaginitis: Apply 2g QHS × 6 weeks. Repeat Pap in 2–3 months

5. With 2 inflammatory Paps, perform colposcopy

C. Atypical squamous cells of undetermined significance (ASCUS)

Action:

1. Colposcopy and endocervical curettage (ECC)—*or* —

2. Low risk patients: Pap smears Q3 months × 1 year, then Q6 months × 1 year—if any of these 6 Paps (over 2 years) is abnormal, then perform colposcopy

3. With 2 ASCUS Paps, perform colposcopy and ECC

D. Atypical glandular cells of undetermined significance (AGCUS)

Action: ECC directed by colposcopy, biopsy and pipelle (cells could be endometrial)

E. Low grade squamous intraepithelial lesion (low grade SIL)

— *See clinical pearls at end of chapter*

1. Mild dysplasia (CIN I)—*or* —

2. HPV

Action:

a. Colposcopy and ECC—*or* —

b. Low risk patients: Pap smears Q3 months × 1 year, then Q6 months × 1 year. If any of these 6 Paps (over 2 years) is abnormal, then perform colposcopy

c. With 2 low grade SILs, perform colposcopy

F. High grade squamous intraepithelial lesion (high grade SIL)

1. Moderate dysplasia (CIN II)—*or* —

2. Severe dysplasia (CIN III)—*or* —

3. Carcinoma *in situ* (CIN III)

Action:

a Colposcopy and ECC to determine distribution of the lesion

b. After colposcopy and ECC, patient should undergo ablative therapy to destroy or remove the entire transformation zone

G. Invasive cancer

Action: Refer to gynecologic oncologist

V. TREATMENT OF SQUAMOUS INTRAEPITHELIAL LESIONS*

A. Indications for surgical excision (Cone)

1. Unsatisfactory colposcopic examination (lesion extends into the cervical canal and is not visualized)

2. Pap and colposcopy do not agree

3. Diagnosis of microinvasive carcinoma based on punch biopsy

B. Cryosurgery

C. Laser vaporization techniques

D. Loop electrosurgical excision procedure (LEEP)/Large Loop excision of transformation zone (LLETZ): Removal of lesion with tissue diagnosis

* After the procedure, all patients will need Pap smears Q3 months × 1 year, Q6 months × 1 year, then Q year if follow-up Paps are WNL

CLINICAL PEARLS

• There were 13,000 cases of cervical cancer and 600,000 cases of CIN in 1991. The incidence of cervical cancer has decreased about 80% in the last 50 years

• 15% of CIN I will progress to CIN III. 60% of CIN I will regress spontaneously. CIN I can be followed expectantly because so many regress spontaneously

• The rate of false negative Pap smears is 15–40%

• There is no "magic formula" to getting repeat Pap smears Q 3 months. The important thing is to perform frequent Paps to decrease the false negative rate. With 2 Paps the false negative rate falls to 2–16%, with 3 Paps it falls to 0.3–6%, and with 4 Paps it falls to 0.05–2.5%

• HPV typing (to determine strains likely to induce dysplasia) generally will not change management

References

Canavan TP, Doshi NR. Cervical cancer. Am Fam Phys 2000;61:1369–76.

Brown AD, Garber AM. Cost effectiveness of 3 methods to enhance the sensitivity of Papanicolaou testing, JAMA 1999;281(4)347–53.

Sawaya GF, et al. New technologies in cervical cytology screening: a word of caution. Cervical screening technologies. Elsevier Science Inc 1999; 94(2):307–10.

Lombard I, et al. Human papillomavirus genotype as a major determinant of the course of cervical cancer. J Clin Oncol 1998;16: 2613–9.

Spitzer M. Cervical screening adjuncts: recent advances. Am J Obstet Gynecol 1998;179:544–56.

American College of Obstetricians and Gynecologists. New pap test screening techniques. ACOG committee opinion no. 206. 1998 Washington, D.C.

Woolf SH. Screening for cervical cancer. U.S. Preventive Services Task Force. Guide to clinical preventive services: report of the U.S. Preventive Services Task Force. 2d ed. Baltimore: Williams & Wilkins, 1996: 105–17.

American College of Obstetricians and Gynecologists. Recommendations on frequency of pap test screening. ACOG committee opinion no. 152. Int J Gynaecol Obstet 1995;49:210–1.

Michael B. Weinstock, MD
Anita Schwandt, MD

23. ABNORMAL UTERINE BLEEDING

I. DIAGNOSIS

    A. Exclude non-uterine causes of bleeding

        1. Lower tract bleeding (vaginal, cervical, urinary bleeding)

        2. Pregnancy (intrauterine, ectopic, molar)

    B. Differentiate between anatomic (normal cycle) **vs. dysfunctional** (irregular cycle) **uterine bleeding**

        1. Anatomic uterine bleeding

            a. Bleeding within normal cycles as a result of a structural abnormality

            b. E.g., Polyps, fibroids, endometriosis, adenomyosis, endometritis, implantation bleeding, cancer

        2. Dysfunctional uterine bleeding (DUB)

            a. Excessive, irregular uterine bleeding without demonstrable organic cause. This usually is a "hormonal problem" of anovulation and unopposed estrogen

            b. Note: During the normal cycle, there will be a progesterone surge after ovulation which allows for cyclic endometrial sloughing. This results in a proliferative endometrium which then sloughs off gradually. In DUB, there is often gradual sloughing of the endometrium as there is no ovulation and no progesterone surge

            c. DUB is a diagnosis of exclusion

II. TERMINOLOGY

    A. Menorrhagia: Prolonged or excessive uterine bleeding occurring at regular intervals

    B. Metrorrhagia: Uterine bleeding occurring at irregular, but infrequent intervals

    C. Menometrorrhagia: Prolonged uterine bleeding occurring at irregular intervals

    D. Polymenorrhea: Uterine bleeding occurring at regular intervals of less than 21 days

    E. Oligomenorrhea: Uterine bleeding in which the interval between bleeding episodes varies from 35 days to 6 months

    F. Amenorrhea: No uterine bleeding for at least 6 months

III. HISTORY

    A. Onset of menarche: The initial cycles after menarche are usually anovulatory due to a delay in the maturation of the hypothalamic-pituitary axis

    B. Menses: Frequency, cyclicity, amount (number pads soaked per day) and duration

    C. Duration of abnormal bleeding

    D. Previous therapy for abnormal bleeding

GYN

E. **Sexual history:** Birth control, vaginal discharge

F. Stress, weight change, exercise

G. **Medications:** Estrogen replacement therapy, oral contraceptives including progestin-only pills, long acting contraceptives (Norplant, Depo-provera)

H. **Past medical history:** Endometriosis, fibroids, polyps, history of abnormal Pap smears, polycystic ovarian syndrome, systemic diseases (especially thyroid, renal, hepatic, and coagulopathies)

I. **Surgery:** Oophorectomy

J. Radiation

IV. PHYSICAL

A. **General exam:** Weight, surgical scars, signs of thyroid abnormalities, hirsutism

B. **Vaginal exam:** Lesions, masses, discharge

C. **Pelvic exam:** Cervical motion tenderness, adnexal mass, pelvic mass

V. LABORATORY: If indicated

A. Pregnancy test

B. CBC

C. Pap smear: If sexually active or if age 18 or older

D. Pelvic cultures (if sexually active): *GC, Chlamydia, Trichomonas*

E. Thyroid (TSH), prolactin, androgen studies (if patient is hirsute)

F. Coagulation studies (PT/PTT, bleeding time)

VI. ABNORMAL UTERINE BLEEDING IN *ADOLESCENTS*

A. **General**

    1. Cycles are often anovulatory and irregular following menarche

    2. The hypothalamic-pituitary-ovarian axis is usually mature within 18 months of menarche

B. **Pelvic exam:** Not necessary if within 18 months of menarche and not sexually active

C. **Management**

    1. If bleeding is not severe: Cycle patients for 3–6 months on oral contraceptive pills

    2. For severe bleeding: Consider further work-up for possible underlying coagulopathy

VII. ABNORMAL UTERINE BLEEDING IN *REPRODUCTIVE AGE* WOMEN

A. **Anatomic uterine bleeding:** Hormonal therapy may be attempted (see below, DUB), but patient will probably need definitive therapy (D&C, surgery, etc.)

B. Dysfunctional uterine bleeding

    1. Endometrial biopsy: Long-term unopposed estrogen stimulation can result in endometrial hyperplasia, consider endometrial biopsy in any women over age 30 with an extended anovulatory period or any women over 20 with prolonged bleeding

    2. Management

        a. Light to moderate flow

            i. Oral contraceptive with 50mcg **Ethinyl Estradiol (Ovcon 50, Demulen 1/50, Ovral)**. Take 1 PO TID × 7 days, allow 7 days off pills for a likely heavy bleed, then start new pack and take as directed 1 PO QD. If patient continues to bleed while using OC's consider changing to an OC with a higher Progestin potency (See Chapter 21, Contraception)

            ii. Provera 10mg PO QD × 7 days

        b. Heavy flow: Hypotensive, anemic, soaking greater than 1 full pad per hour for several hours

            i. **Conjugated Estrogen (Premarin):** 2.5mg PO QID × 7–10 days (bleeding will decrease within several hours to several days) followed by **Progesterone (Medroxyprogesterone Acetate)** 10mg QD × 7–10 days

            ii. For rapid bleeding: **Conjugated Estrogen (Premarin):** 25mg IVP Q3–4hrs for rapid bleeding. Not to exceed 3 doses. Begin Conjugated Estrogens 2.5mg QID for 7–10 days followed by **Progesterone** 10mg QD for 7–10 days

            iii. If bleeding continues, IV **Vasopressin (DDAVP)** or a D&C may be necessary

            iv. **Ferrous Sulfate** 325mg QD to TID

VIII. ABNORMAL UTERINE BLEEDING IN *PERIMENOPAUSAL* WOMEN: Age 35 to menopause
  A. **Anatomic uterine bleeding:** Perform D&C
  B. **Dysfunctional uterine bleeding**
    1. Perform endometrial (pipelle) biopsy to exclude malignancy
    2. If normal, then prescribe hormonal therapy as described above. Use of oral contraceptives that contain Estrogen is contraindicated if patient is a smoker (See Chapter 21, Contraception)
  C. **Diagnosis of DUB vs. menopause** (See Chapter 25, Menopause and HRT)
    1. If patient has 3 months of amenorrhea: To determine if patient is in menopause, then either obtain FSH level or give Provera to stimulate withdrawal bleeding:
      a. Obtain FSH level
        i. If FSH is high (>35mIU/mL), then patient is in menopause. Start hormone replacement therapy (See post-menopausal section below)
        ii. If FSH is low, then patient has DUB. Perform pipelle biopsy to exclude malignancy. Cycle with Provera 10mg × 7 days per month
      b. **Provera:** 10mg QD × 7 days to see if patient has withdrawal bleeding
        i. If there is no withdrawal bleeding, then repeat in 3 months. If she still has no withdrawal bleeding, assume she is in menopause. (See Chapter 25, Menopause and HRT)
        ii. If there is withdrawal bleeding, then patient is not in menopause. Continue workup for sources of abnormal uterine bleeding/amenorrhea
    2. If patient has heavy menses (passing clots or social inconvenience) for 3 months, bleeding between menses for 3–4 months, or 3 consecutive months of menses which last longer than 7 days, then perform pipelle biopsy, consider pelvic ultrasonography to measure the endometrial thickness, or D&C. Manifestations of malignancy (bleeding) must not be dismissed as early menopause.

IX. ABNORMAL UTERINE BLEEDING IN *POST-MENOPAUSAL* WOMEN: Perform pipelle biopsy consider pelvic ultrasonography to measure the endometrial thickness
  A. **If endometrium is hyperplastic:** Perform D&C and hysteroscopy. Hyperplastic endometrium and atypia is associated with malignancy 15% of the time
  B. **If endometrium is atrophic:** Begin HRT
  C. **If biopsy demonstrates polyps:** No further therapy is required
  D. **If biopsy demonstrates cancer:** Refer to gynecologic oncologist

CLINICAL PEARLS
    • All post-menopausal bleeding must be worked up as 7% of post-menopausal bleeding is the result of malignancy!
    • Consider β-hCG in all pre-menopausal women with abnormal bleeding

References
Archer DF, et al. Uterine bleeding in postmenopausal women on continuous therapy with estradiol and norethindrone acetate. Obstet Gynecol Sep 1999; 94:323–9.
Fowler GC, et al. Menstrual irregularities: A focused evaluation. Patient Care Apr 15, 1994; 155–64.
Bayer SR, DeCherney AH. Clinical manifestations and treatment of dysfunctional uterine bleeding. JAMA 1993; 269:1823–8.
Johnson CA. Making sense of dysfunctional uterine bleeding. Am Fam Phys 1991;44:149–57.

GYN

Cathy Greiwe, MD

GYN

24. AMENORRHEA

I. INTRODUCTION: First exclude the most common cause; pregnancy. A history and physical including detailed gynecological exam will guide the evaluation and subsequent lab studies

II. DEFINITION: Amenorrhea (absence of menses) is divided into the following:
- **A. Primary:** No spontaneous uterine bleeding by age 14 in the absence of the development of secondary sex characteristics or by age 16 in otherwise normal development
- **B. Secondary** (more common): Absence of menses for 6 months in woman with prior regular menses or for 12 months in women with prior oligomenorrhea

III. HISTORY
- **A. Medical**
  1. Endocrine or metabolic disorders
  2. Galactorrhea (need to exclude pituitary adenoma)
  3. Past or present serious illnesses
  4. Previous radiation therapy or chemotherapy
  5. Recent weight gain or loss/eating disorder
  6. Psychological disturbance/depression/stress
  7. Athletic training/intense exercise
- **B. Menstrual**
  1. Age at menarche
  2. Date of last menstrual period
  3. Previous menstrual pattern
  4. Events surrounding the onset of amenorrhea
- **C. Reproductive**
  1. Contraceptive use
  2. Gynecologic or obstetric procedures
  3. Pregnancies: outcomes, complications
  4. Pubertal development
- **D. Family**
  1. Age of mother and sister(s) at menarche and menopause
  2. Autoimmune disorders
  3. Congenital anomalies
  4. Endocrinopathies
  5. Infertility
  6. Menstrual dysfunction
  7. Tuberculosis
- **E. Medications:** Associated with amenorrhea
  1. Drugs that increase prolactin
     a. Antipsychotics: Phenothiazines, Haloperidol (Haldol), Pimozide (Orap), Clozapine (Clozaril)
     b. Antidepressants: Tricyclic antidepressants, Monoamine oxidase inhibitors
     c. Antihypertensives: Calcium channel blockers, Methyldopa (Aldomet), Reserpine
  2. Drugs with estrogenic activity: Digitalis, Marijuana, Flavinoids, Oral contraceptives
  3. Drugs with ovarian toxicity: Busulfan (Myleran), Chlorambucil (Leukeran), Cisplatin (Platinol), Cyclophosphamide (Cytoxan, Neosar), Fluorouracil

IV. PHYSICAL
- **A. General:** Body habitus and proportion, obesity, body hair extent and distribution
- **B. HEENT:** Excessive facial hair, acne, funduscopic exam to evaluate for papilledema, visual fields. Assess thyroid for goiter or nodules
- **C. Breast development** and presence of galactorrhea (fat globules visible per microscope exam)
- **D. Abdomen:** Striae in nulliparous women (hypercortisolism)

E. **Genitalia:** Refer to Tanner Stages

V. LABS
  A. Pregnancy test
  B. **See algorithm below** for TSH, Prolactin, FSH, and LH
  C. **Other labs** to consider obtaining to rule out systemic disease include: CBC, Calcium, Phosphorous, TSH, Thyroxine, thyroid antibodies, ESR, total Protein, RF, ANA

GYN

VI. EVALUATION

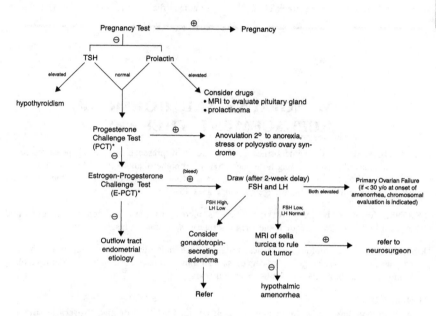

*Refer to text for description of these diagnostic tests

  A. **Progesterone Challenge Test (PCT)**
    1. Method: Give **Medroxyprogesterone Acetate (MPA)** 10mg PO QD × 5 days
    2. Results: The test is positive if there is *any* vaginal bleeding within 2–7 days after the fifth tablet. This confirms a diagnosis of anovulation. There is adequate endogenous estrogen, and the outflow tract is patent
  B. **Estrogen-Progesterone Challenge Test (E-PCT)**
    1. Method: Give **Conjugated Estrogen** 1.25mg PO QD × 21 days, add **MPA** 10mg days 16–21. Repeat cycle if no bleeding by day 28
    2. Results: A positive test indicates menstruation is possible if adequate stimulatory estrogen is available. The workup is depicted in diagram. A negative test requires referral to a gynecologist for further studies

VII. MANAGEMENT
  A. **Anovulation secondary to inadequate Progesterone** (i.e., positive PCT) indicates increased risk of endometrial cancer because of hyperplastic effect of unopposed Estrogen. In addition, there may also be increased risk for breast cancer
    1. To reduce risk of endometrial disease and to provide cycle regularity, give MPA 10mg PO QD for first 7–10 days of each month
    2. If pregnancy is desired, consider ovulation induction
    3. If pregnancy is not desired, then give low dose cyclic oral contraceptives
  B. **Hypoestrogenic women** (i.e. negative PCT and positive E-PCT) should be further evaluated with LH and FSH (see algorithm). Elevated levels are indicative of primary ovarian failure. If onset of amenorrhea is < 30 years old, chromosomal analysis is indicated

CLINICAL PEARLS
- Normally, the arm span and height measures are similar. If the arm span is 5cm greater than the height, suspect hypogonadal disease
- Prevalence of secondary amenorrhea is higher in certain subgroups such as college students, ballet dancers, and competitive endurance athletes

References
Wyngaarden, J.B. et al., ed. Cecil textbook of medicine. 20th ed. Philadelphia:WB Saunders, 1996:Vol. 2, 1302–7.
Kiningham, RB; Apgar BS, Schwenk TL. Evaluation of amenorrhea. Am Fam Phys 1996;53:1185–94.

Michael B. Weinstock, MD
Tina Nelson, MD

25. MENOPAUSE AND HORMONE REPLACEMENT THERAPY

DEFINITION: Menopause is amenorrhea for 12 months in the presence of signs of hypoestrogenemia and a serum follicle-stimulating hormone (FSH) level higher than 40 IU/l. Menopause can also be diagnosed on the basis of subjective symptoms such as hot flushes/flashes, or the result of a progesterone withdrawal. (Mean age 51, range ages 40–58)

I. SIGNS: Menopause begins with skipped periods, increased interval between menses, decreased interval to 23–24 days, frequent and irregular intervals, or long or heavy bleeding

II. SYMPTOMS: Vasomotor (hot flashes, sweating), insomnia, nervousness, vaginal atrophy, urinary atrophy (stress or urge incontinence), skin atrophy (wrinkles), osteoporosis, arteriosclerosis. Symptoms last from several months to several years

III. DIAGNOSIS
    A. If patient has 3 months of amenorrhea: Obtain FSH level or give **Provera** to stimulate withdrawal bleeding
        1. Obtain FSH level: Should be measured on days 2–4 of menses. Sequential measurements may be helpful
            a. *If FSH is high* (>40mIU/mL), then patient is in menopause. The pituitary is trying to stimulate ovulation, but patient is in menopause/ovarian failure. Consider starting hormone replacement therapy (HRT) (See IV below)
            b. *If FSH is low* (< 40mIU/mL), then the patient is not in menopause. Consider pipelle biopsy to exclude malignancy. Cycle with **Provera 10mg QD × 7 days per month**
        2. Withdrawal bleeding: **Provera 10mg QD × 7 days**
            a. If there is no withdrawal bleeding, then repeat in 3 months. If she still has no withdrawal bleeding, assume she is in menopause. Consider starting HRT (See IV below)
            b. If there is withdrawal bleeding, then patient is not in menopause
    B. If patient is having symptoms (hot flushes, etc.) and is not amenorrheic and FSH is elevated (> 20mIU/mL), then she is in the transitional phase and menopause will most likely occur in the next several years
        1. These patients may be placed on low dose oral contraceptives for symptom relief. Patients should be free of the following risk factors: hypertension, hypercholesterolemia, cigarette smoking, previous thromboembolic disorders, cerebrovascular disease or coronary artery disease
        2. Cyclic progestins may be used for women who are not candidates for OCP. One approach is **Medroxyprogesterone** 10mg daily for 10 days each month to induce withdrawal bleeding and decrease the risk of endometrial hyperplasia
    C. If the patient is on oral contraceptives, measure the FSH on the 6th day of the pill-free interval. If FSH > 40 mIU/mL, then change to HRT

D. **If patient has heavy menses** (passing clots or social inconvenience) for 3 months, bleeding between menses for 3–4 months, or 3 consecutive months of menses which last longer than 7 days, then perform pipelle biopsy or D&C. Manifestations of malignancy (bleeding) *must not* be dismissed as early menopause

IV. MANAGEMENT OF MENOPAUSE

A. Hormone replacement therapy (HRT)

1. Advantages of HRT
   a. Control of vasomotor symptoms
   b. Avoid or reverse atrophic vaginitis
   c. Control psychological symptoms
   d. Prevents osteoporosis
   e. Prevents urinary tract atrophy symptoms such as dysuria, urgency, recurrent urinary tract infections and stress urinary incontinence
   f. Estrogen has been shown to improve short-term memory and psychological function in postmenopausal women. There is some evidence to suggest the risk of Alzheimer's disease can be decreased by estrogen therapy

2. Disadvantages
   a. Double the risk of gallbladder disease
   b. Possible small increase in risk of breast cancer
   c. Growth of uterine myomas
   d. Endometrial cancer if not taken with progestins
   e. Cost and inconvenience

3. Contraindications to HRT
   a. Breast cancer that is estrogen receptor positive
   b. Unexplained abnormal uterine bleeding
   c. History of thrombophlebitis, thromboembolic disorders, or stroke
   d. Active liver disease
   e. Known or suspected pregnancy

4. Controversies:Two recent trials (see references below) suggest that there may be an increase in coronary heart disease events in estrogen users who have a history of heart disease

B. Dose: If the patient has had a hysterectomy, Estrogen alone is sufficient

1. Continuous HRT: **Conjugated Estrogens (Premarin)** 0.625mg QD—*plus*—**Provera** 2.5mg QD—*or*—**Prempro (Premarin** 0.625mg/**Provera** 2.5mg—or—**Premarin** 0.625/**Provera** 5mg)
   a. If vasomotor symptoms persist > 3 months, then increase **Premarin** to 0.9mg–1.25mg QD. Continue for several months and then decrease to 0.625mg
   b. Patients will usually have intermittent spotting for the first several months before endometrium becomes atrophic. If patient has *spotting* which does not improve after 3–4 months of therapy, then increase **Provera** to 5mg QD. *Advantage:* Most women will not menstruate with this regime

2. Cyclic HRT
   a. Premarin 0.625mg QD—*plus*—**Provera** 10mg QD × 12 days/month (days 14–25 of cycle)
   b. Premphase PO QD (.625mg of **Conjugated Estrogen** days 1–14, then .625mg **Conjugated Estrogen** and 5mg **Medroxyprogesterone** days 15–28)

3. Patches
   a. **Estrogen** patches: **Climara** and **FemPatch** are applied once weekly; **Alora, Estraderm,** and **Vivelle** are applied twice weekly. These are used in women with hysterectomies
   b. **Estrogen/Progestogen** patch: **Combipatch** is applied twice weekly for women with an intact uterus

4. New HRT products:
   a. **Femhrt (EE** 5mcg/**Norethindrone** 1mg) 1 tab QD
   b. **Ortho-Prefest** 1mg **Estradiol** 1 tab × 3 days then a single tablet of 1mg **Estradiol** combined with 0.09mg **Norgestimate** × 3 days. This regimen is repeated continuously without interruption

5. If the patient had a hysterectomy, then **Estrogen** alone is sufficient

C. **Hot flashes:** May use if patient has contraindications to HRT, for patients with vasomotor intolerance who are not ready for HRT, or concurrently with HRT

1. **Clonidine:** 0.1–0.15mg PO QD or clonidine patch (0.1mg/week). Side effects minimal at these doses, but may include dry mouth, drowsiness, decreased blood pressure

2. Progestins such as **Medroxyprogesterone** (10–30mg orally/day) or **Megestrol Acetate** (20–40mg orally/day) can be used for hot flashes. If either of these result in intolerable side effects, alternative progestins may be given

3. **Black Cohosh** is an herbal supplement that some women use to treat hot flashes and other menopausal symptoms

4. Behavioral techniques: Exercise, relaxation, avoidance of caffeine and alcohol

5. **Bellergal-S** is no longer recommended for treatment of hot flashes. It has a marked sedative effect and potentially can be habit-forming. In addition, studies show little long term effectiveness of this treatment

6. Many women have mild hot flashes that they feel do not need treated. If they are not taking hormone replacement therapy, they should be told that symptoms subside slowly over 3–5 years

D. **Vaginal atrophy/dyspareunia**

1. **Premarin** or **Estrace vaginal cream:** $^1/_8$ applicatorful nightly for 7–10 nights, then every other night or twice weekly

2. **Estring:** Vaginal ring that is replaced every 3 months

E. **Other therapies**

1. **Calcium** 1000–1500mg QD and **Vitamin D$_3$** 400–800 IU QD

2. Exercise and diet

3. Avoidance of smoking, excessive alcohol, and caffeine

F. **For management of osteoporosis**—See Chapter 68, Osteoporosis

G. **Patient Monitoring**

1. Annual Pap smear

2. Annual mammography

3. Endometrial sampling in patients with abnormal uterine bleeding

4. Dual-energy x-ray absorptiometry (DEXA) scan to evaluate for osteoporosis

5. Evaluate calcium intake and recommend 1000–1500mg **Calcium** daily through diet and supplementation. Also, adequate **Vitamin D** intake 200–400 IU/day is necessary for calcium absorption

6. Monitor lipid profile periodically

CLINICAL PEARLS

- 85% of women will have hot flashes and night sweats when they go through menopause
- 10 % of women stop having their menstrual period by 45–46 years of age. 1% enter menopause before age 40. Women live $^1/_3$ to ½ of their lives in menopause
- The Framingham Heart Study found that 10-year incidence of CVD in postmenopausal women age 50–59 was 4-fold higher than in premenopausal women of the same age range. Menopause occurring before age 35 has been associated with a 2- to 3-fold increased risk of myocardial infarction. Oophorectomy (before age 35) increases the risk 7-fold
- Late menopause is a risk factor for breast cancer and uterine cancer
- The most unfavorable factor associated with HRT is breakthrough bleeding
- Choosing a form of HRT that is best suited towards the patient's lifestyle and preference may improve compliance and quality of life
- Women with postmenopausal osteoporosis have a higher bone resorption rate than normal, while the rate of bone formation with osteoporosis is normal
- Postmenopausally body weight increases and total body fat that is unaffected by estrogen administration. There is a distribution of fat from peripheral site to the abdomen. This change of fat distribution is prevented by exogenous estrogen

References

Schairer C, et al. Menopausal estrogen and estrogen-progestin replacement therapy and breast cancer risk. JAMA 2000;283:485–91.

Archer DF, et al. A comparative study of transvaginal uterine ultrasound and endometrial biopsy for evaluating the endometrium of postmenopausal women taking hormone replacement therapy. Menopause Fall 1999;6:201–8.

Archer DF, et al. Uterine bleeding in postmenopausal women on continuous therapy with estradiol and norethindrone acetate. Obstet Gynecol Sep 1999; 94:323–9.

Bachmann GA. Vasomotor flushes in postmenopausal women. Am J Obstet Gynecol 1999;180:312–6.

Chiechi LM, Secreto G. Breast cancer and replacement therapy: which women are at risk? Clin Exp Obstet Gynecol 1999;26:105–8.

Col NF, et al. Individualizing therapy to prevent long-term consequences of estrogen deficiency in postmenopausal women. Arch Intern Med 1999;159:1458–66.

de Aloysio D, et al. The effect of menopause on blood lipid and lipoprotein levels. Atherosclerosis 1999;147:147–3.

Ettinger B, et al. Reduction of vertebral fracture risk in postmenopausal women with osteoporosis treated with raloxifene: results from a 3-year randomized clinical trial. Multiple Outcomes of Raloxifene Evaluation (MORE) Investigators. JAMA 1999;282:637–45.

Grodstein F, et al. Postmenopausal hormones and recurrence of coronary events in the Nurses' Health Study. Paper presented at: the 72nd Scientific Session of the American Heart Association; Nov 7–10, 1999; Atlanta, GA.

Mattsson LA, et al. Continuous, combined hormone replacement: randomized comparison of transdermal and oral preparations. Obstet Gynecol 1999;94:61–5.

Silbergeld EK, Flaws JA. Chemicals and menopause: effects on age at menopause and on health status in the postmenopausal period. J Womens Health 1999;8:227–34.

Stuenkel C, Barrett-Connor E. Hormone replacement therapy: where are we now? West J Med 1999;171:27–30.

Greendale GA, et al. Symptom relief and side effects of postmenopausal hormones: results from the postmenopausal estrogen/progestin interventions trial. Obstet Gynecol 1998;92:982–8.

ACOG Educational Bulletin, Hormone Replacement Therapy. No. 247, May 1998.

Yaffe K, et al. Estrogen therapy in postmenopausal women. Effects on cognitive function and dementia. JAMA 1998;279:688–95.

Burt VK, et al. Depressive symptoms in the perimenopause: prevalence, assessment, and guidelines for treatment. Harv Rev Psychiatry 1998;6:121–32.

Grodstein F, et al. Postmenopausal hormone therapy and mortality. N Engl J Med 1997;336:1769–75.

Huller S, et al. Randomized trial of estrogen plus progestin for secondary prevention of coronary heart disease in postmenopausal women. JAMA 1998;280:605–13.

GYN

Mike Hemsworth, MD
Daniel M. Neides, MD

GYN

26. THE PREMENSTRUAL SYNDROME AND DYSMENORRHEA

Comparative features between PMS and Primary Dysmenorrhea

Feature	PMS	Primary Dysmenorrhea
Time of Onset:	10–14 days before menses	1 day before or on 1st day of menses
Improvement:	Onset of menses	End of menses
Childbirth:	Worsens	Improves

PART I: THE PREMENSTRUAL SYNDROME

DEFINITION: A condition characterized by debilitating affective, behavioral, cognitive, and somatic complaints in the premenstrual period, that interfere with normal functioning, and resolve rapidly at the onset of menstruation

I. PREVALENCE and statistics
   A. Mean age is early 30's
   B. 75% of women have some premenstrual symptoms
   C. 3–8% of cycling women can be diagnosed with PMS
   D. 40–50% of women presenting to the physician with premenstrual complaints will meet criteria for PMS

II. ETIOLOGY: No specific deficiency or abnormality has been identified. Theories include:
   A. Deficiency of Progesterone: Now mostly disregarded
   B. Alterations in ovarian hormone production/derangements in relative amounts of estrogen and progesterone: No abnormal hormone levels found
   C. Alterations at the hypothalamic or suprahypothalamic level: The etiology is most likely as revealed by the effectiveness of the selective serotonin reuptake inhibitors (SSRIs) in treating PMS

III. SYMPTOMS AND SIGNS: There are no diagnostic physical signs of PMS
   A. Affective: Irritability, emotional lability, anxiety, depression
   B. Behavioral: Food cravings, hostility, aggression, altered libido
   C. Cognitive: Forgetfulness, poor concentration, confusion
   D. Somatic: Bloating, fluid retention, weight gain, headache, mastalgia, fatigue, insomnia

IV. DIAGNOSIS based on the following:
   A. Symptom complex consistent with PMS as above
   B. Symptoms must occur exclusively in the luteal phase
   C. Symptoms must be severe enough to interfere with normal functioning
   D. Prospective symptom report over a period of at least 2 or 3 cycles
   E. Exclusion of other psychological and physical disorders by detailed history and physical exam

V. MANAGEMENT: No one treatment is effective for everyone with PMS. It is important to educate and reassure the patient, and tailor the treatment to the individual. It may take some time to find the best option for each patient
   A. Lifestyle changes: Use as an initial approach
      1. Nutrition
         a. Avoid refined sugar, salt, red meat, alcohol, and caffeine

b. A good PMS diet consists of 60% complex carbohydrates, 20% protein, 20% fat
c. Rely more on fish, poultry, whole grains, and legumes for protein, and less on red meats and dairy products
d. Nutritional supplements may be helpful:
   Vitamin B$_6$ 50–500mg QD: Discontinue if no improvement due to risks of neurologic symptoms
   Vitamin E 400 IU QD: May reduce mood symptoms and food cravings
   Magnesium 360mg QD
2. Avoid smoking
3. Exercise: Aerobic exercise which increases heart rate >120 for 30–40 minutes 4–5 times per week may reduce some of the physical symptoms and negative affect
4. Stress management: Identify stressors first, then look for ways to deal with them
5. Adequate sleep
B. Medications: May be directed at the patient's most debilitating symptoms
1. SSRIs: These are becoming a first line drug treatment for PMS. E.g., **Fluoxetine (Prozac)** 20mg QD has been studied most, but all are probably equally effective
2. Oral contraceptive pills: May also worsen symptoms
3. Progesterone: No more effective than placebo, but still used
4. Anxiolytics: **Buspirone (BuSpar)** 10mg TID
5. Tricyclics
   a. **Nortriptyline** 50–125mg QD
   b. **Clomipramine** 25–75mg QD
6. GnRH agonists: Cause a medical menopause, with menopausal side effects. Not recommended for longer than 6 months
7. **Danazol:** May reduce premenstrual mastalgia, but has adverse side effects
8. Diuretics: **Spironolactone** is the only diuretic shown to be effective. May alleviate bloating
C. Surgery: Usually a last resort involving TAH and BSO. GnRH agonists should be used first to predict response to oophorectomy

PART II: PRIMARY DYSMENORRHEA

DEFINITION: Primary dysmenorrhea is painful menstruation without detectable pelvic disease. Secondary dysmenorrhea is painful menstruation associated with an anatomic cause (endometriosis, adhesions, fibroids, other anomalies)

I. PREVALENCE: Dysmenorrhea affects approximately 50% of menstruating women

II. ETIOLOGY: Increased endometrial prostaglandin production causing higher uterine tone and decreased blood flow

III. SIGNS AND SYMPTOMS
Most symptoms begin 6–12 months after menarche
A. Abdominal cramping
   1. Onset usually begins many hours prior to menstruation with most severe cramping occurring on the first day
   2. Cramping may last anywhere from several hours up to 2–3 days
B. Dizziness
C. Nausea and vomiting
D. Diarrhea
E. Depression

IV. DIAGNOSIS: Need to rule out underlying pelvic pathology with thorough history and physical including pelvic exam. Consider chlamydia and gonorrhea studies to exclude subacute salpingo-oophoritis

GYN

V. MANAGEMENT

NSAIDs: Treatment of choice for primary dysmenorrhea, start prior to onset of pain for maximum effect; examples include:

1. **Naproxen (Aleve)** 250–500mg PO Q12hrs
2. **Ibuprofen (Motrin)** 400mg PO Q4–6hrs

CLINICAL PEARLS

- Patients who experience mood swings with PMS can also develop mild to moderate depression, which is known as premenstrual dysphoric disorder (PMDD). Selective serotonin reuptake inhibitors (SSRIs) have been found to be an effective treatment
- Patients who complain of worsening abdominal cramping with each period or who complain of pain not associated with menstruation may have secondary dysmenorrhea (e.g., endometriosis, fibroids)

References

Coco AS. Primary dysmenorrhea. Am Fam Phys 1999;60:489–96.

Barnhart KT. A clinician's guide to the premenstrual syndrome. Med Clin North Am Nov 1995;79:1457–69.

Danford's obstetrics and gynecology. 7th ed. 1995:677–8.

Parker PD. Premenstrual syndrome. Am Fam Phys 1994;50:1309–17.

Michael B. Weinstock, MD

27. EVALUATION OF BREAST MASS, PAIN AND DISCHARGE

I. INTRODUCTION: Breast cancer is the second most frequent cause of cancer deaths

II. HISTORY

- **A.** Nipple discharge
- **B.** Breast pain
- **C.** Breast mass
- **D.** Determine last mammogram and last clinical exam or self exam
- **E.** First degree relative (mother, sister, daughter) with breast cancer (1.4–2.8 times increased risk)
- **F.** Previous biopsy showing atypical hyperplasia
- **G.** History of breast cancer

III. PHYSICAL EXAM

- **A.** Dimpling (peau d'orange appearance)
- **B.** Asymmetry
- **C.** Mass
- **D.** Lymphadenopathy (including axillae) – Late sign
- **E.** Express nipples for discharge

IV. SPECIFIC COMPLAINTS

- **A. Nipple discharge:** 3–10% of breast complaints. Present in 1.8–8.9% of patients with breast disease. Under age 60 ~ 7% cancer. Over age 60 ~ 32% cancer (usually intraductal carcinoma)
    1. History
        a. Duration of symptoms
        b. Unilateral or bilateral (bilateral milky discharge suggests endocrine etiology)
        c. Presence of blood (increases chances of malignancy)
        d. Medication use (oral contraceptives or phenothiazines)
        e. Lactation/breast feeding history
        f. Spontaneous or with stimulation
    2. Physical exam: As above, plus hemoccult the discharge
    3. Evaluation

    a. If discharge is *heme-negative*, then conservative management with follow up in 1–2 months. Obtain mammogram if not up to date. Evaluate for other etiologies. If the discharge is still present in 1–2 months, then proceed as if it were heme-positive

    b. If discharge is *heme-positive*, then consult a surgeon to perform diagnostic mammography followed by galactography (to locate ductal abnormality and locate potential areas for excision or biopsy)

    c. Cytology generally not indicated (won't change management)

B. Breast pain

  1. Differential

    a. Fibrocystic breast disease

    b. Menstrually related pain

    c. Cancer

    d. Costochondritis

    e. Trauma

    f. Mastitis (See Chapter 4, Infant Formula and Breast-feeding)

    g. Causes unrelated to the breast

  2. History

    a. Duration

    b. Location

    c. Trauma

    d. Lumps or discharge

  3. Physical exam—as above

  4. Evaluation

    a. If mass is present, see next section

    b. If < age 35 and no mass, then have patient return for follow up exam in 1–2 months

    c. If > age 35 and no mass, then proceed to breast imaging. If negative, then have patient follow up in 1–2 months for a recheck

C. Breast mass: Less chance in low risk patient with soft or cystic mass with regular borders and freely movable

  1. History

    a. Age of patients (cancer vs. cyst)

    b. Duration

    c. Change in size

    d. Change with menses

    e. Previous biopsies or masses

  2. Physical exam

    a. Cystic or solid

    b. Soft or hard

    c. Regular or irregular borders

    d. Movable or fixed

    e. Enlarged lymph nodes

  3. Evaluation of solitary breast mass: Cystic or solid (determine by exam or ultrasound)

    a. If cystic, then proceed to aspiration (22 gauge needle)

      i. If aspiration is nonbloody and mass disappears, then follow up and imaging per American Cancer Society (ACS) guidelines—cytology not necessary

      ii. If aspiration is bloody or mass does not disappear, then breast imaging and referral for biospy

    b. If solid, then breast imaging and referral for biopsy

V. TESTS

  A. Needle aspiration

  B. Mammography

  C. Ultrasound

  D. Biopsy

VI. INDICATIONS FOR OPEN BREAST BIOPSY

  A. Equivocal cytologic findings on aspiration

B. Bloody cyst fluid on aspiration
C. Failure of mass to disappear completely after fluid aspiration
D. Recurrence of cyst after one or two aspirations
E. Bloody nipple discharge
F. Nipple excoriation (Paget's disease of breast)
G. Skin edema and erythema suggestive of inflammatory breast carcinoma

CLINICAL PEARLS
- Mammography is 75–90% sensitive at differentiating between benign and malignant disease
- The differential diagnosis of a breast mass in a lactating woman includes blocked milk ducts and mastitis. A blocked duct may be relieved by massaging the breast during nursing

References

Barton MB, et al. Breast symptoms among women enrolled in a health maintenance organization: frequency, evaluation, and outcome. Ann Intern Med 1999;130:651–7.

Dixon JM, et al. Risk of breast cancer in women with palpable breast cysts: a prospective study. Lancet 1999;353:1742–5.

Duijm LE, et al. Value of breast imaging in women with painful breasts: observational follow-up study. BMJ 1998;317:1492–5.

Greenberg R, et al. Management of breast fibroadenomas. J Gen Intern Med 1998;339:1021–9.

Morrow M, Wong S, Venta L. The evaluation of breast masses in women younger than forty years of age. Surgery 1998;124:634–41.

Elmore JG, et al. Ten-year risk of false positive screening mammograms and clinical breast examinations. N Engl J Med 1998;338:1089–96.

Conry C. Evaluation of a breast complaint: Is it cancer? Am Fam Phys 1994;49:445.

Gulay H, Bora S, Kilicturgay S, et al.Nipple discharge and rate of malignant breast disease. J Am Coll Surg 1994;178:471–4.

Michael D. Weinstock, MD
Ann Aring, MD

28. VAGINITIS AND SEXUALLY TRANSMITTED DISEASES

DEFINITION: Vaginitis is inflammation of the vagina which results from infection (bacterial, fungal, protozoan), atrophic changes, dermatitis, or mechanical factors

I. HISTORY

A. Vaginal discharge: Color, smell, viscosity
B. Vaginal and vulvar itching
C. Sexual history: New sexual partner, unprotected sex, partner with known STD, previous STDs
D. Predisposing factors: Recent antibiotic use, hot tubs, swimming pools, diabetes, HIV, immunosuppressed state (predisposition to *Candida* infection)
E. Contact dermatitis questions (new clothes, pads, soaps, feminine deodorant soap, latex condoms)

II. PHYSICAL

A. Visually inspect skin, labia, vaginal walls, and cervix for discharge, erythema, lesions, warts
B. Bi-manual examination for adnexal or cervical motion tenderness (CMT)
C. Abdominal examination for suprapubic tenderness (UTI) or bilateral lower abdominal tenderness (PID), unilateral lower abdominal tenderness (cyst, ectopic pregnancy, tubo-ovarian abscess, or PID)

III. LABORATORY

A. *Gonorrhea* and *Chlamydia* cultures if indicated
B. Appearance
  1. White, cottage cheese, yeast smell: *Candida*
  2. Green, bubbly, with "strawberry spots" on vaginal walls and cervix: *Trichomonas*
  3. Grey, low viscosity, adherent to vaginal walls: Bacterial vaginosis

C. Vaginal pH
1. pH 3.5 to 4.5: *Candida*
2. pH > 4.5: Bacterial vaginosis (*Gardnerella*); pH <4.5, it is unlikely patient has BV
3. pH > 6: *Trichomonas*
4. pH > 7: Atrophic

D. Wet mount (KOH and saline): Apply 2 samples to 2 areas of slide, then place 1 drop of KOH to the first and 1 drop of normal saline to the other. Cover with cover slip and examine under microscope

1. Pseudomycelia: *Candida* (there is a significant false negative rate with wet mounts for *Candida*. If the wet mount is negative and *Candida* is suspected, then treat empirically and/or plate specimen on Nickersons agar)
2. Clue cells, positive "whiff" test: Bacterial vaginosis (*Gardnerella*)
   a. Clue cells: Epithelial cells appear stippled due to presence of bacteria
   b. "Whiff test": Bacterial vaginosis infection will give off characteristic fishy odor when saturated with KOH. The presence of *Lactobacillus* or pH < 4.5 excludes the diagnosis of bacterial vaginosis
3. Motile organisms with flagella: *Trichomonas*

GYN

IV. MANAGEMENT OF DISEASES CHARACTERIZED BY VAGINAL DISCHARGE

A. *Candida*
1. Oral
   a. **Fluconazole (Diflucan):** 150mg PO × 1. S*ome clinicians now use as first line* in nonpregnant women due to its low cost, ease of administration. S/E GI upset. Cost is comparable or less than topical medications
   b. **Nystatin:** 100,000 units PO QD–BID × 2 weeks—refractory cases
2. Topical/Intravaginal
   a. **Miconazole (Monistat-3)** vaginal suppositories: 1 intravaginally QHS × 3 days or Miconazole vaginal cream QHS × 7 days
   b. **Clotrimazole (Gyne-Lotrimin):** 2–100mg tablets intravaginally or cream QHS × 3 days
   c. **Terconazole (Terazole)** vaginal cream 0.4%: 1 applicator intravaginally QHS × 7 days—*second line*
   d. **Gentian violet:** Paint vaginal walls Q month in office × 3 months

B. Bacterial vaginosis (*Gardnerella*)
1. **Metronidazole (Flagyl):** 500mg PO BID × 7 days —*or*— 2g PO × 1
2. **Clindamycin Phosphate cream (Cleocin) 2%*:** 1 applicator 5g intravaginally QHS × 7 days
3. **Metronidazole gel 0.75% (Metrogel vaginal)*:** 1 applicator 5g intravaginally BID × 5D
* Topical therapy of BV is slightly less effective than PO

C. *Trichomonas*
Metronidazole (Flagyl): 2g PO × 1 *(Treat partner!)*

D. *Chlamydia trachomatis* (urethral, cervical or rectal). Recommend testing for syphilis and HIV. See Chapter 29, Pelvic Inflammatory Disease for treatment of PID. Also treat partner
1. **Doxycycline (Vibramycin, Doryx):** 100mg PO BID × 7days
2. **Azithromycin (Zithromax):** 1g PO × 1
3. **Ofloxacin (Floxin):** 300mg PO BID × 7days

E. *Gonorrhea* (urethral, cervical or rectal), uncomplicated. Consider testing for syphilis and HIV. See Chapter 31, Pelvic Inflammatory Disease for treatment of PID. Also treat partner
Note: Each of the following is given with **Doxycycline** 100mg PO BID × 7days or **Azithromycin (Zithromax)** 1g PO × 1
1. **Ceftriaxone (Rocephin):** 125mg IM × 1
2. **Cefixime (Suprax):** 400mg PO × 1
3. **Ciprofloxacin (Cipro):** 500mg PO × 1
4. **Ofloxacin (Floxin):** 400mg PO × 1

F. Atrophic vaginitis
1. **Estrogen cream (Premarin** 1–2g, **Ogen** 2–4g) intravaginally QHS. Use for 3 weeks/month
2. **Premarin** 0.625mg PO QD: Add **Provera** if patient still has uterus. See Chapter 25, Menopause and Hormone Replacement Therapy

V. MANAGEMENT OF DISEASES CHARACTERIZED BY GENITAL LESIONS

   A. Herpes simplex virus

   1. First episode: Obtain viral culture to confirm diagnosis

      a. **Acyclovir (Zovirax):** 400mg PO TID for 7–10 days or 200mg PO 5 × day for 7–10 days

      b. **Famciclovir (Famvir):** 250mg PO TID for 7–10 days

      c. **Valacyclovir (Valtrex):** 1g PO BID for 7–10 days

   2. Recurrent episodes

      a. **Acyclovir:** 400mg PO TID for 5 days or 200mg PO 5 × day for 5 days or 800mg PO BID for 5 days

      b. **Famciclovir:** 125mg PO BID for 5 days

      c. **Valacyclovir:** 500mg PO BID for 5 days

   3. Daily suppressive therapy

      a. **Acyclovir:** 400mg PO BID

      b. **Famciclovir:** 250mg PO BID

      c. **Valacyclovir**

         i. For patients with < 10 episodes per year: 500mg PO QD

         ii. For patients with > 10 episodes per year: 1000mg PO QD

   4. Counseling is an important aspect of managing patients who have genital herpes

      a. Patients who have genital herpes should be told about the natural history of the disease with emphasis on the potential for recurrent episodes, asymptomatic viral shedding, and sexual transmission

      b. Patients should be advised to abstain from sexual activity when lesions or prodromal symptoms are present and encouraged to inform their sex partners that they have genital herpes. The use of condoms during all sexual exposures with new or uninfected sex partners should be encouraged

      c. Sexual transmission of HSV can occur during asymptomatic periods. Asymptomatic viral shedding occurs more frequently in patients who have genital HSV-2 infection than HSV-1 infection and in patients who have had genital herpes for less than 12 months. Such patients should be counseled to prevent spread of the infection

      d. The risk for neonatal infection should be explained to all patients, including men. Childbearing-aged women who have genital herpes should be advised to inform healthcare providers who care for them during pregnancy about the HSV infection

      e. Patients having a first episode of genital herpes should be advised that a) episodic antiviral therapy during recurrent episodes might shorten the duration of lesions and b) suppressive antiviral therapy can ameliorate or prevent recurrent outbreaks

   B. Human Papillomavirus (HPV) or Genital Warts

   1. **External genital area**

      a. **Podofilox (Condylox):** 0.5% solution BID for 3 days, wait 4 days and repeat as necessary for 4 cycles

      b. **Imiquimod (Aldara):** 5% cream daily at bedtime 3 times a week for up to 16 weeks

      c. **Cyotherapy** with liquid nitrogen by physician. May be repeated every 1 to 2 weeks

      d. **Trichloroacetic Acid** or **Bichloroacetic Acid** 80 to 90% applied by physician weekly

      e. **Podophyllum** 10 to 25% applied by physician weekly

   2. **Vaginal**

      a. **Cryotherapy** with liquid nitrogen by physician. May be repeated every 1 to 2 weeks

      b. **Trichloroacetic Acid** or **Bichloroacetic Acid** 80 to 90% applied by physician weekly

      c. **Podophyllum** 10 to 25% applied by physician weekly

CLINICAL PEARLS

   • Checking a wet mount and vaginal pH is quick, easy and invaluable in directing therapy

   • Vulvar pruritus is the most common presentation of vulvar dysplasia. If patient has a negative workup for vaginitis then patient should be worked up for vulvar dysplasia by using toluidine blue stain and biopsy or vulvar colposcopy and biopsy

   • Perform the "sniff test" by applying KOH *to the speculum* for better sensitivity for bacterial vaginosis

   • An early manifestation of HIV may be recurrent vaginal yeast infections

References
Woodward C. Drug treatment of common STD's: Part I. Am Fam Phys 1999; 60(5):1387–94.
Woodward C. Drug treatment of common STD's: Part II. Am Fam Phys 1999; 60(6):1716–22.
Eckert LO, et al. Vulvovaginal candidiasis: clinical manifestations, risk factors, management algorithm. Obstet Gynecol 1998;92:757–65.
1998 guidelines for the treatment of sexually transmitted diseases. U S Dept Health & Human Serv. MMWR. Jan 23, 1997;47(RR–1):1–116.
http://wonder.cdc.gov/wonder/STD/STD98TG/STD98TG.HTM

GYN

Michael B. Weinstock, MD
Ann Aring, MD

29. PELVIC INFLAMMATORY DISEASE (PID)

I. CRITERIA FOR DIAGNOSIS OF PID
A. Essential for diagnosis (all must be present)
   1. Lower abdominal tenderness
   2. Cervical motion tenderness (CMT)
   3. Adnexal tenderness
B. Supportive (Additional findings raise likelihood of PID by 5–10%)
   1. Temp > 101°F (38.3° C)
   2. Abnormal cervical or vaginal discharge
   3. Increased ESR or CRP
   4. Positive cultures/DNA probe

II. PATHOGENS
Chlamydia, *N. gonorrhoeæ*, Gram negative facultative bacteria (e.g., *E. coli*), anaerobes, *Streptococcus*, *Mycoplasma*, *Actinomyces*, *G. Vaginalis*, *H. Influenzæ*

III. INDICATIONS FOR HOSPITALIZATION FOR ACUTE PID
A. Diagnosis is uncertain and surgical emergencies (ectopic pregnancy, appendicitis) cannot be excluded
B. Suspected tubo-ovarian abscess
C. Severe vomiting, dehydration, severe illness
D. Pregnancy
E. Patient has failed outpatient therapy
F. AIDS
G. Unable to follow outpatient regimen
H. Failure of oral regimen

IV. MANAGEMENT
A. Outpatient (oral) therapy:
   1. Regimen A
      Ofloxacin: 400mg orally twice a day for 14 days—*plus*—
      Metronidazole: 500mg orally twice a day for 14 days
   2. Regimen B
      Ceftriaxone: 250mg IM once—*or*—
      Cefoxitin: 2g IM plus **Probenecid:** 1g orally in a single dose concurrently once—*or*—
      Other parenteral third-generation Cephalosporin (e.g., Ceftizoxime or Cefotaxime)—*plus*—
      Doxycycline: 100mg orally twice a day for 14 days (Include this regimen with one of the above regimens)
B. Inpatient (parenteral) therapy:
   1. Parenteral Regimen A
      Cefotetan: 2g IV every 12hrs—*or*—
      Cefoxitin: 2g IV every 6hrs—*plus*—

Doxycycline: 100mg IV or orally every 12hrs until improved followed by **Doxycycline:** 100mg PO BID to complete 14 days

2. Parenteral Regimen B

Clindamycin: 900mg IV every 8hrs—*plus*—

Gentamicin: loading dose IV or IM (2mg/kg of body weight), followed by a maintenance dose (1.5mg/kg) every 8hrs. Single daily dosing may be substituted. Followed by **Doxycycline:** 100mg oral BID to complete 14 days

C. **Follow up within 72hrs:** Patients should demonstrate significant clinical improvement within this time. If not, then additional testing or diagnosis need to be assessed

D. **Partner needs to be tested and treated:** Test for HIV, syphilis, and counsel on safe sexual practices

CLINICAL PEARLS

- With 1, 2, or 3 incidences of PID, the chance of infertility is 15, 35, and 55%, respectively
- Risk of ectopic pregnancy is increased 7–10 times; inform patients of increased risk
- A tubo-ovarian abscess will develop in 7–16% of patients who have had PID
- Recurrent infection occurs in 20–25% of patients who have had PID
- A clinical diagnosis of symptomatic PID has a positive predictive value for salpingitis of 65%–90% (compared to laparoscopy)

References

Tukeva TA, et al. MR imaging in pelvic inflammatory disease: comparison with laparoscopy and US. Radiology 1999;210:209–16.

Woodward C. Drug treatment of common STD's: Part II. Am Fam Phys 1999; 60(6):1716–22.

1998 guidelines for the treatment of sexually transmitted diseases. U S Dept Health & Human Serv. MMWR Jan 23, 1997;47(RR–1):1–116.

http://wonder.cdc.gov/wonder/STD/STD98TG/STD98TG.HTM

McGregor JA, et al. Randomized comparison of ampicillin-sulbactam to cefoxitin and doxycycline or clindamycin and gentamicin in the treatment of pelvic inflammatory disease or pendometritis. Obstet Gynecol 1994;83:998–1004.

GYN

IV. Preventive Medicine

PREV

PREV

Preventive Medicine

30. PERIODIC HEALTH EXAMINATIONS

The following information should be used as a guide for disease screening. The frequency of visits will be at the physician's discretion

I. BIRTH—18 MONTHS
Visits should be scheduled at birth and at 2, 4, 6, 12, 15 and 18 months of age
A. History: Medical and family history, feeding schedule, sleeping schedule
B. Physical: Include height, weight and head circumference
C. Laboratory: Specific state screen, Hemoglobin and hematocrit, hearing test and lead levels obtained in high risk patients
D. Immunizations: See Chapter 3, Childhood Immunization Schedule
E. Parent Counseling: emphasis on diet and exercise, dental health and injury prevention

II. 19 MONTHS—6 YEARS
At least once for MMR vaccine (#2—given between ages 4–6), otherwise at physician's discretion
A. History: Updated medical and family history, developmental and behavioral assessment
B. Physical: Height and weight, blood pressure, and eye exam for strabismus and amblyopia (age 3–4 years)
C. Laboratory: Urinalysis (for asymptomatic bacteriuria), lead level, PPD, and hearing test for selected high risk patients
D. Immunizations: See Chapter 3, Childhood Immunization Schedule
  *Hepatitis A should be administered in high risk populations and in children living in states, counties, and communities with rates twice the national average or greater then 20 cases/100,000
E. Counseling: Emphasis on diet and exercise, injury prevention and initiate sex education

III. 7—12 YEARS
Frequency of visits up to physician discretion
A. History: Updated medical and family history
B. Physical: Include height and weight, blood pressure, and Tanner staging
C. Laboratory: Total cholesterol (if parent with blood cholesterol > 240mg/dL), lipoprotein analysis (if parent or grandparent with history of cardiovascular disease < age 55), PPD for high risk patients
D. Immunizations: Verify that all immunizations are up to date. See Chapter 3, Childhood Immunization Schedule
  Hepatitis B vaccine should be administered in previously unvaccinated adolescents ages 11–12. Varicella should be administered to adolescents ages 11–12 if they have not been previously vaccinated and do not have a reliable history of chickenpox infection
E. Counseling: Emphasis on injury prevention, high risk behavior, substance use (alcohol, tobacco, drugs) and sex education

IV. 13—18 YEARS
At least 1 visit for preventive services; otherwise at physician's discretion
A. History: Updated medical and family history; dietary intake; physical activity; tobacco, alcohol and drug use; sexual history
B. Physical: Include height and weight; blood pressure, Tanner staging, testicular exam, pelvic exam and Pap smear (at the onset of sexual activity or age 18, whichever comes first). See Chapter 22, Pap Smears. Explain monthly self breast or testicular exams
C. Laboratory: Total cholesterol and/or lipoprotein analysis for high risk patients as noted above. Consider HIV testing if multiple risk factors present, rubella antibodies for females of child-bearing age lacking immunity, PPD for high risk patients
D. Immunizations: dT (diphtheria tetanus) booster (10 years after last dT); CDC recommendations for menigococcal vaccine in college students who request the vaccine; MMR for those lacking

proof of immunity entering post secondary school education and for those entering medical-related occupations. For high risk patients—influenza vaccine and pneumococcal vaccine, consider Varicella

E. **Counseling:** Emphasis on substance use, sexual practice, preventive health measures (self breast or testicular exams, diet and exercise)

Expert recommendations for preventive care for asymptomatic, low-risk adults

Preventive Service	United States Preventive Services Task Force			American College of Physicians			Canadian Task Force on the Periodic Health Examination		
	Sex	Age	Minimum Frequency	Sex	Age	Minimum Frequency	Sex	Age	Minimum Frequency
Physical examination									
Blood Pressure	MF	18+	q 2 yrs[1]	MF	18+	q 2 yrs	MF	25–64	q 5 yrs
								65+	q 2 yrs
Clinical breast examination	F	50–69[2]	Annually[3]	F	40+	Annually	F	50–69	Annually
Laboratory Tests									
Papanicolaou smear	F	18[4]–65	q 3 yrs	F	20[4]–65	q 3 yrs	F	18[4]–69	q 3 yrs[5]
Stool for occult blood	MF	50+	Annually	MF	50–70/80	Annually[6]	NR	NR	NR
Sigmoidoscopy	MF	50+	q ? yrs[1]	MF	50–70	q 10 yrs	NR	NR	NR
Mammography	F	50–69[2]	q 1–2 yrs	F	50–75	q 2 yrs	F	50–69	Annually
Cholesterol	M	35–65	q 5+ yrs[1]	M	35–65	Once[1]	M	30–59	q ? yrs[1]
	F	45–65		F	45–65				
Immunizations									
Tetanus-diphtheria booster	MF	18+	q 15–30 yrs	MF	18+	q 10 yrs or once at age 50	MF	18+	q 10 yrs
Influenza vaccination	MF	65+	Annually	MF	65+	Annually	MF	65+	Annually
Pneumococcal vacciantion	MF	65+	Once[7]	MF	65+	Once[7]	NR	NR	NR
Counseling[8]	MF	18+	At routine visits	MF	18+	At routine visits	MF	18+	At routine visits

NR = no recommendation; ? = "periodic"
[1] Owing to lack of evidence, the appropriate interval is left to clinical discretion.
[2] The benefits of clinical breast examination and mammography in women age 70 and older have not been determined. Screening decisions in older women should take into account comorbid conditions and life expectancy of each patient.
[3] Studies have also generally employed periodic mammography; the benefit of clinical breast examination alone in women of any age has not been determined.
[4] Or following onset of sexual activity.
[5] After two normal annual smears.
[6] For persons who decline screening sigmoidoscopy, barium enema or colonoscopy.
[7] Reimmunize at age 65 those high-risk individuals who are 5 years or more after primary dose.
[8] Regarding tobacco use, nutrition, exercise, sexual behavior, substance abuse, injury prevention, and dental care.

Tierney LM, et al. Current medical diagnosis and treatment. 37th ed. Norwalk, CT: Appleton & Lange, 1998. © Appleton & Lange. Used with permission.

V. 65 YEARS AND OVER: See Chapter 103, Periodic Health Screening in the Elderly

VI. HIGH RISK PATIENTS

A. Patients defined as **high risk for pneumococcal vaccine** include: chronic cardiac or pulmonary disease, sickle cell disease, nephrotic syndrome, Hodgkin's disease, DM, alcoholism, cirrhosis, multiple myeloma, renal disease, any disease associated with immunosuppression. If vaccine was administered ≥ 5 years ago and patient was < age 65, then revaccinate

B. Patients defined as **high risk for influenza vaccine** include: residents of chronic care facilities, suffering from chronic cardiopulmonary diseases, metabolic disease (including DM), renal diseases, hemoglobinopathies, or any disease associated with immunosuppression

References
CDC. Prevention of hepatitis A through active or passive immunization: recommendations of the Advisory Committee on Immunization Practices (ACIP).MMWR 1999;48 (RR 12);1–37.
CDC. Control & prevention of meningococcal disease: recommendations of the Advisory Committee on Immunization Practices (ACIP). MMWR 1997: modification Oct 21, 1999.
CDC. Prevention of pneumococcal disease: recommendations of the Advisory Committee on Immunization Practices (ACIP). MMWR 1997;46:1–24.

31. CANCER SCREENING

- Cancer is the #2 cause of death in the U.S. after heart disease
- Cancer is the #1 cause of death in women ages 35–75
- Cancer is the #2 cause of death in men ages 35–75
- Cancer is the #2 cause of death in children ages 1–14 after accidents
- 20–25% of Americans will die from cancer
- In 1999—1,221,800 new cancers will have been diagnosed
- In 1999—563,100 Americans will have died from cancer
- 5 million Americans have died from cancer since 1990

The following are guidelines from the American Cancer Society:

I. LUNG CANCER
A. Epidemiology
1. In 1998, 171,500 new cases of lung cancer were diagnosed with 160,000 deaths. 5-year survival rate is < 13%. Tobacco is associated with 87% of all cases of cancer of the lung, trachea, and bronchus
B. Screening
1. Routine screening of asymptomatic persons for lung cancer with yearly roentgenograms is not recommended (has not been shown to effect the mortality rate)
2. Primary prevention: Smoking cessation

II. BREAST CANCER
A. Epidemiology
1. In 1998 there were 178,700 new cases of breast cancer diagnosed and 43,900 deaths. 32% of all newly diagnosed cancers in women are breast cancer. The estimated lifetime risk of dying from breast cancer is 3.6%
2. Factors associated with increased risk include late age of first pregnancy, nulliparity, high socioeconomic status, and a history of exposure to high dose radiation
3. High-risk individuals include those with a first degree relative with breast cancer, previous breast cancer or atypical hyperplasia on biopsy
B. Screening: Average risk
1. Ages 18–39: Self breast exam performed monthly (7–10 days after last day of menstrual period) and a clinical breast exam every 1–3 years
2. Age > 40: Self breast exam every month, clinical breast exam annually, and a mammogram yearly
3. High-risk individuals should follow the same schedule. Screening before age 40 has not shown to effect the mortality rate. Patient preference (and anxiety) may be a reason to screen earlier than age 40 with mammography

III. COLORECTAL CANCER
A. Epidemiology
1. The second most common form of cancer with 131,600 new cases and 56,500 deaths in 1998. A patient's lifetime risk of dying from colon cancer is 2.6%. The 5-year survival is 91% for localized disease, 60% with regional spread, and 6% with distant metastases
2. Persons at highest risk include those with hereditary polyposis and hereditary nonpolyposis colorectal cancer, ulcerative colitis, colorectal cancer or adenomas in a first degree relative, a personal history of large adenomatous polyps or colorectal cancer, and a prior diagnosis of endometrial, ovarian, or breast cancer
B. Screening
1. Average risk: Digital rectal exam yearly beginning at age 40, fecal occult blood testing annually beginning at age 50, and either flexible sigmoidoscopy every 3–5 years or

colonoscopy every 10 years
2. Those individuals at high risk for colorectal cancer should be referred to a gastroenterologist to determine the appropriate time to begin screening

IV. PROSTATE CANCER

A. Epidemiology
1. There were 184,500 new cases and 39,200 deaths due to prostate cancer in 1998
2. After lung cancer, it accounts for more cancer deaths in men than in any other cancer site
3. Ten-year survival rates are 75% when confined to the prostate, 55% with regional extension, and 15% with distant metastases
4. High risk individuals include those with a first degree relative with prostate cancer and African American males

B. Screening
1. Average risk: Annual digital rectal exam (DRE) beginning at age 40. Annual Prostate Specific Antigen (PSA) level beginning at age 50
2. High risk: Annual DRE and PSA beginning at age 40

C. Age specific PSA

Age (Years)	Normal PSA Range
40–49	0–2.5 ng/ml
50–59	0–3.5 ng/ml
60–69	0–4.5 ng/ml
70–79	0–6.5 ng/ml

V. CERVICAL CANCER

A. Epidemiology
1. In 1998 there were 13,700 new cases of cervical cancer with 4,900 deaths
2. High risk individuals include those with a history of an abnormal Pap, smokers, immunosupression, early age of first intercourse, multiple sex partners

B. Screening
1. First intercourse or age 18: Pap smears every 1–3 years after 3 consecutive normal Pap tests (performed yearly)
2. High risk individuals should have Pap tests yearly
3. Patients who have undergone a hysterectomy for benign reasons (e.g., fibroids) and *never* had an abnormal Pap test do NOT require screening for cervical cancer (i.e., vaginal cuff sampling)

VI. OVARIAN CANCER

A. Epidemiology
1. There were 25,400 new cases and 14,500 deaths from ovarian cancer in 1998
2. The 5-year survival is 75% if the cancer is confined to the ovaries and 17% in those diagnosed with distant metastases
3. Symptoms usually do not become apparent until the tumor invades adjacent structures or metastases are determined clinically. $^2/_3$ of all women diagnosed with ovarian cancer have advanced (stage III or IV) disease at the time of diagnosis

B. Screening
1. Average risk: At first intercourse or age 18 up to age 39, Pelvic exam every 1–3 years. Age > 40: Pelvic exam yearly
2. High Risk: nulliparity, history of ovarian cancer, family history of breast, ovary, or endometrial cancer—Pelvic exam annually
3. Less than 0.1% of all women are affected by familial ovarian cancer syndrome but those women may face a lifetime risk of 40% of developing ovarian cancer. Ultrasound and/or tumor markers (CA-125) should be considered
4. The role of lysophosphatidic acid (LPA) is currently being studied at The Cleveland Clinic Foundation. Women with ovarian cancer have higher levels of LPA. Preliminary results show that it is 90% effective in detecting Stage I disease and 100% effective in detecting Stage II. More details to follow

PREV

VII. ENDOMETRIAL CANCER
A. Epidemiology
1. In 1998 there were 36,100 new cases and 6,300 deaths related to endometrial cancer
2. Risk factors include early menarche, late menopause, nulliparity, obesity, unopposed estrogen replacement, and diabetes. Early studies have found Tamoxifen may increase risk of uterine cancer
3. Other risk factors include white race, family history, breast or ovarian cancer, or prior pelvic radiation

B. Screening
1. No organization recommends routine screening in asymptomatic patients. A pipelle biopsy should be considered in those cases where endometrial cancer is a possibility

VIII. TESTICULAR CANCER
A. Epidemiology
1. There were 7,100 new cases and 370 deaths related to testicular cancer in 1995
2. It is the most common form of cancer in men ages 20–35. The incidence in black males is less than $1/5$ that of white males
3. The major predisposing risk factor is cryptorchidism. Other risk factor include previous cancer in the other testicle, history of mumps orchitis, inguinal hernia, or hydrocele in childhood, and high socioeconomic status

B. Screening
1. Age > 14: self exam each month and clinical exam with a physical exam
2. Ages 18–39: self exam each month and clinical exam every 1–3 years with physical exam
3. Age > 40: Clinical exam every year with a physical exam

IX. ORAL CANCER
A. Epidemiology
1. There were 28,700 new cases and 8,000 deaths related to oral cancer in 1998
2. The 5 year survival is 79% for localized disease and 19% if distant metastases occur
3. Risk factors: All tobacco products, alcohol, and advanced age

B. Screening
1. Ages 18–39: Oral exam every 1–3 years (with physical exam). Inquire about tobacco and alcohol use and counsel appropriately
2. Age > 40: Oral exam annually
3. Regular dental exams (annually or semi-annually)
4. Those patients with increased exposure to sunlight should be counseled on wearing sunscreen to protect their lips

X. SKIN CANCER
A. Epidemiology
1. There were 1,000,000 new cases and 1,900 deaths in 1998 related to NONMELANOMATOUS skin cancers (Basal cell or Squamous cell)
2. Malignant melanoma is far deadlier. In 1998, there were 41,600 new cases and 7,300 deaths related to melanoma
3. Risk factors for nonmelanomatous cancers include a history of basal or squamous cell cancers, older age, light eyes, skin, or hair, and substantial cumulative lifetime sun exposure
4. Risk factors for melanoma include white race, atypical moles, certain congenital nevi, many common moles, immunosupression, and a family history of skin cancer. Those with the rare familial atypical mole and melanoma syndrome, the melanoma risk are 100-fold

B. Screening
1. Ages 18–39: Self exam monthly and clinical exam every 1–3 years
2. Age > 40: Self exam monthly and annual clinical exam
3. Avoidance of sun, wearing appropriate clothing when outdoors, and using sunscreens may help decrease the incidence of skin cancer

XI. BLADDER CANCER
A. Epidemiology
1. In 1998 there were 54,400 new cases and 12,500 deaths related to bladder cancer

    2. The incidence is 3–4 times higher in men and twice as high in white men compared to black men

    3. Risk factors include cigarette smoking, occupational exposure to chemicals used in dye, leather, tire, and rubber industries. An association between bladder cancer and coffee and/or artificial sweetener consumption has never been proven

B. Screening

    1. No major organization recommends screening for bladder cancer in asymptomatic adults (including those with risk factors)

    2. Cigarette smokers should be counseled on quitting

XII. THYROID CANCER

A. Epidemiology

    1. In 1995 there were 14,000 new cases and 1,000 deaths related to thyroid cancer

    2. Women account for 77% of new cases and 61% of deaths

    3. Risk factors include exposure to external upper body irradiation during infancy or childhood and individuals with a family history of thyroid cancer or multiple endocrine neoplasia Type 2 (MEN 2) syndrome. Medullary thyroid cancer is inherited in 25% of cases as part of the autosomal dominant MEN 2 syndrome

B. Screening

    1. Ages 21–40: palpation of thyroid every 3 years

    2. Age > 40: palpation of thyroid annually

    3. There are no current recommendations regarding use of ultrasonography, even in higher risk patients

XIII. PANCREATIC CANCER

A. Epidemiology

    1. In 1998, there were 29,000 new cases and 28,900 deaths related to pancreatic cancer

    2. Risk factors include male gender, black race, diabetics, cigarette smokers, and older patients (majority of cases are age >65)

    3. The 5 year survival rate is only 3%

B. Screening

    1. There are no organizations who recommend screening asymptomatic patients

    2. Counsel patients on smoking cessation

CLINICAL PEARLS

- Screening for cancer also includes counseling patients on ways to decrease risks of developing cancer
- Counsel smoking patients regarding ways to quit smoking
- Inform patients about using sunscreen
- Cancer screening highlights the importance of obtaining thorough family and social histories
- Encourage patients to perform monthly *self exams* (breast, testicular, skin)

References

American Cancer Society. Cancer facts and figures, 1998. Atlanta, GA: 1998.

National Center for Health Statistics. Health, United States, 1998 with Socioeconomic status and health chartbook. Hyattsville, MD: Public Health Service, 1998.

U. S. Preventive Services Task Force. Guide to clinical preventive services, 2nd ed. Baltimore, MD: Williams & Wilkins, 1996.

Michael B. Weinstock, MD
Mark Reeder, MD

32. SMOKING CESSATION

I. INTRODUCTION

Smoking is estimated to cause over 400,000 deaths per year in the United States. There is a link between cigarette smoking and cancer, atherosclerotic vascular disease, COPD, gastritis, and skin and connective tissue diseases. There is also evidence that people will be more likely to stop smoking if their *physician* actively encourages it. Smoking cessation is targeted at the physiologic *and* psychologic addiction

II. PHARMACOLOGIC AIDS

Currently there are 5 pharmacologic therapies available (listed below). They are effective without behavioral modification, but are more effective with behavioral modification. Many smokers make multiple attempts before they eventually stop smoking

A. Bupropion (Zyban): Atypical antidepressant that has both dopaminergic and adrenergic actions. Begin 1–2 weeks before stop date. Dose 150mg PO QD for 3 days, then 150mg PO BID for 7–12 weeks. Adverse effects: dry mouth and insomnia. Risk of seizure ~ 1/1000 (increased with history of seizure disorder)

B. Transdermal nicotine patches (OTC)
1. **Nicotrol transdermal:** 15mg/16hrs. Wear for 16hrs daily for 6 weeks then discontinue
2. **Nicoderm CQ**, habitrol patches: 21mg/day × 4–8 weeks, 14mg/d × 2–4 weeks, 7mg/d × 2–4 weeks
3. In patients with CAD, weight < 100 lb. or smoking < 1/2 PPD, start with 14mg/d
4. Change patch each day. Use different site
5. Patients should stop smoking while using patches to prevent nicotine toxicity (possible increased risk of MI)

C. Nicotine nasal spray—Nicotrol NS: Each spray is the equivalent of ½ a cigarette. The patient should use only 1–2 sprays/hr (alternating nostrils) with a maximum of 5 sprays/hr (for heavier smokers) and 40 sprays per day. Each dose delivers 1mg. Use for up to 3 months. The nasal spray delivers nicotine more rapidly than gum, patch, or inhaler but less rapidly than cigarettes. Peak levels occur within 10 minutes and are ²/₃ the level of a cigarette. The large majority of smokers initially experience throat irritation, rhinitis, sneezing, coughing, and watering eyes. Nasal irritation occurs in 100% of users and will occur throughout its use (never improves). Tolerance to the other effects occurs in the first week

D. Nicotine inhaler—Nicotrol inhaler: The inhaler is a plastic rod with a nicotine plug that provides a nicotine vapor when puffed on. The device delivers nicotine bucally. Use 6–16 cartridges per day for up to 12 weeks, then reduce gradually for up to 12 weeks. Adverse effects are mild and consist of throat irritation and coughing

E. Nicotine gum—Nicorette (OTC): Comes in single and double strength (2mg and 4mg). Chew one piece every 1–2hrs, at least 9 per day for 6 weeks, then every 2–4hrs for 3 weeks, then every 4–8hrs for 3 weeks, then stop. Nicotine is released with each chew, so chew only PRN. The proper technique is chew, then cheek the gum

F. Combination therapy: Use **Bupropion** with one of the nicotine agents

III. BEHAVIOR MODIFICATION

Should be used along with medications to prevent recidivism. There are many strategies and it is best to pick one for routine use and to modify it for individual patients. Here is an example of a logical 4 step plan:

A. Set a stop date: Designate a special day (holiday, birthday) and enter into a written contract with patient. Set the date weeks to months in advance to give patient time to anticipate stopping smoking

B. Keep a smoking journal: Record times of day and situations when patient is likely to smoke while patient is still smoking. This will be helpful in determining which situations are likely to lead patient to restart smoking (stress, boredom, after meals, etc.)

C. **Identify alternative behaviors:** To be linked with patient's journal. Since smoking has such a strong oral and manual components, try to find *alternative behaviors* for patient to participate in when he/she has an urge to smoke. Examples are chewing gum cinnamon sticks, and projects involving hands (peeling and eating vegetables, woodwork, etc.)

D. **Establish a reward system:** This will be intimately tied to a patient's follow up and doctor-patient relationship. The physician will view patient's smoking diary and reinforce and encourage patient's continued smoking cessation. It can also involve patient putting money that would have been spent on cigarettes in a glass container to be taken out in three month intervals, marking days off calendar, etc.

E. **Encourage the patient to tell everyone he/she knows** prior to quitting of the patient's intentions. (added pressure—no one wants to appear a failure)

CLINICAL PEARLS

- Most patients will attempt to stop smoking several times before they are ultimately successful. This should not discourage the patient *or* the physician!
- For every 4–5 patients we encourage to stop smoking we will be saving one life
- As with all medicine, our relationship with the patient is a partnership. We can give advice, but it is up to the patient to carry it out. Short term failures are often ultimately successful
- Simply mentioning the importance of quitting smoking (without going into any details) will lead to a quit rate of 7%
- On the average, a 1 PPD smoker will live 5–6 years less than a non-smoker. This translates to ~ 5–6 minutes of life lost per cigarette smoked. More importantly, they will be significantly disabled for years before this
- Nearly 43% of children aged two months to 11 years of age live in homes with at least one smoker. Strong evidence indicates that exposure to environmental tobacco smoke is associated with increased illnesses in children, including lower respiratory disease, middle ear effusion, asthma and sudden infant death syndrome

References

Blondal T, et al. Nicotine nasal sray with nicotine patch for smoking cessation: randomised trial with six year follow up. BMJ 1999;318:285–9.

Hajek P, et al. Randomized comparative trial of Nicotine Polacrilex, a transdermal patch, nasal spray, and an inhaler. Arch Intern Med.1999;159:2035–8.

Hughes JR, et al. Recent advances in the pharmacotherapy of smoking. JAMA 1999;281:72–6.

Covey LS, et al. Major depression following smoking cessation. Am J Psychiatry 1997;154:263–5.

Smoking Cessation Clinical Practice Guideline Panel and Staff. The Agency for Health Care Policy and Research Smoking Cessation Clinical Practice Guideline. JAMA 1996;275:1270–80.

Joseph AM, Norman SM, Ferry LH, et al. The safety of transdermal nicotine as an aid to smoking cessation in patients with cardiac disease. N Engl J Med 1996;335:1792–98.

Hughes JR, et al. American Psychiatric Association practice guideline for the treatment of patients with nicotine dependence. Am J Psychiatry 1996;153(suppl):S1–S31.

33. ENDOCARDITIS PROPHYLAXIS — 1997 AHA RECOMMENDATIONS

I. CARDIAC CONDITIONS
A. Endocarditis prophylaxis recommended:
1. High-risk category
   a. Prosthetic cardiac valves, including bioprosthetic and homograft valves
   b. Previous bacterial endocarditis
   c. Complex cyanotic congenital heart disease (e.g., single ventricle states, transposition of the great arteries, tetralogy of Fallot)
   d. Surgically constructed systemic pulmonary shunts or conduits
2. Moderate-risk category
   a. Most other congenital cardiac malformations (other than above and below)
   b. Acquired valvular dysfunction (e.g., rheumatic heart disease)
   c. Hypertrophic cardiomyopathy
   d. Mitral valve prolapse with valvular regurgitation and/or thickened leaflets

B. Endocarditis prophylaxis not recommended:
1. Negligible-risk category
   a. Isolated secundum atrial septal defect
   b. Surgical repair of atrial septal defect, ventricular septal defect, or patent ductus arteriosus (without residua beyond 6 months)
   c. Previous coronary artery bypass graft surgery
   d. Mitral valve prolapse without valvular regurgitation
   e. Physiologic, functional, or innocent heart murmurs
   f. Previous Kawasaki disease without valvular dysfunction
   g. Previous rheumatic fever without valvular dysfunction
   h. Cardiac pacemakers (intravascular and epicardial) and implanted defibrillators

C. Cardiac risk: Patients at high risk are at much greater risk for developing severe endocardial infection

Source: Dajani, AS, Taubert, KA, et al. Prevention of bacterial endocarditis. Recommendations by the American Heart Association. JAMA 1997;22:1795. Copyright 1997, American Medical Association. Used with permission.

II. PROCEDURES—DENTAL OR SURGICAL
A. Endocarditis prophylaxis recommended (Prophylaxis is recommended for patients with high- and moderate-risk cardiac conditions):
1. Dental extractions
2. Periodontal procedures including surgery, scaling and root planing, probing, and recall maintenance
3. Dental implant placement and reimplantation of avulsed teeth
4. Endodontic (root canal) instrumentation or surgery only beyond the apex
5. Subgingival placement of antibiotic fibers or strips
6. Initial placement of orthodontic bands but not brackets
7. Intraligamentary local anesthetic injections
8. Prophylactic cleaning of teeth or implants where bleeding is anticipated

B. Endocarditis prophylaxis not recommended:
1. Restorative dentistry (operative and prosthodontic) with or without retraction cord. This includes restoration of decayed teeth (filling cavities) and replacement of missing teeth. Clinical judgment may indicate antibiotic use in selected circumstances that may create significant bleeding
2. Local anesthetic injections (nonintraligamentary)
3. Intracanal endodontic treatment; post placement and buildup
4. Placement of rubber dams

5. Postoperative suture removal
6. Placement of removable prosthodontic or orthodontic appliances
7. Taking of oral impressions
8. Fluoride treatments
9. Taking of oral radiographs
10. Orthodontic appliance adjustment
11. Shedding of primary teeth

Source: Dajani, AS, Taubert, KA et al. Prevention of bacterial endocarditis. Recommendations by the American Heart Association. JAMA 1997;22:1797. Copyright 1997, American Medical Association. Used with permission.

III. PROCEDURES—OTHER

A. Endocarditis prophylaxis recommended:
1. Respiratory tract
   a. Tonsillectomy and/or adenoidectomy
   b. Surgical operations that involve respiratory mucosa
   c. Bronchoscopy with a rigid bronchoscope
2. Gastrointestinal tract (Prophylaxis is recommended for high-risk patients; optional for medium-risk patients)
   a. Sclerotherapy for esophageal varices
   b. Esophageal stricture dilation
   c. Endoscopic retrograde cholangiography with biliary obstruction
   d. Biliary tract surgery
   e. Surgical operations that involve intestinal mucosa
3. Genitourinary tract
   a. Prostatic surgery
   b. Cystoscopy
   c. Urethral dilation

B. Endocarditis prophylaxis not recommended († indicates prophylaxis is optional for high-risk patients):
1. Respiratory tract
   a. Endotracheal intubation
   b. Bronchoscopy with a flexible bronchoscope, with or without biopsy†
   c. Tympanostomy tube insertion
2. Gastrointestinal tract
   a. Transesophageal echocardiography†
   b. Endoscopy with or without gastrointestinal biopsy†
3. Genitourinary tract
   a. Vaginal hysterectomy†
   b. Vaginal delivery†
   c. Cesarean section
   d. In uninfected tissue:
      i. Urethral catheterization
      ii. Uterine dilation and curettage
      iii. Therapeutic abortion
      iv. Sterilization procedures
      v. Insertion or removal of intrauterine devices
4. Other
   a. Cardiac catheterization, including balloon angioplasty
   b. Implanted cardiac pacemakers, implanted defibrillators, and coronary stents
   c. Incision or biopsy of surgically scrubbed skin
   d. Circumcision

Source: Dajani, AS, Taubert, KA et al. Prevention of bacterial endocarditis. Recommendations by the American Heart Association. JAMA 1997;22:1797. Copyright 1997, American Medical Association. Used with permission.

IV. PROPHYLACTIC REGIMENS FOR DENTAL, ORAL, RESPIRATORY TRACT, OR ESOPHAGEAL PROCEDURES

SITUATION	AGENT	REGIMEN*
Standard general prophylaxis	Amoxicillin	Adults: 2.0 g; children: 50 mg/kg orally 1 h before procedure
Unable to take oral medications	Ampicillin	Adults: 2.0 g intramuscularly (IM) or intravenously (IV); children: 50 mg/kg IM or IV within 30 min before procedure
Allergic to penicillin	Clindamycin *or*	Adults: 600 mg; children: 20 mg/kg orally 1 h before procedure
	Cephalexin† or cefadroxil† *or*	Adults: 2.0 g; children:50 mg/kg orally 1 h before procedure
	Azithromycin or clarithromycin	Adults: 500 mg; children: 15 mg/kg orally 1 h before procedure
Allergic to penicillin and unable to take oral medications	Clindamycin *or*	Adults: 600 mg; children: 20 mg/kg IV within 30 min before procedure
	Cefazolin†	Adults: 1.0 g; children: 25 mg/kg IM or IV within 30 min before procedure

* Total children's dose should not exceed adult dose
† Cephalosporins should not be used in individuals with immediate-type hypersensitivity reaction (urticaria, angioedema, or anaphylaxis) to penicillins

Source: Dajani, AS, Taubert, KA et al. Prevention of bacterial endocarditis. Recommendations by the American Heart Association. JAMA 1997;22:1798. Copyright 1997, American Medical Association. Used with permission.

V. CLINICAL APPROACH TO DETERMINATION OF THE NEED FOR PROPHYLAXIS IN PATIENTS WITH SUSPECTED MITRAL VALVE PROLAPSE

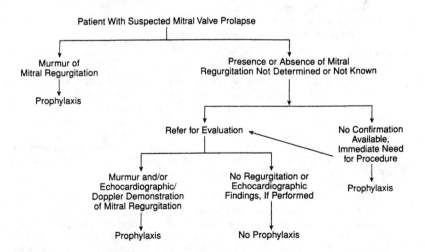

Source: Dajani, AS, Taubert, KA et al. Prevention of bacterial endocarditis. Recommendations by the American Heart Association. JAMA 1997;22:1796. Copyright 1997, American Medical Association. Used with permission.

Diane Minasian, MD
Ivan Wolfson, MD

34. TUBERCULOSIS SCREENING

I. TRANSMISSION

TB is spread primarily through respiratory droplets. By 6–12 weeks most people develop cell-mediated immunity which halts the spread of infection. The PPD (purified protein derivative of TB) test becomes positive by 12 weeks. About 10% of infected people will develop active TB at some time in their life

II. HIGH RISK POPULATION

A. HIV positive
B. Close contacts of people with infectious TB
C. Immigrants from high prevalence countries (Asia, Africa, Latin America, etc.)
D. Medically underserved/low income
E. Certain racial/ethnic groups (African-Americans, Hispanics, Native Americans, etc.)
F. Chronic medical conditions/immunocompromised (chronic steroid use, silicosis, sickle cell disease, end stage renal disease, diabetes, etc.)
G. Homeless persons
H. Alcoholics
I. IV drug users
J. Residents of long-term care facilities (prisons, nursing homes, etc.)
K. Health care workers

III. SCREENING

A. All high risk individuals should be screened annually
B. All pregnant women at high risk should be screened
C. Exceptions to routine screening include:
  1. Documented skin test positive in the past
  2. Prior appropriate treatment for a positive skin test

IV. SKIN TESTING

A. Mantoux test
  1. The Mantoux test is the standard of care. The TINE TEST should not be used in screening
  2. Should be read 48–72hrs after injection, preferably by a health care worker
  3. The measurement is based on the *induration*, not the erythema
  4. The measurement should be 1 number (e.g., 8mm) which should be measured in the transverse plane. Recording "positive" or "negative" is not sufficient
B. Negative skin test: Does *not* exclude TB infection. A reaction may not occur in patients who are immunocompromised, severe febrile illness, virus vaccinations (MMR, OPV), malnutrition, old age, overwhelming TB infections and HIV disease
C. Booster phenomenon
  1. Explanation: Repeated testing of uninfected individuals does *not* sensitize them to tuberculin. However, delayed sensitivity to tuberculin (a positive test) may wane over time. Certain individuals who were exposed to TB early in their life may have no reaction many years later (false negative). In these individuals, it is necessary to do 2 tests, 1 week apart. If the second test (performed 1–2 weeks later) is positive, this represents a booster phenomenon (remote infection) and *not* a recent conversion
  2. Indications: Indicated for the *initial screening* of residents and employees of long-term care facilities and others who will be receiving yearly skin testing. It is done to avoid misinterpreting a boosted reaction as a recent infection

V. CRITERIA FOR A POSITIVE TEST

Positivity is based on a patient's risk and on the fact that the larger the reaction, the greater the

likelihood of infection
  A. **Greater than 5mm**
    1. Patients who have had recent contact with active TB
    2. HIV
    3. X-rays suggestive of previous TB
  B. **Greater than 10mm:** All other *high risk* individuals (See section II, High Risk Population)
  C. **Greater than 15mm:** Everyone else

VI. PRIOR BCG VACCINATION
  A. A history of BCG (Bacille bilié de Calmette-Guérin) vaccination *does not alter the guidelines* for interpreting skin test results
  B. The effectiveness of BCG vaccination varies from 0–76% in major trials

VII. INDICATIONS FOR PREVENTIVE THERAPY
Any patient with inactive disease (a positive skin test and a negative chest x-ray) should be considered for prophylactic therapy. The decision of whether to treat is based on weighing the risk of developing active TB versus the risk of developing toxicity from the treatment (primarily, Isoniazid induced hepatitis)
  A. **Less than age 35**
    1. All patients with positive skin test (See above—criteria for a positive test) and negative chest x-ray
    2. Recent converters: Greater than 10mm increase within a 2-year period
  B. **Greater than age 35** with positive skin test and negative chest x-ray
    1. HIV positive
    2. Close contacts of patients with active TB
    3. Recent converters (greater than 15mm increase within 2 years)
    4. IV drug users
    5. Previously untreated or inadequately treated with abnormal chest x-ray—consider referral
    6. Persons with medical conditions that increase the risk of developing active TB (e.g., end stage renal disease)
  C. **Cases of known TB exposure:** Persons who are close contacts of infectious cases, especially children, should be given preventive therapy regardless of skin test reaction. After 3 months of therapy those who were skin test negative should have the test repeated. If still negative, and close contact with the known case has been broken, treatment can be stopped
  D. **Pregnant women:** If positive skin test then obtain a chest x-ray after 20 weeks of gestation
    1. If the chest x-ray is negative then begin preventive therapy 3 months postpartum. Breast feeding is *not* a contraindication to Isoniazid therapy
    2. High risk women (likely to have been recently infected) should begin therapy after the first trimester. Use **Pyridoxine** with **Isoniazid** during pregnancy to avoid the peripheral neuropathy that may be associated with Isoniazid
  E. **Newborns of skin test positive mothers:** Congenital transmission is very rare. Most newborns who develop TB do so after birth
    1. All household contacts of the skin test positive mother should be tested prior to delivery to identify the active case
    2. CDC recommends that newborns be tested between 3 and 4 months of age

VIII. PREVENTIVE THERAPY TO TREAT INACTIVE DISEASE
  A. **Medications**
    1. Dose: **Isoniazid (INH)** is given once daily at a dose of 10mg/kg/day, up to 300mg/day for 9–12 months
    2. Contraindications: Acute or active liver disease of any etiology or history of previous completion on Isoniazid preventive therapy
    3. Efficacy: **Isoniazid** has been shown to reduce the incidence of clinical TB by 54–88% when taken for 12 months
    4. Persons with conditions in which neuropathy is common as well as pregnant women and persons with a seizure disorder, may be given Pyridoxine (50 mg/day) with Isoniazid
  B. **Labs:** There is a 10–20% chance of mild Isoniazid induced liver function test changes. Some

clinicians check labs only if patient is symptomatic (See below)
1. Age < 20: No baseline or periodic labs are necessary
2. Age 20–35: Baseline SGOT and again at 2 months
3. Age > 35, or persons who use alcohol daily: Check baseline SGOT and then Q month for 3–4 months. If SGOT rises 3–5 times the upper limit of normal, **Isoniazid** should be discontinued

    C. Monitoring: Monthly follow up for questioning for compliance, signs of neurotoxicity (parasthesias), and signs of liver damage (anorexia, weight loss, abdominal pain, nausea, vomiting, jaundice)

References

McColloster P, Neff NE. Outpatient management of tuberculosis. Am Fam Phys 1996;53:1579.
Core curriculum on tuberculosis. 3rd ed. U.S. Dept. of Health and Human Services, Public Health Service, Center for Disease Control, 1994.
U.S. Public Health Service. Tuberculosis in adults. Am Fam Phys 1994;50:811–5.

V. Cardiology & Pulmonary Disorders

CARD

David Sharkis, MD
Daniel M. Neides, MD
Michael B. Weinstock, MD

35. EVALUATION OF CHEST PAIN

I. INTRODUCTION

Failure to diagnose a myocardial infarction represents the most frequent basis of successful litigation against ED physicians

II. DIFFERENTIAL DIAGNOSIS OF CHEST PAIN

(5 life-threatening causes are in **bold italics**)

A. Cardiac: Coronary artery disease (angina, ***myocardial infarction***), ***pericarditis (pericardial tamponade)***, aortic stenosis, hypertrophic cardiomyopathy, aortic regurgitation, mitral valve prolapse

B. Vascular: ***Aortic dissection***, hypertensive crisis, right ventricular strain

C. Pulmonary: ***Pulmonary embolus, pneumothorax***, pneumonia, pleurisy, asthma, bronchitis

D. Gastrointestinal: Esophageal rupture, esophageal reflux or spasm, peptic ulcer disease, Mallory-Weiss tear, pancreatitis, cholecystitis, hepatitis

E. Musculoskeletal: Costochondritis, thoracic outlet syndrome, cervical disc disease, thoracic radiculopathy

F. Psychogenic: Anxiety/panic disorder, depression

G. Other: Herpes zoster, breast disease

III. HISTORY

A. Character of pain

1. Dull pressure, squeezing, burning: Consider CAD or esophageal pain (GERD)
2. Radiation of pain to neck/shoulder/jaw: Consider CAD
3. Radiation of pain to the back: Consider aortic dissection, pancreatitis, or perforated peptic ulcer
4. Sharp, stabbing pain: Consider chest wall (costochondritis), pleurisy, pericardial pain, PE

B. Onset

1. Sudden onset: Consider PE, pneumothorax, or aortic dissection
2. Slow onset (building over 2–5 minutes): Consider CAD

C. Exacerbation/relief

1. Exacerbated by exercise or stress and relieved by rest: Consider CAD
2. Relieved by nitroglycerin: Consider CAD or esophageal spasm
3. Exacerbated by movement or deep inspiration: Consider musculoskeletal, pericardial, or pleuritic disease
4. Worse when lying supine and relieved by upright position: Consider pericarditis

D. Symptoms associated with CAD: Dyspnea, diaphoresis, palpitations, radiation to arm/neck/jaw/shoulder, light-headedness, nausea, vomiting, syncope (orthopnea, nocturnal dyspnea, peripheral edema are associated with CHF)

E. Past medical history

1. Determine risk factors for CAD: Known CAD (history of PTCA or CABG), smoking, HTN, hypercholesterolemia, diabetes, family history, male > age 40, female > age 50
2. Complete past history including childhood illnesses (rheumatic fever)
3. Obtain results of stress tests, cardiac catheterizations, ECHOs, and if PTCA and/or CABG were performed, which vessels were involved
4. Current medications: Including nitrates, anti-hypertensives, H_2 blockers

IV. PHYSICAL EXAM

A. Vital signs: Check BP and heart rate

B. Neck: Assess for midline trachea, JVD, carotid bruits

C. Lungs: Listen for bilateral and equal breath sounds, rales, consolidation

D. Chest: Palpate for tenderness

E. Heart: Inspect chest for presence of surgical scars; palpate for parasternal lift, increased LV

CARD

impulse, point of maximal impulse; auscultate for friction rub, gallops, murmurs, clicks (MVP), distant heart sounds

F. Extremities: Assess for unilateral leg swelling (DVT), cyanosis, clubbing, or edema; palpate femoral pulses (dissection)

V. EVALUATING CHEST PAIN

A. ECG: Important for diagnosing myocardial ischemia or infarction as well as pericardial disease; may show characteristic findings consistent with PE (sinus tachycardia, $S_1 Q_3 T_3$ pattern) (See Chapter 36, ECG Interpretation)

B. Chest x-ray: Will aid in diagnosing pneumothorax, pneumonia, assessing cardiac silhouette, pleural effusion, and determining a widened mediastinum (aortic dissection)

C. Laboratory: Initial labs include CPK with isoenzymes Q8hrs × 3 (CPKs peak at 8–12hrs), Troponin, CBC, Chem 7 & 12

D. Pulse oximetry and arterial blood gas (ABG)

VI. FIVE LIFE THREATENING CAUSES OF CHEST PAIN: PRESENTATION AND DIAGNOSIS

Because the differential diagnosis for chest pain is extensive, it will be imperative to rule out these life threatening causes when a patient presents with chest pain:

Condition	Location of Pain	Quality of Pain	Onset/Duration of Pain	Aggravating/ Relieving	Signs or Symptoms	Diagnosing the Condition
MYOCARDIAL INFARCTION/ UNSTABLE ANGINA	Substernal may radiate to jaw, neck or shoulder	Pressure, heaviness, squeezing, burning	Builds over several mins. to hours	Unable to relieve	SOB, diaphoresis, N/V, dizziness, light-headedness	Serial CPKs ECG. May need LDHs if pain > 24 hours Clinical diagnosis
PNEUMO-THORAX	Unilateral	Sharp, pleuritic	Sudden onset	Painful breathing	Dyspnea; decreased breath sounds; tracheal deviation and tachypnea with tension pneumo	Chest x-ray and physical exam
PERICAR-DITIS (PERICAR-DIAL TAM-PONADE)	Retrosternal and left precodial	Sharp, stabbing, pleuritic	Hours to day	Worse with deep breaths or supine position; better by upright and forward position	Friction rub, pulsus paradoxus, tamponade	ECG; ECHO to rule out tamponade. Consider CXR
PULMONARY EMBOLUS	Substernal	Pleuritic	Sudden onset	Worse with breathing	Dyspnea, tachypnea, tachycardia, rales, hemoptysis	ABG, ECG, Ventilation/ Perfusion scan, Pulmonary angiogram
AORTIC DISSECTION	Anterior chest with radiation to back	Severe pain, tearing sensation	Sudden onset	Unable to relieve	Lower BP in arm, decreased femoral pulses, AR murmur, pulsus paradoxus	Chest x-ray (widened mediastinum), angiography, CT or MRI, TEE

CLINICAL PEARLS

- 10% of acute MI patients state that their chest pain is relieved by antacids. No published data support the use of antacids and viscous lidocaine to rule out an MI
- 10–20% of patients who have an MI will have either a normal ECG or nonspecific changes. A patient with a good history for myocardial ischemia in light of a normal ECG still needs to be admitted and evaluated for coronary artery disease
- If MI/unstable angina is a possibility in a patient with pain > 24hrs duration, obtain Troponin I along with CPKs
- Patients diagnosed with an acute MI (with no known contraindications, i.e., recent surgery, CVA, etc.) should receive thrombolytics within 30–60 minutes after arriving in the ED

• Patients with inferior MI and hypotension may also have right ventricular MI. Diagnosis is made with right sided ECG (See Chapter 36, ECG Interpretation). Approximately 33% of patients with inferior MI have concurrent right ventricular MI, but it is clinically significant about half of the time

References

Zanger D, et al. Contemporary management of angina: Part II. Medical management of chronic stable angina. Am Fam Phys 2000;61:129–38.

Bates ER. Myocardial infarction: fast track evaluation and treatment. Consultant 1994;34(9):1251–63.

Isselbacher KJ, et al., eds. Harrison's principles of internal medicine. 13th ed. New York: McGraw–Hill, 1994:55, 1094–5, 1133–4.

Schlant RC, Alexander RW, eds. The heart: arteries and veins. 8th ed. New York: McGraw-Hill, 1994:460.

Michael B. Weinstock, MD

36. ECG INTERPRETATION

Note: All criteria listed below are not required for diagnosis

I. SEQUENCE TO READ ECG

A. Rate: Rate < 60 = bradycardia, rate > 100 = tachycardia

B. Rhythm: Sinus, junctional, ventricular

C. Axis: Normal axis is -30° to 100°

D. Hypertrophy and heart block: Atrial or ventricular hypertrophy (check P, QRS), heart block (check PR interval, P before each QRS, etc.) and bundle branch block (RBBB, LBBB, LAHB, LPHB)

E. Ischemia/infarction: Check each lead for Q waves, ST elevation or depression, hyperacute or inverted T waves

F. Electrolyte or Digoxin disturbances: Check QT, U waves

II. AXIS

If leads I and II have the largest R waves, or
   the net of I plus aVF is positive,
   the axis can be considered normal

A. Causes of left axis deviation (LAD) (-30 to -120)
   1. Left ventricular hypertrophy (LVH)
   2. Left bundle branch block (LBBB)
   3. Left anterior fascicular block (LAHB)

B. Causes of right axis deviation (RAD) (100 to 180)
   1. Right ventricular hypertrophy (RVH)
   2. Right bundle branch block (RBBB)
   3. Left posterior fascicular block (LPHB)
   4. COPD, pulmonary emboli (PE), cor pulmonale

Normal axis is -30° to 100°

III. HYPERTROPHY

A. Right atrial enlargement (RAE)
   1. ECG diagnosis
      a. Tall P waves in II, III, aVF > 0.12 seconds wide or 3mm tall (P pulmonale)
      b. Large diphasic P wave in V_1 with initial component > 1.5mm
      c. P > 0.11 seconds
   2. Differential diagnosis of RAE
      a. Pulmonary HTN (COPD, PE)
      b. Tricuspid or pulmonic valvular dysfunction (TR, TS, PR, PS)
      c. Congenital disorder

B. Left atrial enlargement (LAE)
   1. ECG diagnosis
      a. P wave in lead I > 0.12 seconds

   b. Terminal negativity of P wave in V_1 > 1mm with duration > 0.04 seconds
   2. Differential diagnosis of LAE
      a. Systemic HTN
      b. Aortic or mitral valvular dysfunction (AR, AS, MR, MS)
      c. Left ventricular failure
C. Right ventricular hypertrophy (RVH)
   1. ECG diagnosis
      a. Right axis deviation > 100°
      b. R > S in right precordium (V_{1-2}) and deep S waves over left precordium (V_{5-6})
      c. ST depression and inverted T wave in V_{1-2}
      d. Associated RAE
      e. Normal QRS
   2. Differential diagnosis of RVH
      a. Pulmonary HTN (COPD, PE)
      b. Pulmonary stenosis, MS, MR, left to right shunt
D. Left ventricular hypertrophy (LVH)
   1. ECG diagnosis: The Estes point system for LVH (95% specific, 50% sensitive)
      a. Amplitude (Any of the following) 3
         i. Largest R or S in limb leads ≥ 20mm
         ii. S in V_1 or V_2 ≥ 25mm
         iii. R in V_5 or V_6 ≥ 25mm
      b. ST segment changes of strain
         i. Without Digitalis 3
         ii. With Digitalis 1
      c. LA abnormality 3
      e. Left axis deviation ≥ -30° 2
      e. QRS duration ≥ 0.09 seconds 1
      f. Intrinsicoid deflection* in V_5 or V_6 > 0.05 seconds 1
         Intrinsicoid deflection is the time to the beginning of the rapid fall from the peak of the R
         Probable LVH = 4 total points
         LVH = 5 total points
   2. Differential diagnosis of LVH
      a. Systemic arterial HTN
      b. AS, AR
      c. Hypertrophic cardiomyopathy
      d. Coarctation of the aorta

IV. HEART BLOCK
   Normal PR = 0.12–0.2 seconds; QRS = 0.08–0.12 seconds; QT_c = < 0.37seconds (males), < 0.40
   seconds (females). QT_c = QT (seconds) / √RR (seconds)
   Note: Small blocks are 0.04 seconds; large blocks are 0.2 seconds
   A. AV block
   1. First degree heart block: PR interval > 0.2 seconds
   2. Second degree heart block
      a. Mobitz I (Wenckebach): PR interval gradually increases until the AV node is not con-
         ducted and a QRS is dropped
      b. Mobitz II: PR is constant with QRS occasionally dropped
   3. Third degree heart block: Complete heart block with no atrial impulses reaching the ven-
      tricles. The P waves and the QRS complexes both independently "march out"
   B. Bundle branch block
   1. Right bundle branch block (RBBB)
      a. Total QRS > 0.12 seconds (QRS = 0.10–0.11 seconds in incomplete RBBB)
      b. RSR' in right precordial leads (V_{1-2})
      c. Terminal broad S in I, V_{5-6}
      d. Right axis deviation (RAD)
   2. Left bundle branch block (LBBB)
      a. Total QRS > 0.12 seconds (QRS = 0.10–0.11 seconds in incomplete LBBB)
      b. Broad R wave in I, V_{5-6}

  c. ST depression and T wave inversion in I, aVL, V_{5-6}
  d. Displacement of the ST segment and T wave in a direction opposite to the major QRS deflection
  e. Left axis deviation (LAD)
  f. Absence of Q wave in I, V_{5-6}
  g. Poor R wave progression
 3. Left anterior fascicular block (LAHB)
  a. LAD (QRS axis -30° to -90°)
  b. Small R in II, III, aVF
  c. S in V_{5-6}
  d. Small Q in I, aVL
  e. Normal QRS duration
 4. Left posterior fascicular block (LPHB)
  a. RAD (QRS axis > 100°)
  b. Small S in II, III, aVF
  c. Small R in I, aVL
  d. Normal QRS duration
  e. Exclude other causes of RAD: RVH, COPD, lateral MI

V. ISCHEMIA/INFARCTION
 A. ECG changes
  1. Ischemia: Horizontal ST segment depression or downsloping ST segment, T waves upright or inverted
  2. Injury: Acute ST segment elevation (convex)
  3. Infarction: Q waves (Q waves must be > 25% of succeeding R wave and > 0.04 seconds)
 B. ECG changes by ischemic/infarction location
  1. Inferior MI: Changes in leads II, III, aVF (right coronary artery or circumflex)
  2. Anterior MI: Changes in leads I, V_{3-4} (left anterior descending artery)
  3. Posterior MI: R wave in V_{1-2}, upright T in V_1, ST depression V_{1-2} (circumflex artery or RCA)
  4. Lateral MI: Changes in leads I, aVL, V_{5-6}
  5. Anterolateral MI: Changes in leads V_{3-6}, aVL
  6. Anteroseptal MI: Changes in leads V_{1-4}
  7. Right ventricular MI: ST elevation in lead V4R seen on a *right sided ECG*

VI. DIFFERENTIAL DIAGNOSIS OF SPECIFIC ABNORMALITIES (ST, QT, ETC.)
 A. Increased PR interval
  1. AV block
  2. Hyperthyroidism
  3. Digitalis effect
  4. Hypothermia
 B. Shortened PR interval
  1. Wolff-Parkinson-White (WPW)
  2. AV junctional rhythm with retrograde P wave conduction
  3. Lown-Ganong-Levine (accessory pathway)
  4. HTN
 C. Increased QRS interval
  1. Hyperkalemia
  2. Bundle branch block
  3. Hypothermia
  4. Quinidine
  5. Procainamide
  6. Tricyclic overdose
 D. ST segment elevation
  1. Q wave MI
  2. Pericarditis (diffuse ST segment elevation)
  3. Ventricular aneurysm (ST segment elevation persists > 2 weeks)

CARD

  4. Early repolarization: Seen best in V_{1-2}, no other ECG abnormalities present, cannot be distinguished from MI. If patient is > age 30, may need to be admitted to exclude MI. Check old ECGs

  5. Prinzmetal's angina

  6. Nonspecific

E. ST segment depression

  1. Ischemia

  2. Non Q wave MI

  3. Ventricular hypertrophy (typically downsloping)

  4. Interventricular Conduction Defect (IVCD)

  5. Digoxin effect, Quinidine effect

  6. Hypokalemia

  7. "Reciprocal" changes in MI

F. Prolonged QT_c: measured from the beginning of the Q to the end of the T wave (> 0.37 seconds in men and > 0.40 seconds in women — due to delayed repolarization of the ventricular myocardium). $QT_c = QT$ (seconds) / $\sqrt{RR}$ (seconds)

  1. Ischemia, CHF

  2. Drugs: Quinidine, Procaine, Norpace, Phenothiazines, Tricyclics, Terfenadine, Cisapride

  3. Hypocalcemia, hypokalemia, hypomagnesemia

  4. Hypothermia

  5. Mitral valve prolapse (MVP)

  6. Ventricular hypertrophy

  7. Intracranial hemorrhage

G. Shortened QT_c

  1. Hypercalcemia

  2. Digoxin

H. Inverted T waves

  1. Ischemia

  2. Non Q wave MI

  3. Chronic pericarditis

  4. Ventricular hypertrophy

  5. Intraventricular conduction defect (IVCD)

  6. Intracranial hemorrhage

  7. Hypokalemia

  8. Pulmonary embolism (PE)

I. Tall/peaked T waves

  1. Hyperkalemia

  2. Acute MI

  3. Intracranial hemorrhage

  4. Normal variant

J. Tall R wave in V_1

  1. Posterior MI

  2. RVH

  3. Incomplete RBBB

  4. Duchenne's muscular dystrophy

  5. WPW

  6. Normal variant (counterclockwise rotation of the heart)

K. RSR' in V_1

  1. Complete or incomplete RBBB

  2. RVH

  3. WPW

  4. Pectus or straight back deformities

  5. Normal variant—occurs in 5% of young people

L. U waves: Considered abnormal when amplitude is > 1.5mm in any lead; best seen in V_3

  1. Bradycardia

  2. Electrolyte imbalance (hypokalemia, hypercalcemia or hypomagnesemia)

3. Drugs (Digitalis, Quinidine, Procainamide, Phenothiazines, Epinephrine)
4. CNS disease
5. LVH
6. Hyperthyroidism
7. Mitral valve prolapse (MVP)
8. Intracranial hemorrhage
9. Negative U waves are suggestive of severe triple vessel disease

M. Poor R wave progression (precordial leads)
   1. COPD
   2. LV dilation
   3. LAHB
   4. Anterior MI

VII. DRUG EFFECTS

A. Digitalis
   1. Digitalis *effect*: Seen in most patients on Digitalis. (Digitalis is often stopped several days before exercise stress testing so that Digitalis effect (ST depression, T wave changes) will not be confused with ischemia)
      a. Increased PR interval
      b. ST segment depression (downsloping ST segment)
      c. Flattening of T waves, diphasic T, inverted T
      d. Shortening of QT interval
      e. Increase of U wave amplitude
   2. Digitalis *toxicity*: This is a clinical and not an ECG diagnosis
      a. Evidence of increased automaticity and impaired conduction
      b. Examples: Bradyarrhythmia, junctional rhythm, AV block, PAT with 2:1 AV block, PVCs, bi-/trigeminy, atrial fib., V. Tach, V. Fib.

B. Quinidine
   1. Quinidine *effect*: Changes seen on ECG
      a. Wide, notched P
      b. Wide QRS (> 0.12 seconds)
      c. ST depression
      d. Prolonged QT_c
      e. U wave
   2. Quinidine *toxicity*: This is a clinical and not an ECG diagnosis
      a. Widening of QRS (> 0.12 seconds)
      b. AV block, sinus bradycardia, sinus arrest
      c. Ventricular arrhythmias, syncope, sudden death
      d. Torsade de pointes

VIII. ELECTROLYTE ABNORMALITIES

A. Hyperkalemia
   1. Tall, narrow, peaked T waves (hyperacute T waves)
   2. Widening of QRS > 0.10 seconds
   3. Wide, flat P waves
   4. Bradyarrhythmias, tachyarrhythmias, AV block, ventricular fibrillation, cardiac arrest

B. Hypokalemia
   1. Flattening and inversion of T wave
   2. Prominent U wave
   3. ST depression
   4. Ventricular ectopy and AV block

C. Hypercalcemia: Decreased QT interval, U waves

D. Hypocalcemia (hypomagnesemia): Increased QT interval

IX. ECG CHANGES ASSOCIATED WITH VARIOUS CONDITIONS
   A. Pulmonary embolism (PE): Sinus tachycardia, S in lead I, Q in lead III, inverted T in lead III,

RAD, ST segment decreased in lead II, transient RBBB, T wave inversion in right precordial leads, right atrial enlargement. Note: the most common is a normal ECG

B. Chronic lung disease: RAD, RVH, right atrial enlargement, low voltage, multifocal atrial tachycardia (MAT), right atrial enlargement

C. Pericardial effusion: Sinus tachycardia, electrical alternans, low voltage (< 5mm), ST segment elevation

D. LV strain: Depressed and wavy ST segment in V_5

E. RV strain: Depressed and wavy ST segment in V_2

F. Wolff-Parkinson-White syndrome (WPW): PR < 0.12, QRS > 0.11, delta wave, ST/T changes, associated with paroxysmal tachycardia

G. Ventricular aneurysm: Persistent ST elevation (> 2 weeks) after MI (usually anterior MI)

H. Early repolarization/normal variant: QRS slurs into ST with high J point and concave up ST segment, most common in lateral and inferior leads

I. Pericarditis: Diffuse ST segment elevation (concave) present in all leads except aVR and V_1, PR segment depression, QRS changes are absent

J. Hypothermia: Prolonged PR, prolonged QT_c, sinus bradycardia syndrome

K. Sick sinus syndrome: Severe sinus bradycardia, sinus arrest, bradycardia alternating with tachycardia, chronic atrial fibrillation, AV junctional escape rhythm

CLINICAL PEARLS
- Reciprocal changes for inferior infarctions may involve I, aVL. Reciprocal changes for a lateral MI may involve II, III, aVF
- Approximately 15% of normal individuals may have a Q wave and/or T wave inversion in lead III
- Q waves may be normal in lead III, V_1 and sometimes V_2

References

Phibbs BP. Advanced ECG: Boards and beyond. 1st ed. Boston: Little, Brown, 1997.

Seelig CB. Simplified EKG analysis. Philadelphia: Hanley & Belfus, 1992.

Marriott HJL. Practical electrocardiography. 8th ed. Baltimore: Williams & Wilkins, 1988.

Dubin D. Rapid interpretation of EKGs. 3rd ed. Tampa, FL: COVER, 1974.

CARD

Beth Weinstock, MD
Michael B. Weinstock, MD
Miriam Chan, PharmD
Dana Nottingham, MD

37. HYPERLIPIDEMIA

I. SIGNIFICANCE
A. A major modifiable risk factor for coronary heart disease, which is the leading cause of death for both women and men in the United States
B. There is a *1% reduction in risk of coronary artery disease (CAD)* for every *1% decrease in LDL*

II. ETIOLOGY
A. **Total cholesterol** is influenced by genetic predisposition, concomitant disease, certain medications, and lifestyle
B. **Genetic connection:** Autosomal dominant familial hypercholesterolemia—present in one in 500 patients with myocardial infarction
  1. Heterozygous: Develop vascular disease in 30's; total cholesterol usually 330–450
  2. Homozygous: Develop vascular disease in teens; total cholesterol usually > 450

III. CHOLESTEROL SCREENING
A. **In adults > age 20 without CAD risk factors,** check a *nonfasting* total cholesterol and HDL level every 5 years
B. **In patients with an abnormal initial screening test** (total cholesterol level > 200 or HDL level < 35) or in patients **with 2 or more risk factors for CAD** (family history, age > 45 in men or age > 55 in women, smoking, HTN, low HDL cholesterol < 35mg/dL, diabetes mellitus) **or history of CAD**, check a *fasting* (>12hrs):
  1. Total cholesterol
  2. HDL
  3. Triglycerides
  4. LDL (LDL = total cholesterol - HDL - triglycerides/5)
C. **If any of the above abnormal,** then recheck in 1–8 weeks and use the average of the two values to guide management
D. **Cholesterol screening in children**
  1. Indications: Children >2 years:
    a. With a parent with total cholesterol > 240mg/dL
    b. With a family history of premature (< age 55) cardiovascular disease
  2. For screening purposes, finger-stick capillary technique is adequate
  3. Recommendations for checking full fasting lipid profile is screening cholesterol > 170mg/dL
E. **Cholesterol screening in the elderly**
  1. The American College of Physicians recommends that total cholesterol measurement be performed at intervals of every 5 years up to age 70
  2. However, elderly patients who are otherwise in good health and who can expect a reasonably long life in the absence of coronary artery disease should not be excluded from cholesterol-lowering therapy. The level of aggressiveness in cholesterol lowering depends on the assessment of CAD risk. Stabilization of atherosclerotic lesions may be very important in elderly patients who inherently have higher risk of coronary events
  3. Despite the lack of data from clinical trials, older patients whose life expectancy is not otherwise limited deserve treatment. Note special nutritional requirements of the elderly, as well as drug-drug interactions
F. **Clinical pearls regarding cholesterol screening**
  1. Patients who are acutely ill, losing weight, pregnant, or breast-feeding should not be screened (results will not be representative)
  2. If patient has had an MI in the last 3 months, cholesterol will be *lower* than the actual value
  3. If full lipid profile is ordered, patient should be fasting 12hrs prior to blood draw (water and black coffee are acceptable)

CARD

4. Cholesterol levels should be measured on *venous* samples
5. Total cholesterol may be 10% higher in winter compared to summer

IV. INDICATIONS FOR THERAPY

A. If patient already has **known CAD**, the goal of therapy should be LDL < 100 (secondary prevention)
B. If patient has **2 or more risk factors for CAD**, the goal of therapy should be LDL < 130
C. In patients **without risk factors for CAD**, the goal of therapy should be LDL < 160
D. In **diabetic patients** (with or without known CAD), the goal of therapy should be LDL <100

INDICATIONS FOR THERAPY BY TOTAL CHOLESTEROL AND LDL:

Cholesterol level	Two or more risk factors for CAD or history of CAD	Action
1. LDL < 130	Present or Absent	Recheck in 5 years
2. LDL 130-160: (Total chol. < 240)	Absent Present	Diet and recheck in 1-2 years Diet and recheck in 3-6 months
3. LDL 160 -190: (Total chol. > 240)	Absent Present	Diet and recheck in 3-6 months Diet *and* Drug therapy
4. LDL > 190:	Present or Absent	Diet *and* Drug therapy

V. MANAGEMENT: Correct secondary causes of lipid disorders

A. Diabetes
B. Obesity
C. Sedentary lifestyle
D. Hypothyroidism
E. Liver (obstructive jaundice)
F. Renal disease (Nephrotic syndrome, dialysis)
G. Smoking
H. Hypertension
I. Alcoholism
J. Menopause
K. Drug induced: Thiazide diuretics, Cimetidine (Tagamet), progestins, steroids (anabolic and corticosteroids), ß-blockers, oral contraceptives, Chlorpromazine, bile salts

VI. LIFESTYLE MODIFICATION

A. The daily American diet usually contains between 400–500mg of cholesterol. Intake of < 200mg/day is needed to reduce total cholesterol through diet alone
B. Saturated fats increase LDL and HDL cholesterol levels. Reducing dietary saturated fats results in greater decrease in total cholesterol than does just restricting overall cholesterol intake
C. Types of diets: Nutrition referral is indicated for all patients with hyperlipidemia—patient can then be given specifics of each diet
  1. Step I diet: reduces cholesterol level up to 4–8% over a 2 to 5 year period, if strictly followed. Reduces intake of the major obvious sources of saturated fat and cholesterol
  2. Step II diet: reduces total cholesterol by 13–16% over 5 years in a select population. Started in patients in whom step I diet is ineffective. Patients with previously diagnosed coronary artery disease should be started initially on step II diet
  3. Fiber: addition of 3g/day of soluble fiber from oat products can lower total cholesterol by 5%
D. Evaluation after dietary management
  1. If total serum cholesterol goal is met and confirmed by an LDL cholesterol, then total cholesterol can be evaluated every 3 months for first year and then every 6 months if stable
  2. If total serum cholesterol goal not reached in 6 months of intensive diet therapy, pharmacologic therapy should be considered. For patients with LDL > 220, shorter follow-up intervals are appropriate and medications should be started sooner
E. Weight loss/Exercise

1. Decreases total cholesterol, decreases triglyceride levels, increases HDL levels, decreases BP, and decreases risk of diabetes mellitus
2. Aerobic activity involving large muscle groups is most beneficial (30 minutes, at least 4 times/week)

VII. TYPES OF LIPID DISORDERS: The most common types of lipid disorders (80–90%) are types IIA, IIB, and type IV. Use this table as a guide to find a logical medication to start with. Always use dietary management concurrently

LAB RESULTS	TYPE	PHARMACOLOGIC MANAGEMENT
Elevated LDL (no change or minimal change in triglycerides or HDL)	Type IIA	1) HMG CoA Reductase Inhibitors 2) Niacin 3) Resins
Elevated LDL (VLDL) and Triglycerides Decreased HDL	Type IIB	1) HMG CoA Reductase Inhibitors 2) Niacin 3) Fibrates
Elevated Triglycerides and LDL (VLDL) Decreased HDL	Type IV	1) Niacin 2) Fibrates
Elevated Triglycerides (chylomicrons) (Treat if > 400 to prevent pancreatitis)	Type I	1) Fibrates 2) Niacin

VIII. DRUG THERAPY

A. HMG CoA Reductase Inhibitors
1. Action: Inhibit rate limiting step in cholesterol biosynthesis. Up-regulates LDL receptors in liver, which increases clearance of LDL. Maximum effect is achieved after approximately 4 weeks of therapy
2. All should be taken QHS
3. Stop treatment in patients with transaminase levels >3× normal
4. On a mg-per-mg basis: 10mg Simvastatin = 20mg Lovastatin or Pravastatin = 80mg **Fluvastatin**
5. Effect: At maximum recommended dose, all decrease LDL by up to 40% (Atorvastatin by 50–60%), increase HDL by 5–10% and decrease TG by 10–20% (except Atorvastatin which decreases TG by 19–37%)

B. Niacin (Nicotinic Acid)
1. Action: Decreases the synthesis of LDL cholesterol by reducing the hepatic synthesis of VLDL cholesterol, by increasing the synthesis of HDL cholesterol, by inhibiting lipolysis in adipose tissue and by increasing lipase activity
2. Effect: Decrease LDL up to 25%, decrease Triglycerides up to 20–50%, increase HDL up to 35%, decrease lipoprotein A up to 50%

C. Bile Acid sequestrants
1. Action: Bind cholesterol-containing bile acids in the intestines, producing an insoluble complex that prevents reabsorption
2. Decrease LDL up to 20%, increase HDL by 3–5%, no effect on Triglycerides
3. Good choice in young patients, women of child-bearing age, and in patients with hepatic disease

D. Fibric Acid derivatives (Fibrates)
1. Action: Increase the clearance of VLDL cholesterol by enhancing lipolysis and reducing hepatic cholesterol synthesis
2. Drug of choice in patients with normal cholesterol and increased Triglycerides
3. Effect: Decreases LDL 10–15%, Decreases Trig 20–50%, Increases HDL 10–15%
4. **Fenofibrate (TriCor)** is the most potent fibrate available to lower Triglycerides and LDL. It is preferred over Gemfibrozil in diabetic patients with combined hyperlipidemia

E. Estrogen replacement
1. Effect: Decreases LDL 10–20%, Increases Triglycerides 0–15%, Increases HDL 10–15%
2. See Chapter 25, Menopause and Hormone Replacement Therapy

CARD

DRUGS	DOSE	SIDE EFFECTS	LABS
HMG CoA REDUCTASE INHIBITORS			
1. Lovastatin (Mevacor)	Begin with 20mg PO QHS – can increase to 40 mg BID (~$65/mo. For 20mg QD)	Mild transient GI disturbances, headache, insomnia, rash, liver dysfunction (risk is dose-related), myopathy, rhabdomyolysis and renal failure * Adverse drug interaction: risk of myopathy increases with concurrent administration of niacin or gemfibrozil. (Also erythromycin, ketoconazole or itraconazole, and cyclosporine)	LFT's @ baseline, 6, and 12 weeks after initiation and increase in dose; then semiannually thereafter
2. Pravastatin (Pravachol)	20mg QHS - may increase to 40mg QD (~$60/mo. for 20mg QD)		LFT's @ baseline and at 12 weeks after initiation or increase in dose
3. Simvastatin (Zocor)	10mg QHS - may increase to 80mg QD (~$60/mo. for 10mg QD)		LFT's @ baseline and semiannually for the first year or after elevation. Additional LFT's @ 12 weeks for 80mg dose
4. Atorvastatin (Lipitor)	10 mg QHS- may increase to 80 mg QD ($55/mo. for 10 mg QD)		LFT's @ baseline, 6, and 12 weeks after initiation and increase in dose; then semiannually thereafter
5. Fluvastatin (Lescol)	20 mg QHS – may increase to 40 mg BID ($40/mo. for 20 mg QD)		LFT's @ baseline, 6, and 12 weeks after initiation and increase in dose; then semiannually thereafter
6. Cerivastatin (Baycol)	0.3mg-0.4mg PO QHS		
NIACIN (NICOTINIC ACID)			
1. Immediate-release Niacin (generic)	100 mg TID with meals, and increase the dosage Q 3d. by 100 mg/dose over 2 weeks until a dose of 500 mg TID is reached. If therapeutic response is not reached, the dose can be increased to 3 – 6 gms/ day in divided doses. May be better tolerated if taken with meals and ASA 325mg is taken 30-60 minutes before each niacin dose (1g TID generic costs ~$7/mo.)	Gastric irritation, increased serum uric acid levels/gout, increased blood sugar (caution in diabetic patients), hepatotoxicity (dose-related, more likely to occur with sustained-release preparations), pruritus, cutaneous flushing – often the reason for d/c	LFT's @ baseline then 3-4 weeks after initiation and again 4 weeks after a dose of 3gm/day is achieved. Once dose stabilized, LFT's every 3-6 months
2. Extended-Release Niacin (Niaspan)	500 mg HS x 1 month, then 2x500 mg HS x 1 month; if needed, may increase to 2x750 mg HS up to 2x1000 mg HS. ASA 325mg is taken 30-60 minutes before each niacin dose. ($45/ 60x500 mg tab)		
BILE ACID SEQUESTRANTS			
1. Cholestyramine (Questran)	4-8g QD-BID, maximum 24 gm/ day (~$55/mo. for 8 gm/d dosage)	Unpleasant gritty taste, bloating, constipation, abdominal pain, flatulence, nausea, bloating and heartburn, decreased absorption of other drugs, including HMG CoA reductase inhibitors	None necessary * May want to check levels of other drugs whose absorption may be affected by resins or ensure these drugs are not taken at the same time as the resins
2. Colestipol (Colestid)	2 gm QD-BID. May increase dose in increment of 2 gm daily q month. Usual dose is 2-16 gm QD-BID (~$95/mo. for 10 gm/d dosage)		
FIBRIC ACID			
Gemfibrozil (Lopid, generic)	600 mg BID before meals ($15-80/mo for 600 mg BID)	GI disturbances (nausea, bloating, flatulence), cholestatic jaundice, myopathy, blurred vision Gemfibrozil potentiates the effects of oral anticoagulants	LFTs should be monitored regularly (e.g., every 2 months)
Fenofibrate (TriCor)	Start with 67 mg capsule QD, increase to 3x67 mg capsules QD if needed; OR 200 mg capsule QD ($65/mo for 67 mg)		
ESTROGEN REPLACEMENT			
Premarin	0.625mg QD	* Need to use with progesterone if pt. still has uterus	None

IX. COMBINATION THERAPY

A. Combination therapy should be considered if cholesterol goals are not met

B. HMG CoA reductase inhibitors should be taken 1hr before or at least 4hrs after the sequestrant (bile acid sequestrant decreases bioavailability of HMG CoA reductase inhibitors)

C. Caution with combination with fibrate-type drugs (Gemfibrozil) and niacin due to risk of myopathy and rhabdomyolysis

POSSIBLE COMBINATION THERAPIES IF SINGLE-AGENT THERAPY IS NOT EFFECTIVE IN REDUCING LIPID LEVELS

Lipid levels	First drug → drug to add
Elevated LDL level and triglyceride level <200 mg per dL	Statin → bile acid-binding resin Nicotinic acid* → statin* Bile acid-binding resin → nicotinic acid
Elevated LDL level and triglyceride level 200 to 400 mg per dL	Statin* → nicotinic acid*‡ Statin* → gemfibrozil (Lopid)† Nicotinic acid → bile acid-binding resin Nicotinic acid → gemfibrozil

LDL=low-density lipoprotein.
*—Possible increased risk of myopathy and hepatitis.
†—Increased risk of severe myopathy.
‡—The combination of nicotinic acid and lovastatin (Mevacor) may induce rhabdomyolysis, a rare adverse drug interaction.

Adapted from National Cholesterol Education Program. Cholesterol lowering in the patient with coronary heart disease. Bethesda, Md.: National Institutes of Health, National Heart, Lung, and Blood Institute, 1997; DHHS publication no. (NIH) 97-3794.

X. XANTHOMAS AND THEIR CLINICAL SIGNIFICANCE

A. Histology: Localized infiltrates of lipid-containing histiocytes

B. Types:

1. Tendinous xanthoma: Firm subcutaneous nodules that arise from tendons, ligaments, and fascia. Usually develop in patients with hypercholesterolemia; most common cause is familial hypercholesterolemia. Should order lipid profile if tendinous xanthoma found on exam

2. Planar xanthoma
   a. Xanthelasma is most common type: typically occur on or around the eyelids. 50% will have associated hypercholesterolemia. Incidence is greater in patients who develop xanthelasmas at age 40–50 years. May be removed with repeated application of trichloroacetic acid. Cholesterol should be followed aggressively
   b. Intertriginous planar xanthoma (web spaces of digits) is pathognomic for homozygous familial hypercholesterolemia

3. Eruptive xanthoma: Appear suddenly in crops of papules on extensor surfaces. May be inflamed and tender; develop almost exclusively in the presence of hypertriglyceridemia, often in the range of 2000mg/dL. Most common cause is uncontrolled DM or ETOH ingestion

XI. LIPOPROTEIN A

A. Specialized form of glycoprotein-LDL-cholesterol complex

B. Independent risk factor for CAD in men if elevated over 30mg/dL (300mg/L)

C. Elevated Lp(a) may be the cause of effect of coronary artery damage (unclear)

D. Reduced by **Nicotinic Acid** (given at dosages of at least 3g/day) and **Estrogen**

CLINICAL PEARLS
- Dietary changes should continue despite initiation of drug therapy
- Use cholesterol lowering drug sparingly in young adult men and premenopausal women who are without risk factors
- The prescription for isolated low HDL is exercise, weight loss and smoking cessation. No benefit exists in increasing *normal* HDL levels

References

American Diabetes Association: Management of dyslipidemia in adults with diabetes (Position Statement). Diabetes Care 23(Suppl. 1):S57–S60, 2000.

Newman TB, Garber AM. Cholesterol screening in children and adolescents. Pediatrics 2000; 105: 637–8.

Shamir R, Fisher EA. Dietary therapy for children with hypercholesterolemia. Am Fam Phys 2000; 61:675–82.

Rader DJ. Pathophysiology and management of low high-density lipoprotein cholesterol. Am J Cardiol 1999; 83(9B):22F–4F.

Corti MC, et al. Clarifying the direct relationship between total cholesterol levels and death from coronary heart disease in older patients. Ann Intern Med 1997;126:753–60.

NCEP (National Cholesterol Education Program) Second Report of the National Cholesterol Education Program Expert Panel on Detection, Evaluation, and Treatment of High Blood Cholesterol in Adults. Bethesda, MD: National Institutes of Health, National Heart, Lung, and Blood Institute. DHHS publication no. NIH 93–3095.

Web site for NCEP second report—updates: http://pharminfo.com/disease/cardio/atpsum.html

National Cholesterol Education Program. Cholesterol lowering in the patient with coronary heart disease. Bethesda, MD: National Institutes of Health, National Heart, Lung, and Blood Institute, 1997; DHHS publication no. (NIH) 97–3794.

Second report of the expert panel on detection, evaluation, and treatment of high blood cholesterol in adults, Executive summary, National institutes of health publication No. 93–3096, Sep 1993 — Updated Aug 1996.

Scandinavian Simvastatin Survival Study Group. Randomised trial of cholesterol lowering in 4444 patients with coronary heart disease: the Scandinavian Simvastatin Survival Study (4S). Lancet 1994; 344:1383–9.

Vinson RP, Harrington, AC. Clinical significance and treatment of xanthomas. Am Fam Phys 1991;44(4):1130.

Daniel M. Neides, MD
Kathy Provanzana, MD

38. HYPERTENSION

I. DEFINITION

    A. Adults: Blood pressure (BP) > 140/90

    B. Children: Guidelines are by age

AGE/YEARS	BLOOD PRESSURE
3–5	116/76
6–9	122/78
10–12	126/82
13–15	136/86

    C. The diagnosis of HTN should not be made by an isolated elevated BP

        1. To diagnose HTN, check BP every 2 weeks for 2 months

        2. If the BP is consistently elevated, the diagnosis is confirmed and treatment should be initiated

II. CLASSIFICATION BY DEGREE

CLASSIFICATION OF BLOOD PRESSURE FOR ADULTS AGED 18 YEARS AND OLDER*

	Blood Pressure, mm Hg		
Category	Systolic		Diastolic
Optimal†	< 120	and	< 80
Normal	< 130	and	< 85
High-normal	130–139	or	85–89
Hypertension‡			
Stage 1	140–159	or	90–99
Stage 2	160–179	or	100–109
Stage 3	≥ 180	or	N≥ 110

* Not taking antihypertensive drugs and not acutely ill. When systolic and diastolic blood pressures fall into different categories, the higher category should be selected to classify the individual's blood pressure status. For example, 160/92 mm Hg should be classified as stage 2 hypertension, and 174/120 mm Hg should be classified as stage 3 hypertension. Isolated systolic hypertension is defined as systolic blood pressure 140 mm Hg or greater and diastolic blood pressure less than 90 mm Hg and staged appropriately (e.g., 170/82 mm Hg is defined as stage 2 isolated systolic hypertension). In addition to classifying stages of hypertension on the basis of average blood pressure levels, clinicians should specify presence or absence of target organ disease and additional risk factors. This specificity is important for risk classification and treatment (see later, IV. D. Risk Stratification and Treatment).
† Optimal blood pressure with respect to cardiovascular risk is less than 120/80 mm Hg. However, unusually low readings should be evaluated for clinical significance.
‡ Based on the average of 2 or more readings taken at each of 2 or more visits after an initial screening.

Source: The Sixth Report of the Joint National Committee on Prevention, Detection, Evaluation and Treatment of High Blood Pressure (JNC-VI). Arch Internal Med 1997;157:2413–46.

RECOMMENDATIONS FOR FOLLOW-UP BASED ON INITIAL BLOOD PRESSURE MEASUREMENTS FOR ADULTS

Initial Blood Pressure, mm Hg*		Follow-up Recommended†
Systolic	Diastolic	
< 130	< 85	Recheck in 2 y
130–139	85–89	Recheck in 1 y‡
140–159	90–99	Confirm within 2 mo‡
160–179	100–109	Evaluate or refer to source of care within 1 mo
≥ 180	≥ 110	Evaluate or refer to source of care immediately or within 1 wk depending on clinical situation

* If systolic and diastolic categories are different, follow recommendations for shorter follow-up (eg, 160/86 mm Hg should be evaluated or referred to source of care within 1 month).
† Modify the scheduling of follow-up according to reliable information about past blood pressure measurements, other cardiovascular risk factors, or target organ disease.
‡ Provide advice about lifestyle modifications.

Source: The Sixth Report of the Joint National Committee on Prevention, Detection, Evaluation and Treatment of High Blood Pressure (JNC-VI). Arch Internal Med 1997;157:2413–46.

SIGNIFICANCE OF BORDERLINE ISOLATED SYSTOLIC HYPERTENSION*

Cardiovascular morbidity and mortality	Incidence in patients with normal baseline blood pressure (N = 2,416) †	Incidence in patients with borderline isolated systolic hypertension at baseline (N = 351) †
All cardiovascular disease, including coronary heart disease	57%	89%
Congestive heart failure	7%	16%
Stroke or transient ischemic attack	9%	16%
Cardiovascular disease mortality	13%	29%
All-cause mortality	38%	59%

Defined as 140–159/<90 mm Hg
† *In patients with normal blood pressure at baseline and patients with borderline isolated systolic hypertension at baseline, 45% and 80%, respectively, progressed to definite hypertension (>160/>90 mm Hg) at 20-year follow-up.*

Source: Adapted from Sagie A, Larson MG, Levy D. The natural history of borderline isolated systolic hypertension. N Engl J Med 1993;329:1912–7. Used with permission.

III. EVALUATION OF PRIMARY AND SECONDARY HYPERTENSION

A. Primary (essential) hypertension: *95%* of hypertensive adults will have no identifiable cause of their HTN after history, physical and labs as indicated below

   1. **History:**
      a. Medication use including OTC medications (decongestants), oral contraceptives and estrogen use
      b. Alcohol and drugs (cocaine, crack, "speed"), caffeine, smoking
      c. Lifestyle (sedentary), exercise, stress, weight
      d. Family history (HTN, stroke, nephropathy, heart disease)
      e. Inquire about current symptoms indicating cardiovascular or peripheral vascular disease, retinopathy, nephropathy or cerebrovascular accident, diabetes, dyslipidemia
      f. Psychosocial and environmental factors which may affect compliance, ability to afford medications, educational level

   2. **Physical examination:** Initial exam includes checking blood pressure in both extremities (coarctation), distal pulses, carotid bruits, retinal exam, cardiovascular exam, signs of heart failure (peripheral edema, JVD, S_3, etc.), thyroid enlargement, lungs (for signs of bronchospasm, rales), abdominal bruits (renal artery stenosis)

   3. **Laboratory tests**
      a. Routine tests: UA, CBC, chemistry (potassium, sodium, creatinine, fasting glucose, total cholesterol, HDL cholesterol), ECG
      b. Optional: Creatinine clearance, microalbuminuria, 24hr urinary protein, blood calcium, uric acid, fasting triglycerides, LDL, glycosolated hemoglobin, TSH, echocardiography

B. Secondary hypertension: The following causes of hypertension account for 5% of the hypertensive population

   1. Consider evaluation for secondary hypertension when:
      a. Patients whose age, history or physical exam, severity of hypertension or initial lab findings suggest a secondary cause. Examples:
         i. Abdominal bruits: Renal artery stenosis (RAS)
         ii. Paroxysms of HTN accompanied by headache, palpitations, perspiration: Pheochromocytoma
         iii. Abdominal or flank masses: Polycystic kidneys
         iv. Delayed or absent femoral pulses: Coarctation of the aorta
         v. Truncal obesity with abdominal striae: Cushings
         vi. Unprovoked hypokalemia: Primary aldosteronism

      vii. Hypercalcemia: Hyperparathyroidism
      viii. Elevated creatinine: Renal parenchymal disease
   b. Poor response to conventional anti-HTN medications after an adequate trial
   c. HTN has suddenly worsened (well controlled hypertension has begun to increase)
   d. Patients with stage 3 HTN
   e. Patients have renal failure after administration of ACE inhibitors/Angiotensin II receptor antagonists
2. In addition to the causes of secondary HTN listed below, evaluate patient for the following causes: oral contraceptives (estrogen), HTN associated with pregnancy, hyper-/hypothyroidism, hyperparathyroidism, hypercalcemia, acromegaly, cocaine or amphetamine use, use of NSAIDs (may blunt action of diuretics, ß-blockers and ACE inhibitors)
3. The following are guidelines for evaluation when secondary HTN is suspected:

DIAGNOSIS	Initial Evaluation	Additional Evaluation
1. Chronic renal failure	Urinalysis, BUN, captopril renography, ultrasound	Renin assay, renal biopsy, IVP
2. Renal artery stenosis	Bruit, captopril renography	Aortogram
3. Coarctation	BP in legs	Aortogram
4. Primary hyperaldosteronism (Conn's syndrome)	Plasma potassium (< 3.5 mEq/L)	Urinary potassium, increased plasma renin, plasma or urinary aldosterone
5. Cushing's Disease	A.M. plasma cortisol after 1mg dexamethasone at bedtime	Urinary cortisol after variable doses of dexamethasone
6. Pheochromocytoma	Spot urine for metanephrine	Urinary metanephrine and catechols; plasma catechols

Source: Adapted from Kaplan NM. Management of hypertension. 4th ed. Durant, OK: EMIS, 1992;22. Used with permission.

C. White coat hypertension
   1. Occurs in up to 20% of patients
   2. In general, *office blood pressure readings* should be used to estimate risk, management, and response to therapy
   3. How to account for "white coat hypertension" is controversial. Studies which show a (cardiovascular, etc.) risk reduction with a lowering of blood pressure used clinic or office blood pressure readings
   4. Consider use of a home blood pressure machine
D. Possible indications for ambulatory blood pressure monitoring
   1. Suspected white coat HTN
   2. Apparent drug resistance
   3. Hypotensive symptoms with medications
   4. Episodic HTN
   5. Autonomic dysfunction

IV. THERAPY

A. Nonpharmacologic treatment of HTN: Weight reduction, quitting smoking, decreasing caffeine, limiting alcohol consumption (2 drinks/day), exercise, behavioral modification (stress management, biofeedback, etc.), stopping medications that increase BP (e.g., OTC decongestants), nutritional guidelines (4g Na^+ diet)
B. Factors influencing initiation of treatment (other than diastolic or systolic blood pressures)
   1. Treatment should be considered sooner in men and postmenopausal women
   2. The presence of cardiovascular disease (left ventricular hypertrophy, ischemic heart disease, aortic aneurysm, or history of cerebrovascular disease) should encourage treatment
   3. Elevated serum creatinine and proteinuria
   4. Presence of diabetes mellitus
   5. The presence of other cardiovascular risk factors: smoking or hyperlipidemia
   6. Family history of HTN, premature stroke, heart disease, or sudden cardiac death

C. The step-care approach
1. The physician starts with 1 drug, titrates up to the maximum tolerated dose, and adds a second, third, or even fourth agent until an adequate response is obtained
2. Initial therapy should be individualized (See table below). A diuretic or ß-blocker should be used as initial therapy unless there are specific reasons for another drug (ACE inhibitor with CHF, etc.) These drugs are preferred for initial therapy because of cost and because they are the only anti-HTN medications that have been proven (at this time) to reduce morbidity and mortality
3. If a patient has a poor response to an initial agent, one could change to another class of antihypertensives before simply adding a second agent (i.e., not all black patients will respond to diuretics and not all elderly patients will respond to ACE inhibitors)

D. Risk stratification and treatment

RISK STRATIFICATION AND TREATMENT*			
Blood Pressure Stages (mm Hg)	**Risk Group A (No Risk Factors; NoTOD/CCD†)**	**Risk Group B (At Least 1 Risk Factor, Not Including Diabetes, NoTOD/CCD)**	**Risk Group C (TOD/CCD and/or Diabetes, With or Without Other Risk Factors)**
High-normal (130–139/85–89)	Lifestyle modification	Lifestyle modification	Drug Therapy§
Stage 1 (140–159/90–99)	Lifestyle modification (up to 12 mo.)	Lifestyle modification‡ (up to 6 mo.)	Drug Therapy
Stages 2 and 3 (≥160/≥100)	Drug therapy	Drug therapy	Drug therapy

*Note: For example, a patient with diabetes and a blood pressure of 142/94 mm Hg plus left ventricular hypertrophy should be classified as having stage 1 hypertension with target organ disease (left ventricular hypertrophy) and with another major risk factor (diabetes). This patient would be categorized as "Stage 1, Risk Group C," and recommended for immediate initiation of pharmacologic treatment. Lifestyle modification should be adjunctive therapy for all patients recommended for pharmacologic therapy.
† TOD/CCD indicates target organ disease/clinical cardiovascular disease
‡ For patients with multiple risk factors, clinicians should consider drugs as initial therapy plus lifestyle modifications.
§ For those with heart failure, renal insufficiency, or diabetes.

Source: The Sixth Report of the Joint National Committee on Prevention, Detection, Evaluation and Treatment of High Blood Pressure (JNC-VI). Arch Internal Med 1997;157:2413–46.

E. Pharmacologic treatment of HTN: The 6th Joint National Committee on Detection, Evaluation and Treatment of high blood pressure (JNC VI) recommends diuretics or ß-blockers as the preferred initial therapy based on the fact that these 2 classes of medications have been shown to reduce mortality and morbidity. Of the following 2 tables, the first makes recommendations on individualizing therapy based on the patient and the second lists side effects and precautions

CARD

Patient Characteristics	Preferred Antihypertensives	Drugs to avoid
Age < 50	α-blocker, β-blocker, ACE	Diuretic
Age > 65	Thiazide, Ca^{+2} channel blocker, ACE	Central α-agonist
African Americans	Monotherapy with diuretics or Ca^{+2} channel blocker	
White race	ACE, β-blocker	
Physically active	α-blocker, ACE, Ca^{+2} channel blocker	β-blocker
Coronary artery disease	β-blocker, Ca^{+2} channel blocker	Direct vasodilator
Asthma/COPD	α-blocker, Ca^{+2} channel blocker, Clonidine	ACE
CHF	ACE, hydralazine and isosorbide dinitrate, carvedilol	Ca^{+2} channel blocker
Migraine	β-blocker, Ca^{+2} channel blocker	Vasodilators
Bradycardia, sick sinus		β-blocker, Diltiazem, Verapamil
Cerebrovascular disease	ACE, Ca^{+2} channel blocker	Central α-agonist
Hyperlipidemia	α-blocker, ACE, Ca^{+2} channel blocker	Diuretic, β-blocker
Depression	α-blocker, ACE, Ca^{+2} channel blocker	Reserpine, β-blocker
Peripheral vascular disease	ACE, Ca^{+2} channel blocker, α-blocker	β-blocker
Renal insufficiency	Loop diuretic, ACE, Ca^{+2} channel blocker	Thiazide, diuretic, K$^+$ sparing agents
Diabetes mellitus	ACE, α-blocker, Ca^{+2} antagonists, diuretics (low doses)	Caution with β-blocker
Gout	α-blocker, ACE, Ca^{+2} channel blocker	Diuretic, β-blocker
Osteoporosis	thiazides	Loop diuretic
Chronic liver disease	Diuretic, α-blocker, Clonidine	β-blocker, Methyldopa
Glaucoma	β-blocker, Clonidine, diuretic	
Impotence	α-blocker, ACE, Ca^{+2} channel blocker	β-blocker, diuretic
Obesity	α-blocker, ACE, Ca^{+2} channel blocker	β-blocker, diuretic
Pregnancy	Methyldopa, Hydralazine	β-blocker, diuretic, Reserpine, ACE
Benign prostatic hypertrophy	α-blocker	

Source: Adapted from Kaplan NM. Management of hypertension. 4th ed. Durant, OK: EMIS, 1992;121–2. Used with permission.

Drugs	Side effects	Precautions
Thiazide diuretics	Hypokalemia, hyperuricemia, glucose intolerance, dyslipidemia	May not help in renal failure; hypokalemia will increase digoxin toxicity
Loop diuretics	Same as for thiazides	Hyponatremia
K$^+$-sparing diuretics	Hyperkalemia, gynecomastia, renal calculi	Monitor K$^+$ closely in patients with renal failure
ACE inhibitors	Cough, rash, hyperkalemia, hypotension, angiodema	Captopril renography for evidence of renal failure; neutropenia may occur in pts. with auto-immune diseases
Ca^{+2} channel blockers	Headache, constipation, flushing, dizzy, lower extremity edema	Caution in pts. with CHF or heart block. Avoid short-acting dihydropyridines. Immediate release nifedipine should only be used with great caution, if at all
β-blockers	Bradycardia, fatigue, insomnia, bizarre dreams, hypertriglyceridemia, lower HDL cholesterol, depression	Avoid in pts. with asthma, COPD, heart block, and sick sinus syndrome; use cautiously in pts. with DM (may mask symptoms of hypoglycemia)
Combined α / β blocker (Labetalol)	Asthma, nausea, fatigue, dizziness	Same as for β-blockers
Vasodilators (Hydralazine, Minoxidil)	Headache, tachycardia, fluid retention, hypertrichosis	**Hydralazine** may cause Lupus-like syndrome; **Minoxidil** may cause pleural/pericardial effusions
Peripheral-acting Adrenergic Inhibitors (Guanethidine, Reserpine)	Orthostatic hypotension, diarrhea, depression	Use cautiously in elderly; Reserpine is contra-indicated in pts. with depression and should be used cautiously if pt. has history of peptic ulcer disease
Central-acting Adrenergic Inhibitors (Clonidine, Guanfacine, Methyldopa)	Drowsiness, dry mouth, fatigue	May see rebound HTN after abrupt discontinuance; Methyldopa may cause liver damage, a direct + Coombs test, autoimmune disorders
α$_1$-adrenergic blocker (Terazosin, Doxazosin, Prazosin)	Orthostatic hypotension, weakness and palpitations	1st dose syncope
Angiotensin II receptor antagonists	Dizziness, insomnia, muscle cramps, GI upset, upper respiratory effects	Hypovolemia, severe CHF, renal artery stenosis, hepatic impairment. Should be used primarily in pts. in whom ACE inhibitors are indicated, but who are unable to tolerate them (ex. cough)

Source: Adapted from Kaplan NM. Management of hypertension. 4th ed. Durant, OK: EMIS, 1992;136–9. Used with permission.

F. Special groups
1. Elderly: See table "Significance of borderline isolated systolic hypertension" at beginning of chapter
   a. Treatment of isolated systolic HTN should be a priority. In the elderly, SBP more closely correlates with morbidity and mortality than DBP
   b. Consider evaluation for secondary causes, especially with new onset of HTN in patients greater than 60 years of age
   c. Goal of therapy should be BP <140/90, but an interim goal of SBP of 160 is acceptable in patients with marked systolic HTN
2. African Americans
   a. Higher incidence of HTN related complications than the general population: 80% higher stroke mortality rate, 50% higher heart disease mortality rate, 320% higher risk of HTN-related ESRD
   b. Lifestyle modifications are particularly important
   c. Monotherapy with diuretics or calcium channel blockers is the preferred initial treatment, but addition of a ß-blocker or ACE to a diuretic may markedly improve response
   d. Many require multidrug therapy
3. Renal failure
   a. In patients with proteinuria greater than 1g/24hrs, BP should be controlled to at least 130/85, and preferable 125/75
   b. Thiazide diuretics are not generally effective with advanced RF (creatinine > 2.5)
   c. Erythropoietin may increase blood pressure 18–45%
4. Left ventricular hypertrophy: Medications shown to decrease mortality: ACE, combination of Hydralazine and Isosorbide Dinitrate, Spironolactone, and ß-blockers
5. Diabetes mellitus
   a. Because of the possibility of autonomic dysfunction, evaluate BP with patients sitting, supine and standing
   b. Ambulatory monitoring may be useful
   c. Goal is BP < 135/85 or 120/70 if microalbuminuria is present
   d. Preferred agents: ACE, α–blockers, calcium antagonists, diuretics (low doses)
6. Women on oral contraceptives: Stop the OC if HTN develops
7. Women on estrogen replacement therapy: Not significantly affected

CLINICAL PEARLS
- Consider immediate therapy in a patient who presents with an initial BP in the moderate-to-severe range (i.e., do *not* wait 2 months to start treatment)
- When drug therapy is started or when any medication change is made, follow-up BP check should be in 4–6 weeks. Once BP is normalized, follow-up can be Q4–6 months
- HTN is "the silent killer" and the goal of treatment is prevention of cardiovascular disease, stroke, nephropathy, and retinopathy
- Compliance is a major factor in treating HTN. Therapy should be individualized
- Patients started on ACE inhibitors should have BP checked in 1 week and serum creatinine checked in 1 month
- Patients with hypertension and *unexplained* hypokalemia (K<3.5) have 50% incidence of primary hyperaldosteronism (Conn's syndrome). Approximately 0.5% of HTN is caused by Conn's syndrome
- When poorly controlled on 2 agents, consider adding a diuretic to the regimen
- Short acting calcium channel blockers should probably not be used in the management of hypertension
- Hypertension affects approximately 50 million adult Americans. 75% aren't controlling BP to below 140/90

References
Guidelines Sub-Committee. 1999 World Health Organization-International Society of Hypertension Guidelines for the management of hypertension. J Hypertens 1999;17(2):151–83.
Moser M. Hypertension treatment & the prevention of coronary heart disease in the elderly. Am Fam Phys 1999;59:1248–56.
Forette F, et al. Prevention of dementia in randomized double-blind placebo-controlled systolic

CARD

hypertension in Europe (Syst-Eur) trial. Lancet 1998;3352:1347.

Muscholl MW, et al. Changes in left ventricular structure and function in patients with white coat hypertension: cross sectional survey. BMJ August 29, 1998;317:565–70.

Whelton PK, et al. Sodium reduction and weight loss in the treatment of hypertension in older persons. A randomized controlled trial of nonpharmacologic interventions in the elderly (TONE). JAMA 1998;279:839–46.

The Sixth Report of the Joint National Committee on Prevention, Detection, Evaluation and Treatment of High Blood Pressure (JNC-VI). Arch Internal Med 1997;157:2413–46.

Psaty BM, et al. Health outcomes associated with antihypertensive therapies used as first-line agents. JAMA 1997;277:739–45.

The Systolic Hypertension in the Elderly Program Cooperative Research Group. Implications of the systolic hypertension in the elderly program. Hypertension 1993;21:335–43.

Michael B. Weinstock, MD
Joe DeRosa, MD
Beth Weinstock, MD
Mrunal Shah, MD

39. CORONARY ARTERY DISEASE

I. RISK FACTORS
A. Absolute
1. Family History (1st degree relative female <65 or male <55)
2. Smoking
3. Diabetes
4. Hypertension
5. Hyperlipidemia (LDL>130, HDL<35)
6. Male
7. Age (male>45, female >55)

B. Relative
1. Obesity
2. Sedentary lifestyle
3. Stress
4. Postmenopausal state

II. ETIOLOGY:
Clinical manifestations are usually caused by fissuring, hemorrhage rupture, and thrombosis of plaque in the epicardial coronary arteries. Plaque is comprised of subintimal collections of abnormal fat, cells, and debris

III. CLINICAL PRESENTATION
A. When ischemic cardiac events are transient, the patient may experience angina pectoris; if prolonged, this can lead to myocardial necrosis and scarring with or without the clinical picture of MI

B. Patients can also present with cardiomegaly and heart failure secondary to ischemic damage of left ventricle; may have caused no symptoms prior to the development of congestive heart failure

IV. HISTORY
A. Description of pain: Character (squeezing vs. stabbing), location, radiation, onset, duration, exacerbating and relieving factors. Ask the patient if they have chest, arm, neck, jaw, or abdominal *discomfort* rather than asking if they have "chest pain"

B. Associated symptoms: Dyspnea, diaphoresis, dizziness, syncope, palpitations, nausea with or without vomiting, pain associated with motion or deep breathing (pleuritic), change in pain with change in position (pericarditis is worse when supine and relieved when sitting forward), peripheral edema, orthopnea, paroxysmal nocturnal dyspnea

C. Risk factors (as above)

D. History of heart disease: CAD/MI, arrhythmia, valvular disease, previous heart catheterization

or stress test, PTCA or CABG. Obtain old EKGs
E. Medications

V. PHYSICAL EXAM
A. **Vital signs:** Blood pressure, heart rate and rhythm, respiratory rate
B. **HEENT:** Hypertensive or diabetic retinopathy, JVD, carotid bruit, thyromegaly
C. **Lungs:** Rales, pleural effusions
D. **Cardiovascular:** Arrhythmia, murmur (MR from papillary muscle dysfunction), rub (pericarditis), gallop (CHF), click (MVP), abnormal apical impulse, third or fourth heart sound
E. **Chest:** Palpation of anterior chest wall (costochondritis)
F. **Abdomen:** Hepatomegaly (CHF, hepatojugular reflux)
G. **Extremities:** Cyanosis, clubbing, edema, shiny hairless legs (PVD)
H. **Skin:** Xanthomas, diabetic skin changes

VI. LABORATORY
A. Lipid profiles: See Chapter 37, Hyperlipidemia
B. CPK peaks at 6–8hrs and then falls within 24hrs
C. Troponin level (most specific; peaks in 2–4hrs and falls in 10–14 days)
Note: For a patient whose ambulatory presentation suggests acute MI, the cardiac enzymes should be ordered in an acute care setting (ED or monitored hospital bed)

VII. CHEST X-RAY:
Check for cardiomegaly, pulmonary edema, pleural effusions, pneumothorax, rib fracture, pulmonary embolus, widened mediastinum (aortic aneurysm or dissection), or infectious etiology of chest discomfort

VIII. EKG
A. A normal EKG does not exclude the diagnosis of CAD; 12-lead EKG recorded at rest is normal in approximately half of patients with angina pectoris
B. With angina, ST segments are usually depressed, but may be elevated in early stages of acute MI and in Prinzmetal's angina
C. T-wave and ST segment changes are nonspecific and may occur in pericardial, valvular, and myocardial disease, or with anxiety, changes in posture, medications, or esophageal disease

IX. DIAGNOSIS
The office diagnosis of angina/CAD is a *clinical diagnosis*, based primarily on the history, physical and ECG. When a cardiac source of pain is suspected, several questions must be answered:
A. **Is the patient currently having symptoms which could be cardiac ischemia?** If so, it is suggestive of acute MI and the patient should be evaluated in an emergency department
B. **Does the patient have unstable angina?** This is defined as angina which is new, occurring at rest, or increasing in intensity, frequency and duration. If so, they may need to be admitted for evaluation. If they are not admitted, a definitive diagnosis should be established and/or definitive therapy should be started
C. **Should medication be started while awaiting a definitive diagnosis?** If stable angina/CAD is suspected, begin aspirin while awaiting a definitive diagnosis. Other medications (ß-blocker, nitrates, etc.) may be started based on the history and physical findings or for associated conditions (HTN, CHF, diabetes, etc.)
D. **What test should be done to make a definitive diagnosis?** There are 2 categories of definitive testing for CAD (See Chapter 43, Cardiac Stress Testing):
1. Stress testing
2. Cardiac catheterization
   Considerations:
   a. If a positive test on an asymptomatic patient will be dismissed as a false positive, do not perform the test
   b. If angina is suspected and a patient with a negative stress test will get a cardiac catheterization anyway, consider proceeding directly to catheterization
   c. Unstable angina is a contraindication to maximal stress testing

X. MEDICAL MANAGEMENT

A. Correction of reversible risk factors (smoking, hypertension, uncontrolled diabetes, obesity, sedentary lifestyle, stress)

CORRECTION OF REVERSIBLE RISK FACTORS		
Intervention	*Cardiovascular event reduction (%)*	*Total mortality reduction (%)*
Smoking cessation	—	43
Lipid lowering	42	30
Exercise	25	20
Blood pressure control	21	12

B. Modification of activity: Reduce energy requirements in AM hours and immediately after meals. Stress management classes may be beneficial

C. Correction of hyperlipidemia: (See Chapter 37, Hyperlipidemia)
1. Primary goal to LDL < 100
2. Secondary goal of HDL > 45 and TG < 200
3. Need to be aggressive in post-menopausal females to reduce cholesterol. In women with hyperlipidemia, lipid lowering agents should be used as first line therapy instead of (or in addition to) HRT
4. Hold oral contraceptives (or get baseline fasting lipid profile) in women > age 35 who smoke

D. Anti-platelet medications
1. **ASA:** 81-325mg PO QD
2. **Clopidogrel (Plavix):** 75mg PO QD. Should be used in those who failed ASA or cannot tolerate ASA

E. ß-Blockers: Proven to prolong survival post-MI. They are believed to promote left ventricular remodeling and decrease myocardial oxygen demand in the post-MI heart. Some ß-blockers also have intrinsic antiarrhythmic properties and may decrease the incidence of ventricular fibrillation. Carvedilol with the same rate of side effects as Metoprolol found to have increased benefit long-term (from vasodilatory and antioxidative effects) with decreased morbidity and mortality. Avoid ß-blocker with intrinsic sympathomimetic activity like Acebutolol and Pindolol
1. **Metoprolol (Lopressor):** 25-50mg PO BID
2. **Atenolol (Tenormin):** 50mg PO BID or 100mg PO QD
3. **Timolol (Blocadren):** 10mg PO BID
4. **Carvedilol:** 3.125mg PO BID, increase gradually to 25-50mg BID
5. **Propranolol (Inderal):** 60-80mg PO TID

F. Nitrates: These have been shown to decrease symptoms of angina, but they do not decrease mortality. May be used in patients with contraindications to ß-blockers, patients who have failed ß-blockers, or who are intolerant to ß-blockers or used in conjunction with ß-blockers
1. Short acting: **Nitroglycerin spray** (0.4mg) or SL **NTG** 1/150 grain (0.4mg), 1/100 grain (0.6mg), or 1/200 grain (0.3mg)—1 SL Q5 minutes × 3 PRN angina. Should be taken 5 minutes before any activity likely to precipitate angina. If pain persists after 3 doses, patient should be evaluated in ED to rule out MI. Patients who require more doses of nitrates or who are not responding as well as they had previously should be re-evaluated
2. Long acting
   a. **Transdermal NTG** 0.1, 0.2, 0.4, 0.6mg/hr—should be removed for 10-12hrs per day
   b. **Isosorbide Dinitrate (Isordil):** 20-80mg PO TID
   c. **Isosorbide Mononitrate**
      i. **Imdur:** 60mg PO QD
      ii. **Ismo:** 20mg PO BID 7hrs apart
3. NTG deteriorates with exposure to air, moisture, and sunlight. If sublingual administration does not cause a slight burning/tingling, the NTG may be inactive

G. Calcium channel blockers: May be used in patients with contraindications to ß-blockers, patients who have failed ß-blockers, or who are intolerant to ß-blockers or used in conjunction with ß-blockers. Should not be the initial anti-anginal medication in most patients. Use with caution in patients with pulmonary congestion or left ventricular dysfunction/decreased ejection fraction, The short acting calcium channel blockers which were found to *increase* the risk of reinfarction in 1 study and should be avoided

1. **Amlodipine (Norvasc):** 5mg PO QD initially, may increase to 10mg QD
2. **Nicardipine (Cardene):** 20mg PO TID initially, may increase to 120mg in 3 divided **doses**
3. **Nifedipine (Adalat CC):** 10mg PO QD, maximum 90mg QD; **(Procardia XL):** 30–60mg PO QD, maximum 90mg QD
4. **Diltiazem (Cardizem):** 30mg PO QID initially, may increase to 360mg QD in 4 divided doses; **(Cardizem SR):** 60–120mg BID; **(Cardizem CD):** 120–300mg QD; **(Dilacor XR):** initially 180–240mg PO QD, maximum 480mg QD
5. **Verapamil (Calan):** 80–120mg PO TID, maximum 480mg QD, elderly or small patients 40mg TID; **(Isoptin):** 80–120mg PO TID, maximum 360mg QD, elderly or hepatic impairment 40mg TID; **(Calan SR):** initially 180mg PO QAM, maximum 480mg QD, elderly or small patients 40mg TID; **(Isoptin SR):** initially 120–180mg PO QAM, maximum 240mg Q12hrs
   - These 5 calcium channel blockers are listed in order of increasing negative inotropic effect (Verapamil is the most, with the greatest chance of heart block)
   - **Short-acting Nifedipine** is the most likely to cause reflex tachycardia and has potential to enhance the risk of adverse cardiac events; therefore it should be avoided

H. Combination therapy: Medications may be additive in effect. Exercise caution in giving a ß-blocker and negative inotropic calcium channel blocker as this has a greater chance of leading to heart block. A particularly potent combination may be a ß-blocker and a calcium channel blocker with a small amount of negative inotropic effect

I. Stress testing: Since the incidence of restenosis after PTCA is minimal after 6 months, some physicians perform the initial post-PTCA stress test at 6 months

XI. INDICATIONS FOR REVASCULARIZATION PROCEDURES (PTCA, CABG)

A. Failed medical therapy (intolerable symptoms despite maximal medical therapy)
B. Left main coronary artery stenosis >50% (with or without symptoms)
C. Triple vessel disease and LV dysfunction (EF <50% or previous MI)
D. Unstable angina symptomatic on stress testing despite maximal medical therapy
E. Post-MI patient continuing to have angina or ischemia
F. Relative indications include patients with anatomically critical lesions (>90%), especially in the LAD, or physiologic evidence of severe ischemia by stress testing or ambulatory monitoring

CLINICAL PEARLS

- Most patients who die suddenly from ischemic heart disease do so as a result of ischemia-induced malignant ventricular tachycardia
- In variant (Prinzmetal's) angina, the chest discomfort characteristically occurs at rest or awakens the patient from sleep. This condition is caused by focal spasm of proximal coronary arteries
- PTCA is more effective than medical therapy for the relief of angina in patients with single-vessel coronary artery disease
- Cholesterol (LDL and TG) are falsely lowered after an acute MI

References
Eikelboom JW, et al. Homocyst(e)ine and cardiovascular disease: a critical review of the epidemiologic evidence. Ann Intern Med 1999;131:363–75.
Ross R. Atherosclerosis—An Inflammatory Disease. N Engl J Med 1999; 340:115–26.
Van der Does R, et al. Comparison of safety and efficacy of carvedilol and metoprolol in stable angina pectoris. Am J Cardiol March 1, 1999;83:643–9.
1999 ACC and AHA update guidelines for coronary angiography and angina available at: http://www.acc.org and at: http://www.americanheart.org).
Parker JD, Parker JO. Nitrate therapy for stable angina pectoris. N Engl J Med 1998;338:520–31.
Smith SC. The challenge of risk reduction therapy for cardiovascular disease. Am Fam Phys 1997;55:491–8.
Clinical practice guideline, unstable angina: diagnosis and management (AHCPR Pub. No. 94–0602) 1994.
Yusuf S, et al. Coronary artery bypass graft surgery and survival rates. Lancet. 1994;344:563.

CARD

Michael B. Weinstock, MD
Joe DeRosa, MD
Melissa Harris, MD

40. AMBULATORY MANAGEMENT OF HEART FAILURE

I. DEFINITION
Dysfunction of the myocardium resulting in decreased cardiac output. The myocardial dysfunction may be systolic (dilated, eccentrically hypertrophied ventricle, EF<45%), or diastolic (thick-walled, concentrically hypertrophied ventricle with normal or small cavity, EF>50%)

II. ETIOLOGY
Disease progression may often be slowed or reversed by appropriate management
A. Ischemic
B. Hypertensive
C. Valvular dysfunction
D. Alcoholic
E. Diabetes
F. Myocarditis
G. Drug induced
H. Hypo-/hyperthyroid
I. Pulmonary hypertension
J. Familial
K. Other: Infiltrative disease (sarcoidosis, hemochromatosis, amyloidosis), TB

III. HISTORY
A. Dyspnea with or without exertion, orthopnea, paroxysmal nocturnal dyspnea (PND), chronic non-productive cough, peripheral edema, nocturia, fatigue, RUQ abdominal pain (liver congestion with right heart failure)
B. Weight gain, medication compliance, diet (including salt), history of HTN, chest discomfort, change in exercise tolerance, diabetic symptoms
C. Assess risk factors for CAD

IV. PHYSICAL EXAM
A. Vitals: Tachypnea, tachycardia, hypotension
B. Neck: Jugular venous distention
C. Pulmonary: Rales (may be difficult to hear in patients with COPD because of decreased lung parenchyma), decreased breath sounds secondary to pleural effusions
D. CV: Murmurs, gallop rhythm, parasternal lift (RVH secondary pulmonary HTN), displaced left ventricular impulse (LV dilation/hypertrophy)
E. Extremities: Dependent pitting edema (pretibial/sacral)
F. GI: Hepatojugular reflux

V. LAB AND OTHER TESTING
A. **Laboratory:** CBC, electrolytes (monitor potassium if patient is on diuretics), TSH, Digoxin level
B. **Chest x-ray:** Cardiomegaly, "fluffy" peri-hilar infiltrates (pulmonary edema), pleural effusion (bilateral or right sided), pulmonary venous congestion
C. **ECG:** Check for evidence of old MI, arrhythmia, bundle branch block (BBB), left ventricular hypertrophy (LVH), Digoxin effects
D. **ECHO:** Suggested for patients with a new diagnosis of CHF to differentiate systolic from diastolic dysfunction, evaluate valvular function, and to check for pulmonary hypertension. ECHO will reveal wall motion abnormalities, old MI, ventricular and atrial hypertrophy or dilation, valvular dysfunction, shunts and pericardial effusion
E. **Cardiac catheterization**: Helpful when valvular disease must be excluded and when determining presence and extent of CAD

VI. NEW YORK HEART ASSOCIATION (NYHA) CLASSIFICATION OF CARDIAC LIMITATION

Class I: No limitation of physical activity. Ordinary physical activity does not cause undue fatigue, dyspnea, or anginal pain

Class II: Slight limitation of physical activity. Ordinary physical activity results in symptoms

Class III: Marked limitation of physical activity. Comfortable at rest, but less than ordinary activity causes symptoms

Class IV: Unable to engage in any physical activity without discomfort. Symptoms may be present even at rest

VII. MANAGEMENT OF HEART FAILURE WITH SYSTOLIC DYSFUNCTION—See Chart
below, Approach to the Patient with Heart Failure

A. Correct reversible causes
1. Prevent new cardiac injury
   a. Smoking cessation
   b. Weight reduction
   c. Control of HTN, hyperlipidemia and DM
   d. Control of alcohol abuse
2. Control of selected cardiac problems: Rate control of atrial fibrillation or SVTs, anticoagulation of atrial fibrillation (if indicated), coronary revascularization or PTCA (if indication)
3. Close follow up to detect early evidence of deterioration
4. Consider influenza and pneumococcal vaccines

B. Diet and activity: Sodium restriction to 3g per day. Fluid restriction should include fluid with meals. Activity should include a regular exercise program such as walking 20–30 minutes a day 4–5 × per week as tolerated. Patients in exacerbations of CHF should remain at rest until symptoms resolve

C. Aspirin: 325mg PO QD should be given if patient has CAD, dilated cardiomyopathy, atrial fibrillation or valvular dysfunction

D. MEDICATIONS WHICH HAVE BEEN SHOWN TO *DECREASE* MORTALITY
1. **ACE inhibitors**
   a. Mainstay of treatment. Significant decrease in mortality. Have been shown to alleviate symptoms, decrease risk of death, and decrease hospitalizations in patients with mild, moderate or severe CHF
   b. Several studies have shown that higher doses result in better clinical outcomes and better survival. Recommendations are to start low and titrate up to a target dose
   c. Not to be used if SBP<80, creatinine>3.0, K>5.5, or bilateral renal artery stenosis present
   d. Use limited by side effect of cough. Early data indicate that ACE II inhibitors have similar efficacy without side effect of cough
   e. Examples include Captopril (Capoten), Enalapril (Vasotec), Lisinopril (Prinivil, Zestril), Ramipril (Altace), Quinapril (Accupril), and Benzepril (Lotensin)
2. **ß-blockers:** New recommendations state the ß-blockers should be used in all patients with stable class II or class III systolic dysfunction, in combination with diuretics and an ACE. Recent large trial indicates ß-blockers can lessen the symptoms of heart failure, decrease the risk of death, and decrease the combined risk of hospitalization and death
   a. Cardiac Insufficiency Bisoprolol Study (CIBIS II) treatment with **Bisoprolol** up to 10mg QD in Class II and III heart failure was associated with a 34% reduction in mortality, 32% decrease in risk of hospitalization for CHF
   b. The US Carvedilol Heart Failure Study Group included 1094 patients with Class II or III heart failure and found 65% reduction in mortality compared to placebo
   c. **Carvedilol:** Dose—Slowly increase from 3.125mg PO BID to 25mg PO BID by doubling every 2 weeks if tolerating well (higher doses appear to be more effective)
   d. The Metoprolol CR/XL Randomized Intervention Trial in Congestive Heart Failure (MERIT-HF) studied 3,991 patients with class II–IV heart failure who had EF's < 40%

CARD

and were optimized on standard therapy who received Metoprolol CR/XL or placebo. The Metoprolol CR/XL group had improved survival, reduced the need for hospitalizations due to worsening heart failure, and improved NYHA functional class

   e. **Metoprolol CR/XL:** The previously mentioned study started with 12.5mg per day in class III and IV failure and 25mg per day in class II failure, and titrated for 6–8 weeks up to a target of 200mg per day

3. **Aldosterone antagonists**
   a. RALES study showed Spironolactone reduced mortality by 27% and decreased hospitalization by 36% in Class IV patients
   b. Current recommendations state that use of this drug merits consideration in patients with Class IV heart failure

4. **Hydralazine and nitrates** combination should only be used in those who cannot take an ACE–I (should not be substituted for an ACE–I)
   a. **Isosorbide Dinitrate (Isordil):** 20–80mg PO Q6–8hrs—*and*—
   b. **Hydralazine (Apresoline):** Initially 10mg PO TID, increase to 25–100mg TID–QID

5. **Heart transplantation**

E. **MEDICATIONS WHICH HAVE BEEN SHOWN TO** *IMPROVE SYMPTOMS*, **BUT HAVE NOT BEEN SHOWN TO IMPROVE MORTALITY**

1. **Diuretics:** Have been shown to improve symptoms, but not mortality
   a. **Furosemide (Lasix):** 20–320mg PO divided QD–QID
   b. **Bumetanide (Bumex):** 1–8mg PO QD or in divided doses
   c. **Aldactone** 25–50mg PO TID. Synergistic with loop diuretics
   d. Concurrent potassium replacement (See Chapter 76, Disorders of Potassium Metabolism)
   e. Note that **Hydrochlorothiazide (HCTZ)** is not effective in severe CHF

2. **Nitrates:** Have been shown to reduce mortality when used with Hydralazine, but not when used alone. Effective for symptom relief. **Isosorbide Dinitrate (Isordil):** 20–80mg PO Q6–8hrs

3. **Digitalis Glycosides**
   a. The Digitalis Investigation Group recently published its results from 6800 patients with ejection fractions of 0.45 or less randomized to Digoxin or placebo, both in addition to diuretics and ACE inhibitors. They conclude:
      i. Digoxin did not reduce overall mortality
      ii. Digoxin did reduce the rate of hospitalization both overall and for CHF
   b. Digoxin has also been shown to decrease CHF symptoms and increase exercise tolerance
   c. **Digoxin (Lanoxin):** 0.125–0.250mg PO QD

4. **Anticoagulants**
   a. Indicated for patients with atrial fibrillation, history of emboli or LV aneurysms (situations where anticoagulation would be used even without history of CHF). Risk of thromboembolism is low in stable patients (1–3% per year) even in patients with very low EF
   b. There are no definitive trials. Anti-coagulation with Coumadin is most justified in patients with atrial fibrillation or a previous embolic event

F. **MEDICATIONS WHICH HAVE NOT BEEN SHOWN TO BE HELPFUL, AND** *MAY BE HARMFUL*

1. **Calcium channel blockers:** Produce little benefit and may accelerate the progression of heart failure. The second generation calcium channel blockers (including Norvasc) may be exceptions

2. **Antiarrhythmic agents** when used to treat asymptomatic arrhythmias. Up to 70% of patients with heart failure can have asymptomatic episodes of nonsustained ventricular tachycardia (VT) less than 30 seconds. Symptomatic ventricular arrhythmias should be treated

3. **Milrinone:** PROMISE study showed that Milrinone at 40mg QD increased mortality by 35% in patients with NYHA class III or IV heart failure

4. **Periodic Dobutamine infusion:** Dose is 5–8mcg/kg/minutes over 1–2 days every 2–4 weeks. Not contraindicated as symptoms may be improved, but mortality is increased

CARD

Approach to the Patient with Heart Failure

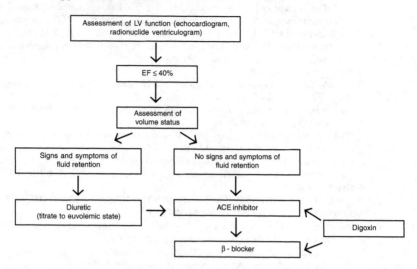

Source: Consensus recommendations for the management of chronic heart failure. On behalf of the membership of the advisory council to improve outcomes nationwide in heart failure. Am J Cardiol Jan 21 1999; 83(2A):24A (Fig 1).

VIII. MANAGEMENT OF HEART FAILURE WITH DIASTOLIC DYSFUNCTION

A. Take patients off Digoxin (unless prescribed for arrhythmia) and ACE inhibitors

B. The goal of therapy is to slow the rate to *allow time for ventricular filling*. Few medications are available to treat diastolic dysfunction, and they should be used with caution

  1. ß-blockers

    a. **Propranolol (Inderal):** 60–80mg PO TID–QID

    b. **Metoprolol (Lopressor):** 50–100mg PO BID

    c. **Timolol (Blocadren):** 10mg PO BID

    d. **Atenolol (Tenormin):** 50mg PO BID or 100mg PO QD

  2. Calcium channel blockers

    a. **Diltiazem (Cardizem, Cardizem SR, Cardizem CD, Dilacor XR):** 60mg PO TID initially, may increase to 360mg QD in 3 divided doses

    b. **Verapamil (Calan, Isoptin, Calan SR, Isoptin SR, Verelan):** 80mg PO TID initially, may increase to 480mg in 3 divided doses

C. The efficacy of therapy will be determined by sequential clinical examination. Medications should be adjusted accordingly

CLINICAL PEARLS

- The most common cause of right heart failure is left heart failure
- Frequent causes of CHF exacerbations are medication non-compliance or change in diet (salt)
- Patients who are bedridden will manifest their edema as sacral (dependent) edema as opposed to edema of the lower extremities
- Patients with stable CHF should continue to exercise as tolerated
- Angiotensin Receptor Blockers: None are currently approved for use in heart failure due to inconclusive results of studies; however, it is considered reasonable to use ARBs instead of ACE-Is in intolerant patients. There are several large studies now in progress to evaluate effect on survival compared to ACE-Is
- Diuretic resistance may be caused by NSAIDs

References

Hjalmarson A, et al. Effects of controlled-release metoprolol on total mortality, hospitalizations, and well-being in patients with heart failure. The Metoprolol CR/XL Randomized Intervention Trial in Congestive Heart Failure (MERIT-HF). JAMA 2000;283:1295–1302.

Belardinelli R, et al. Randomized, controlled trial of long-term moderate exercise training in chronic heart failure. Circulation Mar 9, 1999;99:1173–82.

Brunner-La Rocca HP, et al. Recent insight into therapy of congestive heart failure: focus on ACE inhibition and angiotensin-II antagonism. J Am Coll Cardiol Apr 1999; 33:163–73.

CIBIS II Investigators and Committees. The Cardiac Insufficiency Bisoprolol Study II (CIBIS II): a randomized trial. Lancet 1999:353:9–13.

Consensus recommendations for heart failure. Am J Cardiol 1999;83(2A):1A–38A.

Havranek EP, et al. Dose-related beneficial long-term hemodynamic and clinical efficacy of irbesartan in heart failure. J Am Coll Cardiol Apr 1999;33:1174–81.

Kukin ML, et al. Prospective, randomized comparison of effect of long-term treatment with metoprolol or carvedilol on symptoms, exercise, ejection fraction, and oxidative stress in heart failure. Circulation May 25, 1999;99:2645–51.

Eichhorn EJ, and Bristow MR. Practical guidelines for initiation of beta-adrenergic blockade in patients with chronic heart failure. Amer J Cardiol 1997;79: 794–8.

Garg R, et al. The effect of digoxin on mortality and morbidity in patients with heart failure. N Engl J Med 1997;336:525–33.

Pfeffer MA, et al. ß-adrenergic blockers and survival in heart failure. N Engl J Med 1996;334:1396–7.

The RALES investigators. Effectiveness of spironolactone added to an angiotensin-converting enzyme inhibitor and a loop diuretic for severe chronic congestive heart failure (The Randomized Aldactone Evaluation Study [RALES]). Am J Cardiol 1996;78:902–7.

The US Carvedilol Heart Failure Study Group. The effect of carvedilol on morbidity and mortality in patients with chronic heart failure. New Engl J Med 1996;334:1349–55.

Michael B. Weinstock, MD
Bill Gegas, MD
Darrin Bright, MD

41. ATRIAL FIBRILLATION

I. DEFINITION

Irregularly irregular ventricular rate caused by simultaneous discharges from multiple atrial foci. If the AV node does not block, or if accessory pathways are present there may be a rapid ventricular response (pulse > 100). Note: See IX. Paroxysmal Atrial Fibrillation

II. INCIDENCE

A. Second most common cardiac arrhythmia
B. Incidence Increases with Age
1. 50–59: 0.5%
2. 60–69: 3.8%
3. 70+: 9%

III. ETIOLOGY

An attempt should be made to diagnose the underlying cause, as acute intervention may be necessary even after ventricular rate is controlled

A. Cardiac
1. Cardiac surgery
2. Cardiomyopathy
3. Congenital heart disease
4. Hypertension
5. Lipomatous hypertrophy
6. Myocardial ischemia/infarction
7. Pericarditis
8. Preexcitation syndromes
9. Tachycardia-Bradycardia syndrome
10. Tumors
11. Valvular heart disease: Mitral regurgitation (MR), mitral stenosis (MS), aortic regurgitation (AR), aortic stenosis (AS)

12. Ventricular hypertrophy
13. Ventricular Pacing
B. Systemic
1. Alcohol/"Holiday Heart"
2. Cerebrovascular disease
3. Chronic pulmonary disease
4. Drugs (Ophthalmic Atropine, Digoxin, Theophylline, sympathomimetics, Adenosine, antidepressants, Nicotine gum)
5. Electrocution
6. Electrolyte abnormalities
7. Fever
8. Hypothermia
9. Hypovolemia
10. Pneumonia
11. Pregnancy
12. Sepsis
13. Sudden emotional change
14. Thyrotoxicosis
15. Trauma

IV. HISTORY
A. New onset vs. chronic
B. Chest discomfort
C. Dyspnea
D. Weight loss, sleeplessness, rapid speech, tremor (thyrotoxicosis)
E. Alcohol history: Acute ingestion (holiday heart) vs. alcoholism (alcoholic cardiomyopathy)
F. Medications
G. History of ischemic, valvular or other heart disease

V. PHYSICAL EXAM
A. Vital signs: temperature, O_2 saturation, pulse, blood pressure, and respiration
B. Neck: JVD, thyromegaly
C. Pulmonary: Wheezing, rhonchi
D. CV: Friction rub, murmur, gallop

VI. OTHER TESTS
A. Laboratory
1. Thyroid studies
2. Serial cardiac enzymes
3. Electrolytes
B. ECG: Irregularly irregular rhythm with absence of P waves (special attention to Lead II). Regular vs. rapid rates
C. CXR: Heart size, lung disease
D. Echocardiogram: To evaluate valves, atrial size, hypo-/akinesis, thrombus, pericardial effusion
E. Pharmacologic: To help distinguish between supraventricular tachycardia (SVT) and atrial fibrillation/flutter with RVR, give **Adenosine** 6mg rapid IVP. If unsuccessful then repeat with 12mg rapid IVP. SVT will respond to Adenosine ~90% of the time

VII. MANAGEMENT
A. Hemodynamically unstable: Immediate DC Cardioversion
B. Asymptomatic/minimal symptoms
1. Relieve symptoms
2. Improve cardiac performance
3. Decrease risk of thromboembolism
4. Reduce mortality
C. Rate control
1. **Calcium channel blockers:** Prolongation of AV node conduction. Good if LV function is normal. In elderly patients or patients with decreased LV function, use Diltiazem

      a. Diltiazem (Cardizem): 120–360mg PO QD (use long-acting formulation)

      b. Verapamil (Calan, Isoptin): 120–360mg PO QD (use long-acting formulation)

  2. ß-blockers: Use with caution or use cardioselective agent in COPD, Peripheral Vascular Disease, and CHF

      a. Metoprolol (Lopressor): 25–100mg PO BID

      b. Atenolol (Tenormin): 25–100mg PO QD

      c. Propranolol (Inderal): 40–360mg PO in divided doses

  3. Digitalis Glycosides: Effects include centrally mediated vagal activation and subsequent slowing of the AV nodal conduction and direct action on atrial myocardium. Only 15–20% of patients will convert to NSR with acute therapy—**Digoxin (Lanoxin):** 0.125–0.250mg PO QD

D. Conversion to normal sinus rhythm: Anticoagulation with Warfarin for 3 weeks before and 4 weeks after elective cardioversion is necessary to prevent thromboembolism. Patients alternating between sinus rhythm and atrial fibrillation are at a particularly high risk for thromboembolism and should be converted (chemically or electrically)

  1. Cardioversion: If patient still has RVR (ventricular rate >150 and is hemodynamically unstable (CHF, hypotension, chest pain), then consider emergent cardioversion. Will result in restoration of sinus rhythm in 80–90% of patients

  2. Antiarrhythmics: Consultation with a cardiologist is recommended before initiation of an antiarrhythmic

      a. Class IA—Quinidine (Quinaglute): Inhibits inward sodium channels. Results in prolongation of the action potential and QT interval

      b. Class IC—Propafenone (Rythmol), Flecainide (Tambocor): Inhibits fast sodium channels. Has no effect on the action potential duration or QT interval

      c. Class III—Amiodarone (Cordarone), Sotalol (Betapace): Inhibits outward potassium channels.

VIII. ANTICOAGULATION—See IX. Paroxysmal Atrial Fibrillation

  A. Anticoagulation of patients with chronic atrial fibrillation

    1. The **overall risk of ischemic stroke** in patients with atrial fibrillation varies with age and coexisting risk factors

Factors Increasing the Risk of Stroke in Patients with Atrial Fibrillation
Increasing age
Rheumatic heart disease
Poor left ventricular function or recent congestive heart failure
Enlarged left atrium
Previous myocardial infarction
Hypertension
History of previous thromboembolic events

Source: Akhtar W, Reeves W, Movahed A. Indications for anticoagulation in atrial fibrillation. Am Fam Phys July 1998; 58:131.

Annual Rate of Stroke Based on Five Randomized Studies of Patients with Nonrheumatic Atrial Fibrillation

Category	Rate of stroke per year (%)*	
	Placebo	Warfarin
Independent risk factors		
Age < 65 years		
No risk factors	1.0	1.0
One or more risk factors	4.9	1.7
Age 65 to 75 years		
No risk factors	4.3	1.1
One or more risk factors	5.7	1.7
Age > 75 years		
No risk factors	3.5	1.7
One or more risk factors	8.1	1.2
History of hypertension	5.6	1.9
History of diabetes	8.6	2.8
History of prior stroke or transient ischemic attack†	11.7	5.1
Risk factors in any of the 5 traits‡		
History of congestive heart failure	6.8	1.6
History of angina pectoris	6.7	0.9
History of myocardial infarction	8.2	3.3
History of congestive heart failure, angina pectoris and myocardial infarction	6.1	1.6
Other		
History of peripheral vascular disease	6.0	1.8
Women	5.8	0.9
Paroxysmal or intermittent AF	5.7	1.7
Atrial fibrillation duration > 1 year	4.4	1.5

NOTE: *The five studies are the Atrial Fibrillation, Aspirin, Anticoagulation Study from Copenhagen, Denmark (AFASAK), the Stroke Prevention in Atrial Fibrillation Investigators (SPAFI) study, the Boston Area Anticoagulation Trial in Atrial Fibrillation (BAATAF), the Canadian Atrial Fibrillation Anticoagulation (CAFA) study and the Veterans Stroke Prevention in Nonrheumatic Atrial Fibrillation (SPINAF) study.*

— Rates of stroke are based on the pooled results of five randomized studies the included 3,691 patients with nonrheumatic AF. They received placebo or warfarin.

†— In a separate randomized study of patients with AF who had a stroke or transient ischemic attack within 3 month before enrollment, rate of stroke was 12 percent and 4 percent with placebo and warfarin, respectively (Lancet 1993; 342: 1255-62).

‡— Selection criteria differed somewhat for the randomized trails. These factors were determined to be independent risk factors for stroke in any one of the five randomized studies. The rate of stroke, however, are tabulated from the pooled analysis.

Adapted with permission from Risk factors for stroke and efficacy of antithrombotic therapy in atrial fibrillation. Analysis of pooled data from five randomized controlled trials. Arch intern Med 1994; 154: 1449-57 (Published erratum in Arch Intern Med 1994; 154: 2254) and EAFT (European Atrial Fibrillation Trial) Study Group. Secondary prevention in non-rheumatic atrial fibrillation after transient ischemic attack or minor stroke. Lancet 1993; 342: 1255-62.

Source: Akhtar W, Reeves W, Movahed A. Indications for anticoagulation in atrial fibrillation. Am Fam Phys July 1998; 58:132.

2. **Risks of anticoagulation:** Rate of intracranial hemorrhage in Warfarin-treated patients is 0.3% per year. In the subgroup of elderly patients (mean 80 years) the risk increased to 1.8 % per year from 0.8% for age matched Aspirin controls
3. **Recommendations for anticoagulation of patients in atrial fibrillation**

Recommendations for Anticoagulation of Patients in Atrial Fibrillation		
Age of patient	Other risk factors for stroke	No other risk factors for stroke
< 65 years	Warfarin (Coumadin)	Aspirin or no anticoagulant therapy
65 to 75 years	Warfarin	Aspirin or Warfarin
> 75 years	Warfarin	Warfarin

Source: Akhtar W, Reeves W, Movahed A. Indications for anticoagulation in atrial fibrillation. Am Fam Phys July 1998; 58:130–6.

4. Patients with history of TIA or minor CVA have a 12% risk of CVA per year. The risk is reduced to 4% per year with anticoagulation. The risk of major bleeding is increased 0.3% per year. In absolute terms, for every 1000 patients with a history of TIA or minor CVA treated with anticoagulation, ~80 vascular events (mainly strokes) will be prevented per year. The decrease is 40 per year with Aspirin
5. Inquire about contraindications (recent or scheduled surgery, pregnancy, bleeding tendencies) and medication use which may affect Warfarin levels
6 INR should be kept between 2.0 and 3.0

B. Anticoagulation before cardioversion (Electrical or Chemical)
(TEE) prior to cardioversion
1. Atrial fibrillation of short duration (< 48hrs): The data are unclear. Conservative recommendations include IV Heparin with or without transesophageal echocardiography (TEE) prior to cardioversion
2. Atrial Fibrillation of longer duration (> 48hrs)
a. Warfarin at therapeutic levels for 3 weeks prior to cardioversion
b. Alternative management: IV Heparin for 12hrs followed by TEE. If TEE negative for atrial thrombi then proceed with cardioversion

C. Anticoagulation after cardioversion (Electrical or Chemical)
1. Continued for 4 weeks following cardioversion regardless of the duration prior to conversion
2. Prevents thrombus formation during recovery of atrial mechanical contractility

D. Drugs used for anticoagulation
1. Warfarin: Maintain the International Normalized Ratio (INR) between 2–3. Risk reduction dependent on age and coexisting risk factors
2. Aspirin:
a. Lack of consensus regarding optimal dose. 325mg/day has been tested the most
b. Indicated in patients with lone atrial fibrillation. If Warfarin is contraindicated then consider Aspirin

IX. PAROXYSMAL ATRIAL FIBRILLATION
A. Definition: Intermittent episodes of atrial fibrillation that usually cease spontaneously. When patient is not in atrial fibrillation, the baseline rhythm is usually NSR
B. The risk of thromboembolic disease appears independent of whether atrial fibrillation is chronic or paroxysmal. Several recent trials reported the risk of stroke to be similar in patients with chronic persistent and paroxysmal atrial fibrillation. The SPAF (Stroke Prevention in Atrial Fibrillation) revealed that patients with paroxysmal atrial fibrillation had a stroke rate of 3.7% per year
C. One other consideration is that patients with paroxysmal atrial fibrillation are often

CARD

asymptomatic and episodes occur more frequently and for a longer duration than he/she perceives. Combined analyses (SPAF and Boston Area Anticoagulation Trial for Atrial Fibrillation) show that the annual stroke rate in patients with paroxysmal atrial fibrillation was 5.7% in the control group and only 1.7% in the Warfarin group

D. The use of chronic anticoagulation seems to be supported by this data

CLINICAL PEARLS:
- Atrial fibrillation is the most common arrhythmia encountered in primary care practice
- Prevalence is 0.05% in patients 25–35 years of age and increases to 5% in patients older than 69 years of age
- 70–80% of patients with new onset atrial fibrillation will spontaneously convert to NSR within the first 24hrs
- The sooner atrial fibrillation is converted, the better the chances of success
- The loss of coordinated atrial contraction that occurs with atrial fibrillation causes a 10–20% decrease in cardiac output at a normal rate, and a reduction in diastolic filling time when the response is rapid < 100–120

References

Aronow WS. Management of atrial fibrillation, ventricular arrhythmias and pacemakers in older persons. Management of the older person with atrial fibrillation. J Am Geriatr Soc Jun 1999;47:740–8.

Connolly S. Evidence-based analysis of amiodarone efficacy and safety. Circulation Nov 1999; 100:2025–34.

Ezekowitz M, Levine J. Preventing stroke in patients with atrial fibrillation. JAMA May 1999;281: 1830–5.

Akhtar W, Reeves W, Movahed A. Indications for anticoagulation in atrial fibrillation. Am Fam Phys Jul 1998; 58:130–6.

Jung F, DiMarco J. Treatment strategies for atrial fibrillation. Am J Med Mar 1998; 104:272–86.

Laupacis A, et al. Antithrombotic therapy in atrial fibrillation. Chest 1998;114:579–89.

Wolf P, Singer D. Preventing stroke in atrial fibrillation. Am Fam Phys Dec 1997; 56:2243–50.

Michael B. Weinstock, MD
Mrunal Shah, MD

42. AMBULATORY POST-MI MANAGEMENT

I. IDENTIFY PATIENTS AT HIGH RISK FOR FUTURE EVENTS POST-MYOCARDIAL INFARCTION (MI)*

A. Poor left ventricular (LV) function (EF < 45%): By ECHO or cardiac catheterization. Patients with an EF of 20–44% have a 12% 1-year mortality

B. Positive submaximal stress test (performed prior to hospital discharge)

C. Recurrent ischemia post-MI

D. Multiple cardiac risk factors: Post-MI patients with 4 risk factors have ~ 60% 2-year mortality

E. Location and extent of infarct: Anterior infarct has highest 1-year mortality

F. Ventricular arrhythmias: If a patient has > 10 PVCs/hr compared to < 1 PVC/hr, the 1-year mortality is 18% compared to 3% (indication of poor LV function)

G. Number of vessels with atherosclerotic disease: 1-year mortality is increased from 2% to 12% with triple vessel disease compared to single vessel disease

* Patients at high risk for future events should be strongly considered for cardiology referral, cardiac catheterization, and coronary revascularization (CABG or PTCA) if indicated

II. DIAGNOSTIC TESTING

Most patients will have at least 1 of these 3 tests before hospital discharge:

A. Submaximal stress testing: Performed prior to hospital discharge. This should be followed with a maximal stress test 3–6 weeks post-MI. If either is positive, cardiac catheterization should be strongly considered

B. Cardiac ECHO: To assess LV function and ejection fraction, wall motion, valves, septal defects, papillary muscle function. If the prehospital discharge ECHO shows LV dysfunction (EF < 45%), patients should be strongly considered for cardiac catheterization because of high (12%) 1-year mortality

C. Cardiac catheterization: The gold standard test recommended for patients at high risk of future events (see above) or if above tests are positive

III. INDICATIONS FOR CARDIAC CATHETERIZATION/STATISTICS

Of 100 patients admitted with acute MI:

A. 20 patients will have severe ischemia or severe pump failure during their hospital admission
   Recommendation: Cardiac catheterization

B. 20 patients will become symptomatic during a submaximal stress test prior to hospital discharge
   Recommendation: Cardiac catheterization

C. 10 patients will become symptomatic during maximal stress testing 3–6 weeks post-discharge
   Recommendation: Cardiac catheterization

D. The remaining 50 patients will be at low risk with a 0–5% 1-year mortality. One half of the remaining 50 patients will undergo cardiac catheterization within 1 year. Medical management and risk factor modification should be aggressively pursued

IV. MANAGEMENT

A. Risk factor modification post-MI: Strongly encourage treatment, compliance, and/or behavioral modification of the following risk factors. Patients with 4 risk factors have a 2-year mortality which is 60% compared to 5% in patients with 1 risk factor (See separate chapters on smoking, hypertension, diabetes, cholesterol management, and depression)
   1. Smoking
   2. Hypertension: Reduction of mortality by 20% with successful reduction of blood pressure
   3. Diabetes: Presence of diabetes increases 1-year mortality post-MI by 25%
   4. High cholesterol: Target LDL post-MI is < 100mg/dL
   5. Sedentary lifestyle
   6. Obesity
   7. Depression

B. Cardiac rehabilitation: Most post-MI patients will benefit, although the extent of rehabilitation will have to be tailored to a patient's specific situation. Mortality may be decreased by up to 25% with participation in cardiac rehab

C. Medical management post-MI (Medications with proven efficacy include aspirin, ß-blockers, ACE inhibitors and anti-coagulants)

   1. Aspirin: Indicated for all patients unless allergic. Peptic ulcer disease is *not* a contraindication
      a. The *ISIS 2* trial showed that Aspirin reduced vascular death by 23% and reduced non-fatal infarctions by 49% post-MI
      b. **Aspirin** would save 5,000 lives a year if given to all post-MI patients, yet as many as 28% of post-MI patients do not receive it. Aspirin has an approximate cost of $13 per life saved
      c. Dose at 160–325mg PO QD with meals

   2. ß-blockers: Indicated for all patients except those with *severe* CHF or second/third degree heart block. Although their efficacy is proven, only 20–30% of post-MI patients are prescribed ß-blockers
      a. The ß-blocker Heart Attack Trial (BHAT) showed that ß-blockers (which reduce the heart rate) reduced sudden death by 32%, recurrent infarction by 27%, and overall cardiac mortality by 22% post-MI. The benefit is more pronounced in patients with co-morbid factors of angina, prior heart failure or arrhythmia
      b. Should be administered *within hours* post-MI
      c. **Metoprolol (Lopressor):** 50mg PO Q6hrs started 15 minutes after last IV dose, then 100mg PO BID if tolerated. Start with 25mg PO Q6hrs in patients who do not tolerate full IV dose
      d. **Atenolol (Tenormin):** 50mg PO BID or 100mg PO QD
      e. **Propranolol (Inderal):** 60–80mg PO TID–QID

CARD

  f. **Timolol (Blocadren):** 10mg PO BID

  g. Avoid Labetalol and intrinsic sympathomimetics such as Acebutolol and Pindolol

 3. Angiotensin converting enzyme (ACE) inhibitors: New studies suggest a reduction in the incidence of sudden cardiac death and nonfatal subsequent infarctions following myocardial infarction. Indicated for post-MI patients with clinical signs and symptoms of congestive heart failure and/or an EF<40%, as long as the systolic blood pressure is >100 mm Hg

  a. The *SAVE* study used oral Captopril in patients with EF < 40%, 3–16 days post-MI and showed that total mortality was decreased by 19%, re-infarction by 24%, and subsequent hospitalizations for CHF decreased by 19%

  b. Several other studies (i.e., *AIRE, GISSI-3, SMILE*) have also indicated benefit from ACE inhibitors post-MI in patients with LV dysfunction

  c. The proposed mechanism of action is by reducing ventricular dilation, remodeling, wall stress and thinning

  d. Should be *administered 1 to 3 days post-MI* and *only oral routes of administration* should be used. The *CONSENSUS II* study failed to demonstrate any advantage to starting oral /intravenous Enalapril within 24hrs after the onset of MI

  e. **Captopril (Capoten):** Begin with 25mg PO TID and increase to 50–100mg PO TID. Do not use with renal artery stenosis. Check serum creatinine before and 4 weeks after initiating therapy

  f. **Enalapril (Vasotec):** 5–20mg PO QD in 1–2 divided doses. Same cautions as with Captopril

  g. **Lisinopril (Prinivil, Zestril), Ramipril (Altace):** Proven in clinical trials. Less expensive than Captopril and Enalapril

  h. **Quinapril (Accupril), Benzepril (Lotensin):** Not proven in clinical trials, but thought to have same efficacy as Captopril and Enalapril at lower cost

 4. Statins

  a. The goal for post-MI patients with hypercholesterolemia is LDL< 100mg/dL

  b. The *Scandinavian Simvistatin Survival Study (4S)* included 4,444 patients with angina or previous MI and hypercholesterolemia (i.e., 213–310mg/dL) who were treated with Simvistatin (Zocor) or placebo and followed for a median of 5.4 years. The treated group had a 30% risk reduction in overall mortality and a 42% risk reduction in coronary death

  c. Pooled data from the PLAC I and PLAC II trials demonstrated a 67% reduction in non-fatal MI and 40% reduction in the mortality rate among patients treated with Pravastatin (Pravachol) compared with placebo over a follow-up 3-year period

  d. For further guidelines and drug doses/side effects, etc., See Chapter 37, Hyperlipidemia

 5. Anticoagulants: Indicated when there are other conditions that would benefit from treatment with oral anticoagulation (atrial fibrillation)

 6. Nitrates: If a patient has to use PRN nitrates post-MI, strong consideration should be given to cardiac catheterization if it has not been performed

 7. Calcium channel blockers

  a. Should not be used for secondary prevention post-MI except possibly in non-Q-wave MI where the EF has been preserved and there is no evidence of CHF. A Danish study *(DAVIT II)* suggested that Verapamil may be used for Q wave MIs without associated heart failure

  b. Nifedipine should not be used post-MI as it has been shown to *increase* mortality

  c. Although calcium channel blockers are not beneficial post-MI, they *are* beneficial for hypertension and angina (See Chapter 39, Coronary Artery Disease)

 8. Antiarrhythmics: Although effective at suppressing ventricular ectopy, the *CAST* study showed that certain antiarrhythmics increased mortality post-MI. Therefore, they should not be routinely used post-MI

References

Domanski MJ, et al. Effect of angiotensin converting enzyme inhibition on sudden cardiac death in patients following acute myocardial infarction. A meta-analysis of randomized clinical trials. J Am Coll Cardiol 1999;33:598–604.

Freemantle N, et al. ß Blockade after myocardial infarction: systematic review and meta regression analysis. BMJ 1999;318:1730–7.

Marchioli R, et al., of the GISSI-Prevenzione Investigators. Dietary supplementation with n-3 polyunsaturated fatty acids and vitamin E after myocardial infarction: results of the GISSI-Prevenzione trial. Lancet 1999;354: 447–55.

Gottlieb SS, et al. Effect of beta-blockade on mortality among high-risk and low-risk patients after myocardial infarction. N Engl J Med 1998;339:489–97

Cody RJ. ACE inhibitors: myocardial infarction and congestive heart failure. Am Fam Phys 1995;52 (6):1801–6.

AHCPR guidelines #17. Cardiac rehabilitation as secondary prevention. Rockville, MD; 1995.

Havranek EP. Managing patients with myocardial infarction after hospital discharge. Am Fam Phys 1994;49(5):1109–19.

Pfeffer MA, et al. Results of the Survival and Ventricular Enlargement Trial (SAVE): effect of captopril on mortality and morbidity in patients with left ventricular dysfunction after myocardial infarction. N Engl J Med 1992;327:669–77.

Beta-blocker Heart Attack Trial (BHAT) Research Group. A randomized trial of propranolol in patients with acute myocardial infarction. JAMA 1982;247:1707–14.

Michael B. Weinstock, MD

43. CARDIAC STRESS TESTING

I. INDICATIONS FOR CARDIAC STRESS TESTING*

A. Evaluating chest pain

B. Evaluating a patient after myocardial infarction (submaximal or maximal)

C. Generating an exercise prescription (See below)

D. Evaluating dysrhythmias

E. Determining functional capacity

F. Establishing the severity/prognosis of ischemic heart disease

G. Evaluating anti-anginal or anti-hypertensive therapy

H. Screening for ischemic heart disease in asymptomatic patients. This should only be done for those patients with high risk (multiple or strong risk factors) or those whose occupations place others at risk (airline pilots, etc.)

* It is important to think of how the test result will change your management of the patient. If a positive test on an asymptomatic patient will be dismissed as false, then don't perform it. If a patient with symptoms of angina and multiple risk factors has a negative test and catheterization will be performed anyway, consider proceeding directly to the catheterization

II. CONTRAINDICATIONS TO MAXIMAL STRESS TESTING

A. Possible acute myocardial infarction in progress

B. Unstable angina

C. Uncontrolled hypertension

D. Significant ventricular arrhythmias

E. Recent systemic or pulmonary embolism (within 3 months)

F. Severe uncontrolled CHF or pulmonary HTN

G. Active myocarditis, dissecting aneurysm, IHSS, aortic stenosis (AS), pericarditis

III. PRE-EXERCISE TESTING

INDICATIONS FOR PRE-EXERCISE TESTING IN ASYMPTOMATIC PATIENTS

	1. HEALTHY PATIENTS		2. HIGH RISK PATIENTS*		3. PATIENTS WITH HEART DISEASE
	Young (Men ≤ 40, women ≤ 50)	Older patients	No angina symptoms	Symptomatic for CAD	
Moderate exercise	no	no	no	yes	yes
Vigorous exercise	no	yes	yes	yes	yes

*Patients with risk factors for CAD (i.e., family history, smoking, diabetes, etc.)

Source: Adapted from American College of Sports Medicine. Guidelines for exercise testing and prescription. 4th ed. © Williams & Wilkins. Philadelphia: Lea & Febiger, 1991:8. Used with permission.

IV. SENSITIVITY AND SPECIFICITY

Exercise EKG testing is 60–80% sensitive and 70–80% specific for coronary artery disease (CAD). These statistics can be misleading because they do not take into account the patient's pretest likelihood of significant CAD. Stress testing should generally not be carried out in individuals at very low risk for CAD because of the cost of "false positive" results. In patients at high risk for CAD, consideration should be given to proceeding directly to cardiac catheterization as a positive test will add little to the information already known, and a negative test will still leave an unacceptably high chance of CAD

V. TESTS TO EVALUATE ANGINA

A. Myocardial perfusion scintigraphy

1. Radionuclide is injected after the patient is "stressed" and images are examined for perfusion defects (ischemia). Patients who are unable to exercise because of COPD, PVD, or physical limitations will have a chemical stress thallium test.
2. *Sensitivity is 80–90% for clinically significant CAD.* False positive rate is ~20%. Compared to stress ECHO, radionuclide stress tests have a higher sensitivity and lower specificity for clinically significant CAD
3. Indications
   a. Difficulty interpreting resting ECG (BBB, baseline ST/T changes, Digitalis effect, LVH with strain, low voltage, etc.)
   b. Follow-up of abnormal exercise stress test (if results don't correlate with clinical impression)
   c. To distinguish between ischemia and infarction or to localize a region of ischemia; visualization of an old infarct
   d. To determine prognosis in patients with angina or prior MI
   e. Persantine thallium for risk stratification for vascular patients pre-op

B. Stress ECHO: *Exercise stress ECHO, Dobutamine stress ECHO*

1. Imaging of wall motion, valves, and ejection fraction before and after the heart is being stressed by exercise or Dobutamine. Changes in wall motion (hypokinesis, akinesis) suggest myocardial ischemia. A Dobutamine ECHO should be performed on patients unable to exercise
2. Compared to stress thallium, stress ECHO has a higher specificity and a lower sensitivity for clinically significant CAD
3. Less expensive than stress thallium
4. Indications: Similar to stress thallium

C. Coronary angiography (cardiac catheterization)
  1. Mortality ~ 0.1%, morbidity 0–5%
  2. Indications
    a. Patients being considered for PTCA or CABG who have failed ambulatory treatment of angina
    b. Patients being considered for PTCA or CABG who have unstable angina
    c. Patients being considered for PTCA or CABG whose non-invasive testing suggests high risk for CAD
    d. To assess post-MI patients who have severe ischemia, pump failure, positive pre-hospital discharge submaximal stress test or positive maximal stress test (performed 3–6 weeks after hospital discharge) (See Chapter 42, Ambulatory Post-MI Management)
    e. Reassess post-CABG or post-PTCA patients with recurrence of symptoms
    f. To diagnose patients with undiagnosed chest pain

References
Younis LT, Chaitman BR. The prognostic value of exercise testing. Cardiology Clinics 1993; 11(2):229–39.
American College of Sports Medicine. Guidelines for exercise testing and prescription. 4th ed. Philadelphia: Lea & Febiger, 1991:8.

CARD

David Sharkis, MD
Michael B. Weinstock, MD
Daniel M. Neides, MD
Loren Leidheiser, DO

44. EVALUATION OF SHORTNESS OF BREATH

I. DIFFERENTIAL DIAGNOSIS
  A. Upper airway causes
    1. Angioedema/anaphylaxis
    2. Retropharyngeal abscess
    3. Tracheal obstruction (cancer, foreign body, mucous plug)
    4. Infectious: epiglottitis, croup
  B. Pulmonary causes
    1. Infection (pneumonia, bronchitis, TB)
    2. Obstructive lung disease (COPD: asthma, chronic bronchitis, emphysema)
    3. Restrictive lung diseases
      a. Extrathoracic: Chest wall restriction (kyphoscoliosis, obesity, pregnancy, ascites), diaphragmatic dysfunction, abdominal distention
      b. Intrathoracic: Infiltrate, infiltrative process (sarcoidosis, amyloidosis, pulmonary fibrosis), pneumonectomy, parenchymal process
    4. Pneumothorax
    5. Pleural effusion
    6. Lung masses, metastatic disease
    7. Pulmonary embolism
    8. Pulmonary hypertension
    9. Adult respiratory distress syndrome (ARDS)
    10. Carbon monoxide toxicity
    11. Cystic fibrosis
  C. Cardiac causes
    1. Congestive heart failure (pulmonary edema)
    2. Acute MI/anginal equivalent/myocardial ischemia
    3. Pericarditis/pericardial tamponade
    4. Cardiac valvular disease
    5. Cardiac arrhythmias (atrial fibrillation, ventricular tachycardia)
  D. Systemic causes

    1.Noncardiogenic pulmonary edema: Drug OD, pancreatitis, trauma, sepsis, inhalation of toxic chemicals
    2. Anemia
    3. Diabetic Ketoacidosis (DKA)
    4. Gastroesophageal reflux (GERD)
    5. Hyper-/hypothyroidism
    6. Deconditioning
    7. Carbon monoxide poisoning

E. Central causes
    1. Panic disorder/anxiety
    2. Acute hyperventilation
    3. Cheyne-Stokes: Seen in coma from intracerebral pathology
    4. CNS/systemic neuromuscular disorders
    5. Multiple sclerosis
    6. Phrenic nerve dysfunction

II. HISTORY

A. History of Present Illness (HOPI): Fever, cough (productive vs. non-productive), hemoptysis, association with orthopnea/paroxysmal nocturnal dyspnea/peripheral edema (CHF), chest discomfort (MI/angina, pericarditis), exacerbating/relieving factors, sore throat/dysphonia/dysphagia, acuity of onset (acute onset: PE, MI, pneumothorax, foreign body, ruptured valve), work and travel exposures, anxiety/depression

B. PMH: Inquire about history of shortness of breath, cardiac or pulmonary disease, medications, smoking history, CAD risk factors, history of diabetes (silent MI), history of previous DVT/PE, prolonged immobility, cancer or use of oral contraceptives (risk factors for DVT/PE), history of TB, supplemental home oxygen

III. PHYSICAL EXAMINATION

A. Vital signs

B. HEENT: Assess JVD (CHF, valvular dysfunction, pericardial tamponade, pulmonary HTN), tracheal deviation (pneumothorax), periorbital cyanosis, glossal deviation, erythematous/edematous pharynx, retropharyngeal abscess, whispered pectoriloquy, egophony, tactile fremitus (See Chapter 45, Community Acquired Pneumonia for further discussion and definitions)

C. Chest: Rales (CHF), rhonchi/rales (pneumonia), increased A-P chest wall diameter (COPD), dullness to percussion/decreased breath sounds (effusion/consolidation), wheezing (asthma, pulmonary edema, foreign body), stridor (upper airway obstruction), palpable crepitus (PTX)

D. Cardiac: Gallop, murmur, rub, distant heart sounds (pericardial tamponade), loud P_2 (pulmonary HTN)

E. Extremities: Clubbing, cyanosis, edema, unilateral edematous/tender leg (DVT)

IV. TESTS

A. Radiology: Obtain PA and lateral CXR
    1. Pleural effusions are best seen at the costophrenic angle on the lateral film
    2. Pneumonia is a *clinical diagnosis* as CXR findings of pneumonia may lag behind clinical findings
    3. Assess for presence of pneumothorax, heart size, rib fracture, or free air under the diaphragm
    4. *Lateral neck films* may be obtained when upper airway compromise is considered

B. ABG

C. Pulse oximetry: *Measures oxygenation only.* Rest and exercise oximetry may reveal oxygen desaturation (early finding in interstitial lung disease and pulmonary HTN). In most patients with undiagnosed SOB, an ABG determination provides the most information. The pulse oximetry may be limited by certain conditions (severe vasoconstriction, hypothermia, nail polish, methemoglobinas or carboxyhemoglobins)

D. ECG: Should be performed in any patient > age 30 and all patients with history of CAD or diabetes with undiagnosed dyspnea. In addition to signs of ischemia/infarction and arrhythmias, look for signs of pericarditis (diffuse ST segment elevation and PR depression in lead II), pericardial effusion/tamponade (decreased QRS amplitude and electrical alternans), PE (sinus tachycardia and $S_1 Q_3 T_3$), and COPD (P-pulmonale, multifocal atrial tachycardia (MAT))

E. Pulmonary function testing
  1. Indications
     a. Evaluation of pulmonary dysfunction: Obstructive vs. restrictive impairment
     b. Evaluation of dyspnea and cough
     c. Evaluation of response to therapy
     d. To determine if there is bronchial reactivity: Methacholine challenge
     e. To determine if there is a reversible component to obstructive lung disease
     f. Preoperative evaluation in selected patients (See Chapter 98, Preoperative Evaluation)
     g. Evaluation of upper airway obstruction with a flow-volume loop
  2. Examples of changes in PFTs with various pulmonary disorders:

Tests*	Obstructive†	Emphysema	Restrictive†
FEV_1 (Liters)	↓↓	↓↓	↓
FVC (Liters)	↓	↓	↓↓
FEV_1 / FEV%	↓	↓	Normal or ↑
RV (Liters)	↑	↑↑	↓
TLC (Liters)	Normal or ↑	↑↑	↓
DL_{CO}	Normal or ↑	↓↓	Normal or ↓

† For examples of obstructive/restrictive lung diseases, See Section I, Differential Diagnosis
FEV_1 (forced expiratory volume in 1 second), FVC (functional residual capacity), RV (residual volume), TLC (total lung capacity), DL_{CO} (diffusing capacity of carbon monoxide)

*Source: Adapted from Williams DO, Cugell DW. Pulmonary function tests: indications and Interpretation. Hosp Med 1988;24(5):48.

F. Chest CT: Used primarily as a follow-up of abnormal CXR
G. Ventilation-perfusion (V/Q) scan: If diagnosis of pulmonary embolism is suspected based on clinical presentation or prior studies
H. Pulmonary angiogram: If V/Q scan is indeterminate or low probability in a patient with a high pre-test probability of PE
I. Laboratory (if indicated)
  1. CBC (anemia)
  2. Thyroid functions tests
  3. Electrolytes (hypokalemia may cause weakness of respiratory muscles)
  4. Carbon monoxide level
  5. Cardiac enzymes
J. Bronchoscopy: Indications
  1. Evaluation of hemoptysis
  2. Diagnosis and staging of bronchogenic carcinoma, biopsy of tracheal or main stem bronchus tumors
  3. Diagnosis of lung infiltrates and certain pulmonary infections including PCP and TB
  4. Removal of foreign bodies
K. Cardiopulmonary exercise stress testing: If clinical presentation suggests cardiac etiology or if workup is negative

V. INDICATIONS FOR MECHANICAL VENTILATION
  A. Inability to protect airway (drug ingestion, CVA, trauma, decreased mental status, etc.)
  B. Impending airway obstruction (retropharyngeal abscess, epiglottitis, massive mediastinal adenopathy)
  C. Hypoxia (pO_2 < 50–60): Despite supplemental oxygen
  D. *Symptomatic* hypercarbia (pCO_2 > 50): This criteria must be individualized as an asthmatic in distress may be intubated for a pCO_2 of 40, whereas a patient with COPD may be a chronic

CO_2 retainer ($CO_2 > 90$–100). A patient with chronic CO_2 retention will have a *normal pH* and elevated HCO_3, whereas a patient with acute CO_2 retention will have a *pH which is decreased* and a near normal HCO_3

CLINICAL PEARLS

- Tachypnea is the most common sign of pneumonia in the elderly and in children
- In immunocompromised patients, dyspnea is often the initial manifestation of *Pneumocystis* pneumonia (PCP)
- Subcutaneous Epinephrine or Terbutaline should be used with caution in patients > age 30
- With asthmatics steroids should be given early to minimize their chances of hospital admission
- Orthopnea may be seen in patients with severe dyspnea regardless of etiology as diaphragmatic mechanics are improved in the upright position
- Retropharyngeal abscess and epiglottitis are emergency situations requiring immediate pharyngeal examination by ENT specialists
- Patients with alcoholism and seizure disorders are at risk for aspiration
- A normal pulse oximetry does not exclude the possibility of pulmonary emboli

References

American Thoracic Society. Dyspnea. Mechanism, assessment, and management: a consensus statement. Am J Respir Crit Care Med 1999;159:321–40.

Gillespie DJ. Unexplained dyspnea. Mayo Clin Proc 1994;69:657–63.

Williams DO, Cugell DW. Pulmonary function tests: indications and interpretation. Hospital Med 1988;24(5):23–53.

Beth Weinstock, MD

45. COMMUNITY–ACQUIRED PNEUMONIA

I. DEFINITION

A. An acute infection of the pulmonary parenchyma associated with:
1. Symptoms of acute infection—*and*—
2. The presence of an acute infiltrate on chest x-ray or auscultatory findings consistent with pneumonia

B. Pneumonia is considered nosocomial (not community-acquired) if the patient has been hospitalized or treated in a nursing home for 14 days prior to presentation of current illness

II. SIGNIFICANCE

A. Approximately 500,000 adult hospitalizations per year

B. Annual incidence of pneumonia in patients older than 65 years is about 1%

C. The combination of community acquired pneumonia (CAP) and influenza ranks as the sixth leading cause of death in the U. S. Mortality has remained fairly constant at about 25% over the last 4 decades, despite antibiotic advances, although mortality among outpatients is less than 1%

III. ETIOLOGY—Note: A definitive pathogen is found only in about $^1/_3$ of patients

A. Neonate
1. Group B *Streptococcus*
2. *Listeria monocytogenes*
3. Gram negatives—*E.Coli, Klebsiella*
4. *Chlamydia Trachomatis* (neonate to 3 months)
5. CMV, HSV, Rubella

B. < 1 year
1. *Streptococcus pneumoniae*
2. *Haemophilus influenzae*
3. *Staphylococcus aureus*

4. RSV, Parainfluenza virus

C. > 1 year
1. *Streptococcus pneumoniae*
2. *Haemophilus influenzae*
3. *Staphylococcus aureus*
4. Influenza virus
5. Rhinovirus, Parainfluenza, Adenovirus
6. *Chlamydia Pneumoniae, Mycoplasma* (school-age)

D. Adult
1. *Streptococcus pneumoniae* (13.4%)
2. *Haemophilus influenzae* (2.5%)
3. *Mycoplasma pneumoniae* (1.5%)
4. Gram-negative bacilli
5. *Staphylococcus aureus*
6. *Moraxella catarrhalis*
7. *Legionella pneumophila*
8. *Chlamydia pneumoniae*
9. Viruses
10. *Mycobacterium tuberculosis*
11. *Pneumocystis carinii*

E. Elderly, extended-care facility
1. *Streptococcus pneumoniae*
2. *Haemophilus influenzae*
3. *Klebsiella pneumoniae*
4. *Pseudomonas aeruginsoa*
5. Anaerobes (if aspiration suspected)

F. Immunocompromised patient: All of the above—plus—
1. Fungal organisms: Histoplasmosis, coccidioidomycosis, *cryptococcus*, etc.
2. *Pneumocystis carinii, mycobacterium* spp., CMV

IV. DIAGNOSIS
   A. History: Note—Elderly do not often present with classic pneumonia symptoms; confusion is a common symptom in the elderly
   1. Symptoms
      a. General: Rigors, chills, fever
      b. Lungs: Cough, sputum production, dyspnea
      c. Chest: Pleuritic chest pain
      d. Musculoskeletal: Myalgias and arthralgias
   2. Timing and preceding symptoms: Sudden onset (indicative of "classic" pneumococcal pneumoniae), recent influenza infection
   3. Risk Factors: Extremes of age, smoking history, debilitating illness or immunocompromised state, nursing home resident, history of influenza-like illness, alcoholism, HIV risk factors, risk factors for aspiration (syncope, loss of consciousness, CVA, sedative drugs)

   B. Physical exam
   1. Vitals: Fever, tachypnea, tachycardia
   2. State of hydration: Skin turgor, mucous membranes, urine output
   3. Immunocompromised state: Lymphadenopathy, thrush, Kaposi's sarcoma, wasting
   4. Lung exam
      a. Inspection: Retractions, use of accessory muscles, asymmetry in inspiration due to splinting
      b. Auscultation
         i. Crackles (rales) are most common finding in patients with CAP
         ii. Bronchial breath sounds due to consolidation
         iii. Whispered pectoriloquy: Increased clarity of patient's whispered voice due to consolidation
         4) Egophony: Change in tone of patient's voice from "e" to "a"
      c. Palpation: Tactile fremitus (detects asymmetry in the "voice buzz" while patient is

speaking)

    d. Percussion: Asymmetry between the hemithoraces

  5. Clubbing

C. X-ray

  1. Recommended for all patients suspected of pneumonia (T > 37.8° C, HR >100, rales, locally decreased breaths sounds)

  2. Helps to predict severity of disease: Multilobar infiltrates and pleural effusions are associated with increased mortality

  3. CXR may be falsely negative in dehydrated patients

  4. "Classic" findings

    a. Diffuse bilateral infiltrates: *Pneumocystis carinii*

    b. Cavity with air-fluid level: Anaerobic lung abscess

    c. Upper lobe cavitary lesion: *Mycobacterium tuberculosis*

    d. Nodular or reticular infiltrates: Mycoplasma or Chlamydial atypical organisms

    e. Pleural effusions: Staphylococcal or streptococcal infection

    f. Lobar infiltrate: Most commonly *streptococcus pneumoniae*

D. Laboratory

  1. Oxygenation

    a. Pulse oximetry helpful in outpatient setting. Consider admitting patients with oxygen saturation < 90%

    b. Arterial blood gas: Consider ordering when admitting patients, especially with a history of COPD or suspicion of pulmonary embolism. pO_2 <60 mmHg is predictive of increased mortality

  2. Sputum stain and culture: Not necessary or helpful in outpatients diagnosed with CAP

  3. Blood cultures: Not necessary for outpatient therapy. Only 11% of hospitalized patients with CAP will have positive blood cultures

  4. CBC: Leukocyte count should not be used in decision-making; has not been shown to affect mortality

  5. Electrolytes

    a. Hyponatremia occurs in CAP, most commonly *Legionella pneumonia*. Na <130 mEq/L predictive of increased mortality

    b. BUN > 30mg/dL, and serum glucose >250mg/dL also predictive of increased mortality

  6. HIV: Consider if patient has any risk factors

V. OUTPATIENT VS. INPATIENT THERAPY—Consider admission for the following:

  A. Age greater than 50 with co-morbid conditions

  B. Social

    1. Elderly patients with poor social support

    2. Alcoholics

    3. Psychiatric illnesses

    4. Homelessness

  C. Abnormalities on physical exam

    1. Altered mental status

    2. Pulse >125 bpm

    3. RR >30/minute

    4. SBP < 90 mmHg

    5. T < 35° C or > 40° C

  D. Abnormal lab findings:

    1. pH < 7.35

    2. BUN > 30mg/dL

    3. Na < 130 mEq/L

    4. Glucose > 250mg/dL

    5. Hematocrit < 30%

    6. pO_2 < 60 mmHg

    7. Pleural effusion

VI. TREATMENT (OUTPATIENT)

  A. Macrolides: Cover gram-positive bacteria, as well as atypical organisms. Clarithromycin and

Azithromycin have enhanced activity versus H. flu
1. **Azithromycin (Zithromax):** 500mg PO QD × 1, then 250mg PO QD × 4 days
2. **Clarithromycin (Biaxin):** 500mg PO BID × 10–14 days
3. **Erythromycin:** Don't use if patient has high probability of H. flu infection (COPD)
   a. **EES:** 400mg QID × 10–14 days
   b. **Erythromycin base:** 250mg–500mg QID × 10–14 days
B. **Flouroquinolone:** Older quinolones (Ciprofloxacin) ineffective against pneumococcus
   a. **Levofloxacin (Levaquin):** 500mg PO QD × 10–14 days
   b. **Gatifloxacin (Tequin):** 400mg PO QD × 10–14 days
   c. **Moxifloxacin (Avalox):** 400mg PO QD × 10–14 days
   d. **Sparfloxacin (Zagam):** 400mg PO QD × 1, then 200mg PO QD × 10–14 days
   Note: Photosensitivity reactions are common with Sparfloxacin. Prolongation of the QT interval has been reported in patients receiving Sparfloxacin and Moxifloxacin
C. **Doxycycline:** 100mg PO BID × 10–14 days

VII. FOLLOW-UP: FOR OUTPATIENT TREATMENT
A. Advise patient to return to office for high fever >102° F (38.9° C), worsening shortness of breath, inability to swallow medications or keep down liquids, failure to improve after 2 days of antibiotics, chest pain, or hemoptysis
B. Consider admission for elderly patients with poor social support, alcoholics, psychiatric illnesses, homelessness, etc.
C. Follow-up CXR is not necessary: initial x-ray findings may take weeks—months to clear. However, follow-up x-ray may be advisable if any suspicion of underlying malignancy

VIII. PREVENTION
A. Pneumococcal polysaccharide antigen vaccine: Risk for acquiring complications of pneumonia is reduced by ²/₃ following vaccination
B. Influenza vaccine: Yearly for all patients at risk for pneumonia

CLINICAL PEARLS
- Pneumococcus remains the number–one agent of bacterial pneumonia in children and adults
- Think HIV; always check the mouth for thrush or oral hairy leukoplakia
- The presence of dementia or confusion in an elderly patient increases the likelihood ratio of a chest film being positive for pneumonia
- Treat early; delay in antibiotics is associated with increased mortality
- Treat empirically: gram stains are not helpful

References
Bernstein JM. Treatment of community-acquired pneumonia. IDSA guidelines. Chest Mar 1999:115:9S–13S.
Bartlett JG, Breiman RF, Mandell LA, et al. Community- acquired pneumonia in adults: Guidelines for management. Clin Infect Dis 1998;26:811–38.
Fine MJ, Auble TE, Yealy DM, et al. A prediction rule to identify low-risk patients with community-acquired pneumonia. N Engl J Med 1997;336(4):243–250.
Fine MJ, Hough LJ, Medsger AR, et al. The hospital admission decision for patients with community-acquired pneumonia. Results from the pneumonia Patient Outcomes Research Team cohort study. Arch Intern Med 1997;157(1):36–44.
Gleason PP, Kapoor WN, Stone RA, et al. Medical outcomes and antimicrobial costs with the use of the American Thoracic Society guidelines for outpatients with community-acquired pneumonia. JAMA 1997;278(1):32–9.

Daniel M. Neides, MD
Ann M. Aring, MD

46. OUTPATIENT MANAGEMENT OF ASTHMA

I. DEFINITION: Obstructive lung disease manifested by recurrent wheezing
  A. Obstruction is secondary to inflammation, mucosal edema, mucous hypersecretion, and smooth muscle contraction
  B. Asthmatic airways are hyperresponsive and airway inflammation increases this level of hyperresponsiveness

II. DIAGNOSIS
  A. Signs and symptoms
    1. Dyspnea, chest tightness or pain, cough, decreased exercise tolerance
    2. Wheezing, prolonged expiratory phase, tachypnea, tachycardia, use of accessory muscles, decreased intensity of breath sounds
    3. May also note nasal polyps, eczema, rhinorrhea, post-nasal drip
  B. Laboratory evaluation
    1. PFTs: Pre- and post-bronchodilator (spirometry and peak expiratory flow rates (PEFR))
    2. O_2 saturation: May need ABG if severe disease or to assess treatment

Clinical appearance	pH	PaO_2	$PaCO_2$
mild	increased	normal	decreased
moderate	normal	decreased	normal
severe	decreased	decreased	increased

    3. Consider CBC, chest x-ray, sinus x-ray, allergy testing

III. MANAGEMENT OF THE ADULT ASTHMATIC PATIENT

STEPWISE APPROACH FOR MANAGING ASTHMA IN ADULTS AND CHILDREN OVER 5 YEARS OLD

Goals of asthma treatment

- Prevent chronic and troublesome symptoms (e.g., coughing or breathlessness in the night, in the early morning, or after exertion)
- Maintain (near) "normal" pulmonary function
- Maintain normal activity levels (including exercise and other physical activity)
- Prevent recurrent exacerbations of asthma and minimize the need for emergency
- Provide optimal pharmacotherapy with minimal or no adverse effects
- Meet patients' and families' expectation of and satisfaction with asthma care

CARD

Classification of Severity: Clinical Features Before Treatment*

	Symptoms**	Lung Function	Long-Term Control (preferred treatments are in bold print)	Quick Relief (preferred treatments are in bold print)
STEP 4 Severe Persistent	• Continual symptoms • Limited physical activity • Frequent exacerbations • Frequent nighttime symptoms	FEV_1 or $PEF \leq 60\%$ predicted; PEF variability > 30%	Daily medications: • **Anti-inflammatory: inhaled cortico-steroid (high dose)** and • Long-acting bronchodilator; either long-acting inhaled $beta_2$-agonist, sustained-release theophylline, or long-acting $beta_2$-agonist tablets AND • Corticosteroid tablets or syrup long term (2mg/kg/day, generally do not exceed 60mg/day).	• Short-acting bronchodilator: **inhaled $beta_2$-agonists as needed for symptoms** • Intensity of treatment will depend on severity of exacerbation; see "Managing Exacerbations of Asthma" • Use of short-acting inhaled $beta_2$-agonists on a daily basis, or increasing use, indicates the need for additional long-term-control therapy.
STEP 3 Moderate Persistent	• Daily symptoms • Daily use of inhaled short-acting $beta_2$-agonist • Exacerbations effect activity • Exacerbations ≥ twice a week; may last days • Nighttime symptoms > once a week	FEV_1 or $PEF > 60\%$ $\leq 80\%$ predicted; PEF variability > 30%	Daily medication: • Either — **Anti-inflammatory: inhaled corticosteroid** (medium dose) OR — Inhaled corticosteroid (low-medium dose) and add a long-acting bronchodilator, especially for nighttime symptoms: either **long-acting inhaled $beta_2$-agonist,** sustained-release theophylline, or long-acting $beta_2$-agonist tablets. • If needed —Anti-inflammatory: inhaled corticosteroids (medium-high dose) AND — Long-acting bronchodilator, especially for nighttime symptoms; either **long-acting inhaled $beta_2$-agonist,** sustained-release theophylline, or long-acting $beta_2$-agonist tablets	• Short-acting bronchodilator: **inhaled $beta_2$-agonists as** needed for symptoms. • Intensity of treatment will depend on severity of exacerbation; see "Managing Exacerbations of Asthma" • Use of short-acting inhaled $beta_2$-agonists on a daily basis, or increasing use, indicates the need for additional long-term-control therapy.
STEP 2 Mild Persistent	• Symptoms > twice a week, but < once a day • Exacerbations may effect activity • Nighttime symptoms > twice a month	FEV_1 or $PEF \geq 80\%$ predicted; PEF variability 20–30%	Daily medication: • **Anti-inflammatory:** either **inhaled corticosteroid** (low doses) or **cromolyn or nedocromil** (children usually begin with a trial of cromolyn or nedocromyl) • Sustained-release theophylline to serum concentration of 5–15mcg/mL is an alternative. Zafirlukast or Zileuton may also be considered for patients ≥ 12 years of age, although their position in therapy is not fully established.	• Short-acting bronchodilator: **inhaled $beta_2$-agonists as** needed for symptoms. • Intensity of treatment will depend on severity of exacerbation; see "Managing Exacerbation of Asthma" • Use of short-acting inhaled $beta_2$-agonists on a daily basis, or increasing use, indicates the need for additional long-term-control therapy.
STEP 1 Mild Intermit-tent	• Symptoms ≤ twice a week • Asymptomatic and normal PEF between exacerbations • Exacerbations brief (from a few hours to a few days); intensity may vary • Nighttime symptoms ≤ twice a month	FEV_1 or $PEF \geq 80\%$ predicted; PEF variability < 20%	• No daily medication needed	• Short-acting bronchodilator: **inhaled $beta_2$-agonists as** needed for symptoms. • Intensity of treatment will depend on severity of exacerbation; see "Managing Exacerbation of Asthma" • Use of short-acting inhaled $beta_2$-agonists more than twice a week may indicate the need to initiate long-term therapy.

* The presence of one of the features of severity is sufficient to place a patient in that category. An individual should be assigned to the most severe grade in which any feature occurs. The characteristics noted in this figure are general and may overlap because asthma is highly variable. Furthermore, an individual's classification may change over time.
** Patients at any level of severity can have mild, moderate or severe exacerbations. Some patients with intermittent asthma experience severe and life-threatening exacerbations separated by long periods of normal lung function and no symptoms.

↓ Step down
  Review treatment every 1–6 months; a gradual stepwise reduction in treatment may be possible

↑ Step up
  If control is not maintained, consider step up. First, review patient medication technique, adherence, and environmental control (avoidance of allergens or other factors that contribute to asthma severity)

Notes:
• The stepwise approach presents general guidelines to assist clinical decision making; it is not intended to be a specific prescription. Asthma is highly variable; clinicians should tailor specific medication plans to the needs and circumstances of individual patients
• Gain control as quickly as possible; then decrease treatment to the least medication necessary to maintain control. Gaining control may be accomplished either by starting treatment at the step most appropriate to the initial severity of their condition or by starting at a higher level of therapy (e.g., a course of symptomatic corticosteroids or higher dose of inhaled corticosteroids)
• A rescue course of systemic corticosteroid may be needed at any time and at any step
• Some patients with intermittent asthma experience severe and life-threatening exacerbations separated

by long periods of normal lung function and no symptoms. This may be especially common with exacerbations provoked by respiratory infections. A short course of systemic corticosteroids is recommended
- At each step, patients should control their environment to avoid or control factors that make their asthma worse (e.g, allergens, irritants); this requires specific diagnosis and education
- Referral to an asthma specialist for consultation or co-management is recommended if there are difficulties achieving or maintaining control of asthma or if the patient requires step 4 care. Referral may be considered if the patient requires step 3 care (see also component 1 — Initial Assessment and Diagnosis)

Adapted from the NIH Guidelines for the diagnosis and management of asthma, 1997

IV. MANAGEMENT OF THE PEDIATRIC ASTHMATIC PATIENT

STEPWISE APPROACH FOR MANAGING INFANTS AND YOUNG CHILDREN (5 YEARS OLD AND YOUNGER) WITH ACUTE OR CHRONIC ASTHMA SYMPTOMS

Classification of Severity: Clinical Features Before Treatment*

	Symptoms**	Long-Term Control	Quick Relief
STEP 4 Severe Persistent	• Continual symptoms • Limited physical activity • Frequent exacerbations • Frequent nighttime symptoms	Daily anti-inflammatory medicine — High-dose inhaled corticosteroid with spacer/holding chamber and face mask — If needed, add systemic corticosteroids 2mg/kg/day and reduce to lowest daily or alternate-day dose that stabilizes symptoms	Bronchodilator as needed for symptoms (see step 1) up to 3 times a day
STEP 3 Moderate Persistent	• Daily symptoms • Daily use of inhaled short-acting beta$_2$-agonist • Exacerbations effect activity • Exacerbations ≥ twice a week; may last days • Nighttime symptoms > once a week	Daily antiinflammatory medication. Either: — Medium-dose inhaled corticosteroid with spacer/holding chamber and face mask OR, once control is established: — Medium-dose inhaled corticosteroid and Nedocromil OR: — Medium-dose inhaled corticosteroid and long-acting bronchodilator (theophylline)	Bronchodilator as needed for symptoms (see step 1) up to 3 times a day
STEP 2 Mild Persistent	• Symptoms > twice a week, but < once a day • Exacerbations may effect activity • Nighttime symptoms > twice a month	Daily anti-inflammatory medication. Either: — Cromolyn (nebulizer is preferred; or MDI) or Nedocromil (MDI only) TID–QID — Infants and young children usually begin with a trial of Cromolyn or Nedocromil OR — Low-dose inhaled corticosteroid with spacer/holding chamber and face mask	Bronchodilator as needed for symptoms (see step 1)
STEP 1 Mild Intermittent	• Symptoms ≤ twice a week • Asymptomatic and normal PEF between exacerbations • Exacerbations brief (from a few hours to a few days); intensity may vary • Nighttime symptoms ≤ twice a month	• No daily medicine needed	• Bronchodilator as needed for symptoms < twice a week. Intensity of treatment will depend on severity of exacerbation. Either: — Inhaled short-acting beta$_2$-agonist by nebulizer or face mask and spacer/holding chamber OR: — Oral beta$_2$-agonist for symptoms • With viral respiratory infection: — Bronchodilator Q 4–6 hours up to 24 hours (longer with physician consult) but, in general, repeat no more than once every 6 weeks — Consider systemic corticosteroid • If current exacerbation is severe OR: • If patient has history of previous severe exacerbations.

* The presence of one of the features of severity is sufficient to place a patient in that category. An individual should be assigned to the most severe grade in which any feature occurs. The characteristics noted in this figure are general and may overlap because asthma is highly variable. Furthermore, an individual's classification may change over time.

** Patients at any level of severity can have mild, moderate or severe exacerbations. Some patients with intermittent asthma experience severe and life-threatening exacerbations separated by long periods of normal lung function and no symptoms.

CARD

↓ Step down
Review treatment every 1–6 months. If control is sustained for at least 3 months, a gradual stepwise reduction in treatment may be possible

↑ Step up
If control is not achieved, consider step up. But first: review patient medication technique, adherence, and environmental control (avoidance of allergens or other precipitant factors)

Notes:
• Gain control as quickly as possible; then decrease treatment to the least medication necessary to maintain control. Gaining control may be accomplished by either starting treatment at the step most appropriate to the initial severity of their condition or by starting at a higher level of therapy (e.g., a course of systemic corticosteroids or higher dose of inhaled corticosteroids)
• A rescue course of systemic corticosteroid (Prednisolone) may be needed at any time and step
• In general, use of short-acting β_2-agonist > 3–4 times in 1 day or regular use on a daily basis indicates the need for additional therapy
• It is important to remember that there are very few studies on asthma therapy for infants
• The stepwise approach presents guidelines to assist clinical decision making. Asthma is highly variable; clinicians should tailor specific medication plans to the needs and circumstances of individual patients
• Consultation with an asthma specialist is recommended for patients in this age group requiring step 3 or step 4 care. Consider consultation for patients in this age group requiring step 2 care

Adapted from the NIH Guidelines for the diagnosis and management of asthma, 1997.

V. TREATMENT OPTIONS
A. Nonpharmacologic
    1. Educating patients and families is essential; their understanding of the disease and recognition of warning signs allows early intervention
    2. Avoidance of known allergens or other irritants: Tobacco smoke, cold air, strong odors or fumes, keeping pets out of bedroom
    3. Immunotherapy (if strong allergic component)
        a. Understanding asthma as *Increased Airway Hyperreactivity* yields a new therapeutic approach to treating and preventing exacerbations, not only relieving immediate symptoms
        b. Regular use of anti-inflammatory agents reduces the need for bronchodilators and decreases the airway's response to viruses, allergens, and irritants
        c. Avoid allergens by removing pets and/or stuffed animals from the home (or at least the bedroom) and *avoid cigarette smoke*
        d. Consider chronic sinusitis, allergies, and reflux as clinical conditions that may increase airway hyperreactivity
        e. Avoid ß-blockers and NSAIDs
        f. The patient should use a *peak flow meter* as an objective measure of disease control
B. Pharmacologic
    1. **Anti-inflammatory agents**
        a. Corticosteroids (oral or inhaled)—Act by reducing inflammation
            i. Long-term side effects of oral steroids include osteoporosis, hypertension, cataracts, Cushing's syndrome, immunosuppression. Thrush is common with inhaled steroids and can be avoided by rinsing mouth after use
            ii. Inhaled: Beclomethasone (Vanceril, Beclovent), Triamcinolone (Azmacort), Fluticasone (Flovent), others
            iii. Oral—**Prednisone** or **Prednisolone**: 1–2mg/kg/day (maximum 40–60mg QD)
            iv. Oral steroids are usually given for 3–5 days for an exacerbation of asthma. Tapering is unnecessary if used in short bursts (3–5 days) but may be needed for persistent symptoms or frequent exacerbations. A 10–14 day tapered course of oral steroids should be considered if the patient has moderate to severe asthma or has frequent exacerbations
        b. **Cromolyn Sodium (Intal)** or **Nedocromil Sodium (Tilade)**
            i. Act by decreasing airway hypersensitivity, inhibiting mast cell degranulation and inhibiting early and late asthmatic responses

ii. Side effects: None. Allow *4–6* week trial to determine effectiveness

iii. Dose: MDI (1mg/puff) 2 puffs BID–QID
> Dry powder inhaler (20mg/capsule) 1 capsule BID–QID
> Nebulizer solution (20mg/2mL ampule) 1 ampule BID–QID

2. **Bronchodilating agents:** Morbidity results from failure to recognize and treat asthma exacerbations:
   - Regular use of bronchodilators may exacerbate the airway hyperreactivity that exists in all asthmatics. Patients who escalate use of bronchodilators during acute exacerbations gain only temporary relief of symptoms and have a false sense of disease control. This has led to an *increased mortality* from asthma
   - Determine how often bronchodilators are used and recognize that increased use may reflect a deterioration of control and should call for an initiation or increase in anti-inflammatory therapy

   a. β_2**-agonists (Albuterol, Metaproterenol):** Act by relaxing smooth muscle. Provide symptomatic relief but do not alter disease state. Useful for prevention of exercise-induced asthma
      i. Inhaled
         aa. Metered dose inhaler (MDI)
            Albuterol (Proventil, Ventolin), Metaproterenol (Alupent): 2 puffs Q4–6hrs
            Salmeterol (long-acting): 2 puffs Q12hrs (For long-term maintenance treatment, should not be used for acute exacerbation)
         bb. Dry powder inhaler
            1. **Serevent Diskus:** 1 inhalation Q12hrs (for long-term maintenance treatment only)
            2. **Ventolin Rotacap:** 1 capsule Q4–6hrs
         cc. Nebulizer
            Albuterol (5mg/mL): 1.25–5mg in 2mL saline Q4–6hrs. Maximum adult dose is 5mg
            Metaproterenol (50mg/mL): 10–15mg in 2mL saline Q4–6hrs. Maximum adult dose is 15mg
            Note: MDIs are technically difficult to use. Spacers are recommended
      ii. Oral
         aa. **Albuterol:** Liquid 0.1–0.15mg/kg Q4–6hrs; tablets (2, 4mg) 1 tab Q4–6hrs (liquid, 2mg/5cc)
         bb. **Metaproterenol:** Liquid 0.3–0.5mg/kg Q4–6hrs; tablets (10, 20mg) 1 tab Q4–6hrs (liquid 10mg/5cc)

   b. **Theophylline:** Acts by inhibiting breakdown of cAMP by phosphodiesterase and improving diaphragmatic and respiratory muscle contractility. Use with caution in patients with CHF or hepatic failure
      i. Cimetidine, antibiotics (Erythromycin), and anti-convulsants decrease elimination and may increase toxicity
      ii. Side effects: Nausea/vomiting, headache, tachycardia, arrythmias, or seizures
      iii. Dose: Available in liquid, tablets and capsules. Dose given should achieve the therapeutic window of *5–15mcg/mL*

3. **Leukotriene inhibitors:** Act by inhibiting chemical mediators LTC4, LTD4, LTE4 in the arachidonic acid pathway. These chemical mediators are known to be responsible for bronchoconstriction, mucus secretion, inflammatory cell infiltration and microvascular permeability
   a. **Zafirlukast (Accolate):** LTD4 receptor antagonist
      i. Dose: 20mg PO BID 1hr before or 2hrs after in adults and children over 12 years of age
      ii. Drug interactions: Warfarin concentration is increased. Terfenadine, Theophylline, and Erythromycin decrease Zafirlukast serum concentrations
      iii. Side effects: Gastrointestinal disturbances, headache, increased aminotransferase activity. Churg-Strauss syndrome has occurred rarely
   b. **Zileuton (Zyflo):** Blocks 5-lipoxygenase
      i. Dose: 600mg PO QID for adults and children more than age 12
      ii. Drug interactions: Theophylline, Warfarin, Propranolol, Terfenadine decrease elimination and may increase toxicity

iii. Side effects: Increased ALT 5% patients, headache, dyspepsia, nausea

c. **Montelukast (Singulair)**

i. Dose: ages 2–5, 4mg chewable tab PO QD in the evening

ages 6–14, 5mg chewable tab PO QD in the evening

> age 15— adult: 10mg tab PO QD in the evening

ii. Drug interactions: Phenobarbital or Rifampin may increase Montelukast elimination

iii. Side effects: fatigue, fever, dyspepsia, gastroenteritis, headache, dizziness, and rash

4. HOME TREATMENT

MANAGEMENT OF ASTHMA EXACERBATIONS: HOME TREATMENT

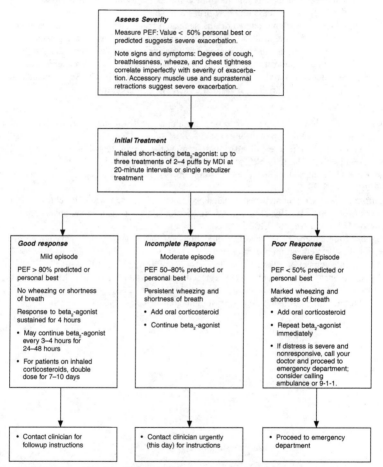

Assess Severity

Measure PEF: Value < 50% personal best or predicted suggests severe exacerbation.

Note signs and symptoms: Degrees of cough, breathlessness, wheeze, and chest tightness correlate imperfectly with severity of exacerbation. Accessory muscle use and suprasternal retractions suggest severe exacerbation.

Initial Treatment

Inhaled short-acting beta$_2$-agonist: up to three treatments of 2–4 puffs by MDI at 20-minute intervals or single nebulizer treatment

Good response	*Incomplete Response*	*Poor Response*
Mild episode	Moderate episode	Severe Episode
PEF > 80% predicted or personal best	PEF 50–80% predicted or personal best	PEF < 50% predicted or personal best
No wheezing or shortness of breath	Persistent wheezing and shortness of breath	Marked wheezing and shortness of breath
Response to beta$_2$-agonist sustained for 4 hours	• Add oral corticosteroid	• Add oral corticosteroid
• May continue beta$_2$-agonist every 3–4 hours for 24–48 hours	• Continue beta$_2$-agonist	• Repeat beta$_2$-agonist immediately
• For patients on inhaled corticosteroids, double dose for 7–10 days		• If distress is severe and nonresponsive, call your doctor and proceed to emergency department; consider calling ambulance or 9-1-1.
• Contact clinician for followup instructions	• Contact clinician urgently (this day) for instructions	• Proceed to emergency department

Adapted from the NIH Guidelines for the diagnosis and management of asthma, 1997.

VI. PEAK EXPIRATORY FLOW RATE (PEFR) MONITORING

Useful to monitor treatment in patients with moderate to severe asthma

A. Frequency

1. During acute exacerbations, patients ideally should measure PEFR before and after bronchodilator therapy BID

2. Once asthma is under control, patients can monitor PEFR 2–3 times/week

B. Proper measurement

1. Patients > age 5 can perform PEFR

2. Instructions should be given and the patient should practice prior to leaving the office

    3. The patient should perform the process 3 times (with each measurement) and record the *highest number achieved*

C. Interpretation

    1. Predicted values are based on height and age

    2. PEFR values analogous to stop light:

        a. Green light: PEFR is more than 80% patient's personal best

        b. Yellow light: PEFR is 50–80% patient's personal best

        c. Red light: PEFR is below 50% patient's personal best. The physician should be notified

CLINICAL PEARLS

- The incidence of asthma and morbidity and mortality are *increasing* despite our understanding of the disease and new drugs available
- Risk factors of asthma-related deaths: teenager, black race, underestimation of symptoms, poor access to medical care, depression, and previous life-threatening asthma attack
- Physicians can decrease morbidity by educating patients about asthma and asthma medications
- Long acting β_2-agonists (Salmeterol) should not be used for acute exacerbations
- Inhaled steroid is first line therapy followed by ß-agonist PRN. Use Serevent and leukotriene inhibitors, Theophylline, if needed to achieve good control

References

Harding SM, et al. 24-h esophageal pH testing in asthmatics. Respiratory symptom correlation with esophageal acid events. Chest 1999;115:654–9.

Kemp JP, et al. Therapeutic effect of zafirlukast as monotherapy in steroid-naive patients with severe persistent asthma. Chest 1999;115:336–42.

Lockey RF, et al. Nocturnal asthma. Effect of salmeterol on quality of life and clinical outcomes. Chest 1999; 115:666–73.

Malmstrom K, et al. Oral montelukast, inhaled beclomethasone, and placebo for chronic asthma. Ann Intern Med March 16, 1999;130:487–95, and Smith LJ. Newer asthma therapies [Editorial]. Ann Intern Med March 16, 1999;130:531–2.

Highlights of the expert panel report 2: guidelines for the diagnosis and management of asthma. National asthma education program. Bethesda, MD. NIH Pub. No. 97–4051A; May 1997.

Moffitt JE. Management of asthma in children. Am Fam Phys 1994;50:1039–50.

Podell RN. National guidelines for the management of asthma in adults. Am Fam Phys 1992;46:1189–95.

Barnes PJ. Current therapies for asthma. Chest 1997;11(2):17S–26S.

Hay DW. Pharmacology of leukotriene receptor antagonists. Chest 1997;11(2):35S–45S.

CARD

47. CHRONIC OBSTRUCTIVE PULMONARY DISEASE (COPD)

DEFINITION: Classically defined as asthma, chronic bronchitis and emphysema. This section will focus on chronic bronchitis and emphysema

I. HISTORY

Patients commonly have a long history of cigarette smoking, cough and increased sputum production (chronic bronchitis), and dyspnea (emphysema). **Chronic bronchitis** is defined as *productive cough for 3 months or more in 2 consecutive years without another explanation.* **Emphysema** is characterized as having abnormal, permanent enlargement or air spaces distal to the terminal bronchiole with destruction of their walls and without obvious fibrosis

II. PHYSICAL EXAMINATION

Increased A-P diameter, decreased lung sounds, prolonged expiration, dyspnea at rest, pursed lip breathing, periorbital cyanosis, use of accessory muscles to breath, rales and rhonchi. Pink puffer (emphysema) vs. blue bloater (chronic bronchitis)

III. CHEST X-RAY

Shows flattening of diaphragms, increased lung volumes, bullae and blebs, small heart (secondary to vertical orientation), increased retrosternal clear space

IV. LABORATORY

A. ABG: Useful for patients suspected of having moderate to severe lung disease

B. α-1 antitrypsin levels: Obtain if patient presents with emphysema at < age 50 or if there is a family history of early onset emphysema

V. PULMONARY FUNCTION TESTING

Perform spirometry and/or DLCO and lung volumes in selected patients

VI. MANAGEMENT OF COPD*

The management should follow a step-care approach starting with Steps I and II (usually used concurrently)

A. STEP I: Smoking cessation (See Chapter 32, Smoking Cessation)

B. STEP II: Bronchodilators: *First line therapy* is **Ipratropium Bromide** MDI (metered dose inhaler). If this is unsuccessful then consider adding a ß$_2$-agonist MDI. If unsuccessful, an oral **Methylxanthine** may be added in selected patients

  1. **Ipratropium Bromide MDI (Atrovent)** 2 puffs QID: Not to exceed 12 puffs per day. Agent of choice in COPD as there is almost no systemic absorption. Patients must be instructed on MDI use. Peak effect occurs in 1½–2hrs, therefore must be used on a continuous basis

  2. β$_2$-adrenergic agonists: *Second line.* Usually will be added to **Ipratropium**

    a. **Albuterol MDI (Proventil, Ventolin):** 1–2 puffs Q4–6hrs

    b. **Albuterol** nebulized solution **(Ventolin nebules):** 2.5mg TID–QID

    c. **Metaproterenol MDI (Alupent, Metaprel):** 2–3 puffs Q3–4hrs

    d. **Metaproterenol** nebulized solution **(Alupent, Metaprel inhalant solution):** 0.2–0.3mL of 5% solution in 2.5mL of normal saline TID–QID

    e. **Pirbuterol MDI (Maxair):** 2 puffs every 4–6hrs

    f. **Terbutaline MDI (Brethaire):** 2 puffs every 4–6hrs

    g. **Salmeterol (Serevent)** MDI or diskus for long-term maintenance therapy, 2 puffs Q12h only

  3. **Combination Ipratropium** (21mcg) and **Albuterol** (120mcg)—**Combivent Inhaler,** Dose: 2 puffs QID, max 12 puffs/24hrs

  4. **Oral Methylxanthine:** For use in selected patients. Target Theophylline levels should be *10–15µg/mL* to minimize side effects

CARD

     a. **Theophylline** immediate release tablets: 10mg/kg/day in 4 divided doses

     b. **Theophylline** sustained release tablets: 10mg/kg/day in 1–3 doses

C. STEP III: Corticosteroids: Should be used concurrently with Step II if patient has not shown sufficient improvement with Step II approach

  1. Give trial of oral corticosteroid: **Prednisone** 40mg PO QD for 7–14 days

     a. If there is no improvement in FEV_1 (at least 20–30%) then discontinue steroid without tapering and continue bronchodilator therapy

     b. If there is an improvement, then taper to the lowest possible dosage and switch to an inhaled corticosteroid

  2. Inhaled steroids: Are less helpful in patients with COPD than asthma. If there is no improvement on inhaled corticosteroid, then consider switching back to PO corticosteroid

     a. **Beclomethasone (Beclovent, Vanceril):** MDI 2 puffs BID–QID

     b. **Flunisolide (Aerobid):** MDI 2 puffs BID

     c. **Triamcinolone (Azmacort):** MDI 2 puffs BID–QID

D. Adjunctive therapy: Consider use of mucolytic-expectorant as adjunct to chronic or acute COPD if the history suggests thick or viscous sputum or difficulty with expectoration. Examples are **Iodinated Glycerol** 60mg PO QID and **Guaifenesin (Robitussin, Humibid LA)** 1–2 PO BID

* Source: Adapted from Bone MD, Roger C. A step-care approach to managing COPD. J Resp Diseases, 1991; 12(8):727–40. Used with permission.

VII. VACCINATIONS

  A. Influenza vaccine: Annually

  B. Pneumococcal vaccine: Perform once; if given ≥5 years ago when patient ≤ age 65, then repeat

VIII. INDICATIONS FOR SUPPLEMENTAL OXYGEN

  Goal: PaO_2 60–80mm Hg

  A. Resting PaO_2 ≤ 55mm Hg or O_2 saturation ≤ 89% at rest, with exercise or during sleep

  B. PaO_2 56–59mm Hg with concurrent cor pulmonale or polycythemia or CHF

IX. PULMONARY REHABILITATION

  Shown to decrease hospital admissions and increase quality of life. No change in mortality

X. AMBULATORY MANAGEMENT OF ACUTE EXACERBATIONS

  See Chapter 48, Bronchitis, under Part Two (Acute Exacerbation of Chronic Bronchitis)

CLINICAL PEARLS

    • For patients requiring chronic oral corticosteroids, remember to monitor them for osteoporosis and DM

References

Freidman M, et al. Pharmacoeconomic evaluation of a combination of ipratropium plus albuterol compared with ipratropium alone and albuterol alone in COPD. Chest Mar 1999;115:635–41.

Iqbal F, et al. Declining bone mass in men with chronic pulmonary disease. Chest 1999;116:1616–24.

Celli BR. Standards for the optimal management of COPD: A summary. Chest 1998;113:283s.

Fein AM. Lung volume reduction surgery: Answering the crucial questions. Chest 1998;113:277S.

Heath JM, Mangia R. Chronic bronchitis: primary care management. Am Fam Phys 1998;57:2365–72.

Nieferman MS. Mechanisms and management of COPD. Chest 1998;113:233S

Ferguson GT, Cherniak RM. Management of chronic obstructive pulmonary disease. N Engl J Med 1993;328:1017–22.

Bone MD, Roger C. A step-care approach to managing COPD. J Resp Diseases, 1991;12(8):727–40.

Diane Minasian, MD
Daniel M. Neides, MD

48. ACUTE BRONCHITIS / EXACERBATIONS OF CHRONIC BRONCHITIS

— PART ONE: ACUTE BRONCHITIS—

DEFINITION: An inflammatory condition of the tracheobronchial tree

I. ETIOLOGY
  A. **Viral** (most common): Influenza A & B, parainfluenza, RSV, adenovirus, and rhinovirus
  B. **Bacterial:** *Mycoplasma pneumoniæ, Chlamydia pneumoniæ, Moraxella catarrhalis, Bordetella pertussis,* or *Legionella pneumophila*
  • Cigarette smokers are predisposed to the development of acute bronchitis secondary to direct injury to airway epithelium, less cilia present, and delayed mucociliary clearance; smokers also tend to have infections that are more frequent, more severe, and last longer

II. CLINICAL FEATURES
  Symptoms may vary depending on etiologic agent and host factors including age of host and coexisting pulmonary disease (asthma or COPD) and whether the patient smokes
  A. **Cough:** May have sputum production as well; usually has persisted longer than usual course following a URI
  B. **Chest congestion and substernal chest pain**
  C. **Fever**
  Note: Chills, myalgias, dyspnea and fatigue are uncommon complaints and if present may suggest pneumonia

III. DIAGNOSIS
  Usually based on symptoms and physical examination
  A. Lung examination may reveal diffuse wheezing, but in general is without other adventitial sounds
  B. Do not culture sputum, as the majority of cases will have a viral etiology

IV. TREATMENT: SYMPTOMATIC (See Chapter 116, Symptomatic Medications)
  A. **Albuterol (Proventil, Ventolin) MDI:** 2 puffs QID
  B. **Cough suppression:** A codeine-based antitussive will help; if daytime sedation is a concern, **Tessalon Perles** 1 PO TID PRN or **Dextromethorphan**/expectorant (e.g., **Robitussin DM** 5–10mL Q4h PRN) is a good alternative
  C. **Expectorants/Mucolytics:** Widely prescribed but probably do not alter the course of the disease
  D. **Adequate hydration**
  E. **Encourage smoking cessation**
  Note: If symptoms persist longer than 7–10 days, consider treating for a bacterial etiology:
  Erythromycin 250mg PO QID × 10 days

— PART TWO —
ACUTE EXACERBATION OF CHRONIC BRONCHITIS

DEFINITION: Chronic bronchitis is the presence of a productive cough 3 months of the year for 2 consecutive years, excluding other causes of chronic sputum production (TB, bronchiectasia) often associated with cigarette smoking

I. ETIOLOGY
  A. **Viral** (50% of acute exacerbations): Influenza A & B, parainfluenza, RSV, rhinovirus, coronavirus
  B. **Bacterial:** *Streptococcus pneumoniæ, Hemophilus influenzæ* (non-typeable), *Moraxella catarrhalis, Chlamydia pneumoniæ*
  • Bacterial colonization of the tracheobronchial tree is usually a pre-existing feature of chronic bronchitis

II. CLINICAL FEATURES
  A. Persistent cough

B. Change in amount, color, and consistency of sputum
C. Worsening dyspnea and fatigue
  • Note: Hemoptysis is rare. Fever and chills are less commonly seen and suggest the possibility of pneumonia

III. DIAGNOSIS
Usually a clinical diagnosis based on symptoms and physical exam
A. Gram stain of sputum is usually not helpful secondary to bacterial colonization of the tracheobronchial tree
B. A chest x-ray may be beneficial if ruling out an underlying pneumonia or if the symptoms persist despite adequate treatment (consider lung cancer a possibility)

IV. TREATMENT
A. Adequate hydration
B. Antibiotics: Since a bacterial etiology is seen in many cases, antibiotics are indicated (see below)
C. Mucolytics (**Organidin:** 60mg PO QID)
D. Postural drainage to clear secretions
E. Consider oral steroids (**Prednisone:** 40mg PO QD × 5 days)
F. β_2-agonists (**Proventil inhaler**)
G. Ipatropium Bromide (Atrovent)
H. Smoking cessation
Note: Hospitalization should be based on the degree of respiratory distress. Most patients can be treated as outpatients

V. ANTIBIOTICS FOR ACUTE EXACERBATION OF CHRONIC BRONCHITIS
A. First line agents
  Trimethoprim-Sulfamethoxazole (Bactrim, Septra): 1 DS tablet PO BID × 10 days
  Doxycycline: 100mg PO BID × 10 days
B. Second line agents
  Amoxicillin-Clavulanate (Augmentin): 500mg PO TID × 10 days
  Azithromycin (Zithromax): 500mg PO day #1, then 250mg PO QD × 4 days
  Clarithromycin (Biaxin): 500mg PO BID × 10 days
  Cefuroxime (Ceftin): 250–500mg PO BID × 10 days
  Loracarbef (Lorabid): 400mg PO BID × 7 days
  Levofloxacin (Levaquin): 500mg PO QD × 7 days
  Gatifloxacin (Tequin): 400mg PO QD × 7–10 days

VI. PREVENTIVE MEDICINE
A. Pneumococcal vaccine once; repeat if initially given ≥ 5 years ago and patient ≤ age 65
B. Influenza vaccine every year
C. Smoking cessation

CLINICAL PEARLS
  • Pertussis, which can be confirmed by nasopharyngeal cultures, should be considered in adolescents and adults with a prolonged cough
  • A PPD skin test to rule out TB is indicated in a patient with persistent respiratory symptoms
  • Most cases of acute bronchitis are viral in origin. One study (a meta-analysis of 9 randomized, controlled, double blind studies) found the number needed to treat (NNT) patient was 18. The NNT to cause 1 additional effect was 14

References
Gonzales R, et al. The relation between purulent manifestations and antibiotic treatment of upper respiratory tract infections. J Gen Intern Med 1999;14(3):151.
Gonzales R, et al. Factors associated with antibiotic use for acute bronchitis. J Gen Intern Med Aug 1998;13:541.
O'Brian K, et al. Cough illness/bronchitis: principles of judicious use of antimicrobial agents. Pediatrics 101 Jan 1998;101(1 Suppl):178.
Smucny JJ, et al. Are antibiotics effective treatment for acute bronchitis? A meta-analysis. J Fam Pract- ice Dec 1998;47(6):453.
Griffith DE, Kronenberg RS. Chronic bronchitis: choosing the optimal treatment. Postgrad Med 1993;94(8):93–100.
Orr PH, et al. Randomized placebo controlled trials of antibiotics for acute bronchitis: a critical review of the literature. J Fam Practice 1993;36(5):507–12.

VI. Management of Common Ambulatory Conditions

GEN

Steve Markovich, MD
Daniel M. Neides, MD
Rugen Alda, MD

49. MANAGEMENT OF DIABETES MELLITUS

I. GENERAL
A. Currently 20 million people in the U.S. will have a form of diabetes mellitus, and only about ½ are diagnosed
B. By the year 2010, the number of people with diabetes worldwide will double. The increased prevalence of diabetes mellitus in the United States stems largely from an increase in type 2 diabetes, which is a result of an aging population, an increasing prevalence of obesity, and a more sedentary population
C. Control of blood sugar decreases complications in both Type 1 and Type 2 diabetes
D. In the U.S., it is has been estimated that $100 billion, or 1 out of every 7 health care dollars, is spent on patients with diabetes

	Type 1 — IDDM	Type 2 — NIDDM
Age of onset	Usually Type 1 < 30 yr.	Usually Type 2 > 40 yr.
Ketosis	Common	Rare
Body weight	Nonobese	Obese (80%)
Prevalence	0.2–0.3%	2–4%
Genetics		
HLA association	Yes	No
Monozygotic twin studies	Concordance rate 40–50%	Concordance rate near 100%
Associated other autoimmune diseases	Occasional	No
Treatment with insulin	Always	Sometimes
Insulin secretion	Severe deficiency	Variable; mild-moderate deficiency to hyperinsulinemia
Insulin resistance	Less common	Usually

II. SUGGESTIVE SYMPTOMS
A. Symptoms of marked hyperglycemia include polyuria, polydipsia, polyphagia, weight loss, fatigue, abdominal pain, reactive hypoglycemia, myopia, recurrent vaginitis or urinary tract infection and hyperesthesia (burning feet).
B. Impairment of growth and susceptibility to certain infections may also accompany chronic hyperglycemia

III. CLINICAL PICTURE
A. **Type 1 Insulin-dependent diabetes mellitus (IDDM)**
    1. Uncomplicated onset: Progressive osmotic diuresis causes dehydration, thirst, and if glucose losses are extensive, weight loss despite polyphagia. In children, the onset of these symptoms often occurs over a short period
    2. Acute decompensation: Diabetic Ketoacidosis (DKA)
B. **Type 2 Non-insulin-dependent diabetes mellitus (NIDDM)**
    1. Uncomplicated onset: Most patients are asymptomatic and the diagnosis is made by the detection of hyperglycemia or glycosuria on routine exam
    2. Acute decompensation: Nonketotic hyperosmolar coma (a syndrome of extreme hyperglycemia and dehydration). Hyperosmolar coma most frequently occurs in older patients in whom an intercurrent illness increases glucose production secondary to stress hormones and impairs the capacity to ingest fluids

IV. TESTING AND DIAGNOSIS

A. The gold standard for making the diagnosis of DM is a fasting (8hrs) plasma glucose >126mg/dL on at least 2 occasions

B. American Diabetes Association: Clinical Practice Recommendations 2000

1. Suggested criteria for testing for diabetes in the asymptomatic, undiagnosed individual

---

Table 6 — *Criteria for testing for diabetes in asymptomatic, undiagnosed individuals*

1. Testing for diabetes should be considered in all individuals at age 45 years and above and, if normal, it should be repeated at 3-year intervals.
2. Testing should be considered at a younger age or be carried out more frequently in individuals who:
   - are obese (≥ 120% desirable body weight or a BMI ≥ 27 kg/m²)
   - have a first-degree relative with diabetes
   - are members of a high-risk ethic population (e.g. African-American, Hispanic-American, Native American, Asian-American, Pacific Islander)
   - have delivered a baby weighing > 9 lb or have been diagnosed with GDM
   - are hypertensive (≥ 140/90)
   - have a HDL cholesterol level ≤ 35 mg/dL (0.90 mmol/L) and/or a triglyceride level ≥ 250 mg/dL (2.82 mmol/L)
   - on previous testing, had IGT or IFG

The OGTT or FPG test may be used to diagnose diabetes, however, in clinical settings the FPG test is greatly preferred because of ease of administration, convenience, acceptability to patients, and lower cost.

---

2. Suggested criteria for diagnosis of diabetes mellitus

Table 3 — *Criteria for diagnosis of diabetes mellitus*

1. Symptoms of diabetes plus casual plasma glucose concentration ≥ 200 mg/dL (11.1 mmol/L). Casual is defined as any time of day without regard to time since last meal . The classic symptoms of diabetes include polyuria, polydipsia, and unexplained weight loss.

or

2. FPG ≥ 126 mg/dL (7.0 mmol/L). Fasting is defined as no caloric intake for at least 8h.

or

3. 2-h PG ≥ 200 mg/dL (11.1mmol/L) during an OGTT. The test should be performed as described by WHO (2), using a glucose load containing the equivalent of 75-g anhydrous glucose dissolved in water.

In the absence of unequivocal hyperglycemia with acute metabolic decompensation, these criteria should be confirmed by repeat testing on a different day. The third measure (OGTT) is not recommended for routine clinical use.

Source: American Diabetes Association: Clinical Practice Recommendations 2000. Report of The Expert Committee on the Diagnosis and Classification of Diabetes Mellitus. Diabetes Care Jan 2000; 23 (Suppl. 1):S4–S19, Tables 3 & 6. Copyright© 2000, American Diabetes Association.

Note: HgbA1C is not recommended for diagnosis

C. Gestational diabetes see Chapter 15, Prenatal Care, IV. C.

V. TREATMENT

A. Goals

1. Blood glucose levels
   a. Ideal 80–120mg/dL, up to 140 in the elderly or those at risk of hypoglycemia
   b. Postprandial hyperglycemic peak 100–160mg/dL
2. Achieve and maintain normal weight
   a. Ideal body weight (IBW) for women=100 lbs + 5 lbs/inch over 5 feet tall
   b. Ideal body weight (IBW) for men=106 lbs + 6 lbs/inch over 5 feet tall
3. Avoid hypoglycemia
4. Enjoy a "modified" normal lifestyle—consider the patient's health care beliefs, education level, cultural background, support system, and financial circumstance

GEN

    5. Minimize complications: HTN, hyperlipidemia, albuminuria, retinopathy, neuropathy, nephropathy, CAD, PVD (see section VIII)

B. Diet
1. Caloric requirements can be estimated by multiplying IBW × 10
2. Arrange a consultation with a dietician if available
3. Follow guidelines established by the American Diabetes Association (ADA) for caloric restriction
4. Reassure patients that weight loss may decrease the need for medication

C. Exercise
1. An EKG stress test is recommended before prescribing a vigorous exercise program
2. Exercise helps with glycemic control. Diabetics should try to exercise 20–30 minutes 3 × /week
3. Patients requiring insulin should be warned of the danger of exercise-induced hypoglycemia. Insulin or medication requirements may decrease with exercise
4. Careful monitoring of blood glucose levels before and after exercise is essential

D. Glucose monitoring: Essential in Type 1 and Type 2 DM although the frequency on monitoring will differ
1. Finger stick (capillary glucose) most helpful although they can be expensive
2. Check AC and HS in new diabetics, when adjusting medications or insulin
3. The patient should be educated on the use of the home monitor and it should be regularly checked for proper calibration
4. If the patient is uncomfortable performing the finger stick, an alternative is to monitor their urine for glucose and ketones. This is somewhat inaccurate and is not quantitative
5. Monitor control over the last 2–3 months via HgbA1C (Glycosylated hemoglobin). Goal is < 8%, optimal is < 7% while avoiding symptomatic hypoglycemia
    a. 4.5–6.4%: Normal
    b. 6.4–7.5%: Excellent control
    c. 7.5–8.5%: Very good control
    d. 8.5–10%: Fair control
    e. >10%: Poor control

E. Examination (See section IX, diabetic flowchart)
1. Every 3 months check BP, urine dip, foot exam, HgbA1C, review BS records
2. Every year perform a complete physical, funduscopic exam (or referral), Chem 12, and lipid profile
3. Every 2–3 years check a thyroid panel
4. Maintain BP<135/85

VI. ORAL MEDICATIONS USED IN THE TREATMENT OF TYPE 2 DIABETES

A. Sulfonylureas (1ˢᵗ and 2ⁿᵈ Generation):
1. **Mechanism of action:** Increase insulin production in response to glucose and increase tissue sensitivity by increasing receptors. Typically lowers fasting plasma glucose by 60–70mg/dL and the HgbA1C by 1.5%–2%
2. **Complications and contraindications:** Hypoglycemia is the most common and severe side effect. Another potential side effect of sulfonylureas is worsening myocardial ischemia or damage during an acute ischemic event, when energy sensitive potassium channels must open to dilate the coronary arteries and increase intracellular energy levels. Other side effects include weight gain, hemolytic anemia, skin rashes, headache, blurred vision, and dizziness. Chlorpropamide has been shown to induce a disulfiram-like reaction, reversible SIADH, and exacerbate fluid retention in patients with congestive heart failure

B. Biguanides
1. **Mechanism of action:** Approximately 75% of the antihyperglycemic effects are mediated through inhibition of gluconeogenesis, which results in decreased hepatic glucose production. In addition, in the presence of insulin, it increases sensitivity and responsiveness in skeletal muscle, erythrocytes, adipose tissue and intestinal tract. Helps prevent weight gain and decreases triglycerides and LDL cholesterol. As monotherapy, does not cause hypoglycemia. Decreases HgbA1C in average of 1%–2%. Probably best first line agent in obese individuals
2. **Complications and contraindications**
    a. Lactic acidosis (3 cases/100,000 patients); should not be used in patients with renal

insufficiency—creatinine in women > 1.4, creatinine in men > 1.5. Creatinine clearance (see Chapter 115, Formulas) is suggested to be a better measurement to follow; a clearance of less than 60mL/min is a contraindication to use. This might benefit clinicians when considering using biguanides in patients with elevated creatinine levels

    b. Should be discontinued 2 days prior and 2 days following IV contrast

    c. Metallic taste, GI side effects and decreased B_{12} levels can also occur

C. α-Glucosidase inhibitors

    1. Mechanism of action: Inhibits α-glucosidase in the small intestine, thus inhibiting the break down of sucrose, which causes decreased glucose absorption proximally. The terminal ileum produces new carbohydrate-metabolizing enzymes, which ultimately delays the absorption of glucose. The result is a smoother, prolonged carbohydrate absorption curve and a smaller peak in postprandial glucose concentrations. Decreases HgbA1C an average of 0.5%–1.0%

    2. Complications and contraindications: Bloating and flatulence

D. Thiazolidinedione

    1. Mechanism of action: At low levels attaches to receptors to help facilitate entry of glucose into the cell. At high doses, hepatic glucose production is suppressed and free fatty acids are reduced. They also increase HDL. Decreases HgbA1C an average of 1.5%

    2. Complications and contraindications: Weight gain, fluid retention and dilutional anemia are common. LFTs should be performed every 2 months during the first year of therapy. Thiazolidinediones should not be started if any liver enzyme is found to be elevated. If LFTs are elevated, withdraw medicine

E. Megltinides

    1. Mechanism of action: Similar to the sulfonylureas. It is dependent in part to the presence of glucose, because it may affect a different type of pancreatic ß-cell. Main effects are on postprandial plasma glucose concentrations. Stimulates the pancreas for only a short time, thus decreasing the total insulin and thus decreasing weight gain and hypoglycemic episodes

    2. Complications and contraindications: Hypoglycemia is the most common side effect, but less frequent. Similar profile to the sulfonylureas

	Generic Name	Brand Name	Usual Daily Dosage	Duration	Supply
Sulfonylureas	**First Generation**				
	Acetohexamide	*Dymelor*	500 to 750 mg QD or BID	12-24 hrs	250, 500 mg
	Chlorpropamide	*Diabinase*	250 to 375 mg QD	60 hrs	100, 250 mg
	Tolazamide	*Tolinase*	250 to 500 mg QD or BID	10-18 hrs	100, 250, 500 mg
	Tolbutamide	*Orinase*	1000 to 2000 mg BID	12-24 hrs	500 mg
	Second Generation				
	Glimepiride	*Amaryl*	1 to 4 mg QD	24 hrs	1, 2, 4 mg
	Glipizide	*Glucotrol*	10 to 20 mg QD or BID max 40 mg	18-30 hrs	5, 10 mg
	Glipizide Extended Release	*Glucotrol XL*	5 to 20 mg QD	24 hrs	5, 10 mg
	Glyburide	*Diabeta*	5 to 20 mg QD or BID	10-30 hrs	1.5, 2.5, 5 mg
		Micronase	5 to 20 mg QD or BID	10-30 hrs	1.5, 2.5, 5 mg
		Glynase Prestabs	3 to 12 mg QD or BID	24 hrs	1.5, 3, 6 mg
Biguanides	Metformin	*Glucophage*	1500 to 2550 mg BID or TID	18 hrs	500, 850, 1000 mg
α-Glucosidase Inhibitors	Acarbose	*Precose*	50 to 100 mg TID with meals	Not absorbed	25, 50, 100 mg
	Miglitol	*Glyset*	50 to 100 mg TID with meals	Not absorbed	25, 50, 100 mg
Thiazolidinediones	Rosiglitazone	*Avandia*	4 to 8 mg QD or 2 to 4 mg BID	24 hrs	2, 4, 8 mg
	Pioglitazone	*Actos*	15 to 45 mg QD	16-24 hrs	15, 30, 45 mg
Megltinides	Repaglinide	*Prandin*	1 to 4 mg TID take within 30 minutes of meals	1 hr	0.5, 1, 2 mg

F. Oral hypoglycemics are contraindicated in pregnancy: Pregnant patients need to be treated with insulin

G. With failure of monotherapy, add a drug (up to 3) instead of substituting
   1. With continued fasting hyperglycemia, then add Metformin or a Thiazolidinedione
   2. With continued postprandial hyperglycemia add Acarbose or a sulfonylurea or Repaglinide

VII. INSULIN

A. Types
   1. Human (recombinant), Beef-Pork, Pork
   2. Generally classified by onset and duration of action
   3. May be mixed to provide variations in onset and duration and ease of use

B. Properties of various insulin types

CLASS	BRAND	ONSET	PEAK	DURATION
Rapid Acting	Humalog	15 min	30–90 min	1.5–3 hrs
	Humulin/Novolin R (human)	0.5–1 hrs	2–4 hrs	6–12 hrs
	Iletin I R (beef-pork)			
Intermediate Acting	Humulin/Novolin N (human)	1–2 hrs	4–6 hrs	18–24 hrs
	Humulin/Novolin L (human)	2–3 hrs	8–12 hrs	16–24 hrs
	Lente (pork)			
	NPH (Pork			
Long Acting	Humulin U (Ultralente)	4–6 hrs	10–14 hrs	23–36 hrs
	Protamine Zinc (PZI)			
Mixed	Novolin/Humulin 50/50	30 min	2–4 hrs	24 hrs
	Novolin/Humulin 70/30	30 min	3–4 hrs (1st)	24 hrs
			10–12 hrs (2nd)	

C. Insulin Regimens: Consider formal diabetes education from the ADA or local hospital prior to initiating
   1. Type 1 Diabetics
      a. Physiologic insulin secretion is 20–40 U per day
      b. Start with 0.25–1.0 U/kg per day human N insulin (peds less, adolescents more)
   2. Type 2 Diabetics
      a. **B**edtime **I**nsulin (NPH) plus **D**aytime **S**ulfonylurea (**BIDS**)
         i. Begin with 10–20 U NPH 30 min before bedtime
         ii. Adjust by 2–4 U per day as needed
         iii. Check blood glucose QAC and HS
      b. 70/30 QAM, Humalog at dinner and NPH at HS
      c. 70/30 QAM and before dinner
      d. Custom split dosing with intermediate N and short acting R insulin
         i. AM dose: $^2/_3$ daily dose. Of this $^2/_3$ will be NPH and $^1/_3$ will be regular
         ii. PM dose: $^1/_3$ daily dose. Of this $^2/_3$ will be NPH and $^1/_3$ will be regular

D. Considerations
   1. If a patient is hospitalized with new-onset DM, place the patient on *a sliding scale* to determine what the daily insulin requirement will be (once the patient is stable)
   2. If a previously diagnosed patient is admitted to the hospital and hyperglycemia is detected, place the patient on a sliding scale of regular insulin until they are stable and then try to reinstitute their previous insulin doses
   3. Dosing adjustments may be needed for changes of activity, stress, change in diet, or infection
   4. For morning hyperglycemia, check a 2 AM glucose to rule out the Somogyi effect (rebound hyperglycemia secondary to hypoglycemia)

VIII. COMPLICATIONS

A. Diabetic Ketoacidosis
B. Nonketotic Hyperosmolar Coma
C. Nephropathy
   1. ACE inhibitors (e.g., **Captopril** 50mg PO BID) decrease proteinuria and should be considered in the IDDM population even without the presence of HTN
   2. Check 24hr urine for microalbuminuria every year. If present, start ACE inhibitor as above

GEN

3. Cough occurs in 10–30% of patients on ACE inhibitors. Try to maintain even a small dose, or may consider angiotensin II receptor blockers (renal protective effects with ACE II blockers have not been established)

D. Neuropathy: There are various forms of diabetic neuropathy
1. Mononeuropathy involving peripheral or cranial nerve (e.g., CN VI palsy, foot drop)
2. Symmetrical peripheral polyneuropathy (the most common—e.g., "burning feet")
3. Autonomic neuropathy (e.g., gastroparesis, orthostatic hypotension)

E. Retinopathy
1. The leading cause of new blindness in the U.S.
2. Ophthalmologic exams
   a. NIDDM: Perform at time of diagnosis, yearly thereafter
   b. IDDM: First exam within 5 years of diagnosis, yearly thereafter

F. Arteriosclerosis
1. Occurs more extensively and earlier than in the general population
2. Encourage smoking cessation, treat HTN aggressively, monitor and treat elevated lipids

G. The Diabetic Foot
1. Best therapy is prevention
2. Patients should be instructed to examine their feet daily for calluses, blisters, skin breakdown, and erythema
3. Shoes should be properly fitted. Patient should look inside shoes each time before putting on
4. If there is any evidence of infection, cultures (including anaerobic cultures) should be obtained. Antibiotic therapy should be effective against gram positives and gram negatives as well as anaerobes (e.g., **Augmentin** 875mg PO BID)

H. Infections
1. Secondary to decreased phagocytosis of immune cells
2. Pneumonia, osteomyelitis, and vaginitis are examples of infections seen in DM patients

IX. THE DIABETIC FLOW SHEET: A flow sheet on the front of the patient's chart can make each visit easier and help avoid overlooking potential problems

DIABETIC FLOW SHEET

Name: _____
Date of onset: _____
Age of onset: _____

Parameter and Frequency	Date	Date	Date	Date	Date
History					
Weight (each visit)					
BP (each visit)					
Heart and Lung exam (each visit)					
Feet (each visit)					
Fundi & Neuro (every other visit)					
Lab					
Random BS (each visit)					
Urine Dipstick (each visit)					
HgbA1C (Q 3–6 months)					
BUN/Cr (Q year)					
Lipid profile (Q year)					
TSH/T4 (Q 2–3 years)					
Referrals (including Ophtho)					
Medications					
Oral agent and dose					
Insulin: A.M.					
P.M.					
Diet					
Education/Questions					

GEN

CLINICAL PEARLS

- Diabetic nephropathy accounts for close to half of the patients receiving long-term renal dialysis in the U.S. 20–30% of Type 2 diabetes will develop nephropathy
- Between 1–5 % of patients with impaired glucose tolerance will go on to develop symptomatic diabetes or diagnostically abnormal glucose tolerance per year. Treatment with oral hypoglycemics does not delay the development of diabetes, but weight loss and exercise may
- Gestational diabetes occurs in 1–2% of pregnancies. These patients have a 30% risk of developing diabetes within 5–10 years postpartum
- Up to 20% of Type 2 diabetics have retinopathy when they are diagnosed

References

American Diabetes Association. Standards of medical care for patients with diabetes mellitus (Position Statement). Diabetes Care 2000; 23(1) Supp: S32–S42.

American Diabetes Association. Care of children with diabetes in the school and day care setting (Position Statement). Diabetes Care 23 2000; (Suppl.1):S100–S103.

American Diabetes Association. Consensus Statement: Type 2 diabetes in children and adolescents. Diabetes Care 2000; 23(3):381–389.

Vigan S, et al. Cost-utility analysis of screening intervals for diabetic retinopathy in patients with type 2 diabetes mellitus. JAMA 2000;283:889–96.

American Diabetes Association. Diabetic nephropathy (Position Statement). Diabetes Care 2000; 23 (Suppl. 1):S69–S72.

American Diabetes Association. Preventive foot care in people with diabetes (Position Statement). Diabetes Care 2000; 23 (Suppl. 1):S55–S56.

American Diabetes Association. Smoking and diabetes (Position Statement). Diabetes Care 2000; 23 (Suppl. 1):S63–S64.

The Expert Committee on the Diagnosis and Classification of Diabetes Mellitus: Report of the Expert Committee on the Diagnosis and Classification of Diabetes Mellitus. Diabetes Care 1999; 22 (Suppl. 1):S5–S19.

Bell DS, et al. Advances in therapy for type 2 diabetes. Patient Care 1999;33(16):189–200.

Davidson MB, et al. Relationship between fasting plasma glucose and glycosylated hemoglobin. Potential for false-positive diagnoses of type 2 diabetes using new diagnostic criteria. JAMA April 7, 1999;281:1203–10, and Vinicor F. When is diabetes diabetes? JAMA April 7, 1999;281: 1222–4.

Feinglos MN, Bethel MA. Oral agent therapy in the treatment of type 2 diabetes. Diabetes Care April 1999;22 (suppl 3):C61–3.

Florence JA. Treatment of type 2 diabetes mellitus. Am Fam Phys 1999;59(10):2835–44.

Gæde P, et al. Intensified multifactorial intervention in patients with type 2 diabetes mellitus and microalbuminuria: the Steno type 2 randomised study. Lancet February 20, 1999;353:617–22.

Hoogwerf BJ, et al. Effects of aggressive cholesterol lowering and low-dose anticoagulation on clinical and angiographic outcomes in patients with diabetes. The Post Coronary Artery Bypass Graft Trial. Diabetes June 1999;48:1289–94.

Link N. Dietary management of type 2 diabetes mellitus. West J Med July 1999;171:25–6.

Ritz E, Orth SR. Nephropathy in patients with type 2 diabetes mellitus. N Engl J Med October 7, 1999;341:1127–33.

Smieja M, et al., for the International Cooperative Group for Clinical Examination Research. Clinical examination for the detection of protective sensation in the feet of diabetic patients. J Gen Intern Med July 1999;14:418–24.

Weinstock RS, et al. Diet and exercise in the treatment of obesity: effects of 3 interventions on insulin resistance. Arch Intern Med Dec 1998;158:2477–83.

Viberti G, et al. Effect of captopril on progression to clinical proteinuria in patients with insulin-dependent diabetes mellitus and microalbuminuria. JAMA 1994;271:275–9.

Havas S. Educational guidelines for achieving tight control and minimizing complications of type 1 diabetes. Am Fam Phys 1999;60:1985.

GEN

Geoffrey Eubank, MD
Elizabeth Walz, MD
Charles Levy, MD
Kathy Provanzana, MD
Kim Martin, PA

50. HEADACHE: DIAGNOSIS AND MANAGEMENT

I. EPIDEMIOLOGY

Most common pain problem seen in the ambulatory setting (greater than 10 million office visits per year). Over 4 billion dollars are spent annually on over-the-counter medications for headaches. This does not include time missed from work, prescription medications, or physician visits

II. HISTORY

The cornerstone of diagnosis is to determine which headaches are more dangerous (secondary to medical problems) by classifying as a primary (migraine, tension, cluster, etc.) or secondary (CNS mass lesions, infections/meningitis, etc.) headache

A. Headache characteristics: Age of headache onset, location, frequency, severity, quality, speed of onset, or triggers (foods, stress, hunger, menstrual cycle, cough/exertion, position changes, etc.)

B. Associated symptoms: Photophobia, phonophobia, nausea/vomiting, sinus complaints (congestion, nasal discharge), fever, stiff neck, focal neurologic complaints, visual changes

C. Medications: Past and present medications and response to treatment. Consider both abortive and prophylactic therapies. Pay close attention to OTC medications, caffeine use, and foods which may be triggers (MSG, red wine)

Chronic analgesic use/abuse may lead to rebound headaches. Look for medications that can cause headaches (nitrates, Reserpine, Indomethacin, Minoxidil, Apresoline, oral contraceptives)

D. Past medical and surgical history: Especially malignancy, stroke, head trauma, neurosurgery, psychosocial history, hypertension, hematologic abnormalities, polymyalgia rheumatica

E. Family History: Migraines tend to be hereditary and begin in childhood or early adult life; other headaches less so

III. PHYSICAL EXAM

A. Vital signs: Fever (may indicate meningitis, sinusitis, viral syndromes), BP (diastolic BP greater than 110 can cause hypertensive headache)

B. Ophthalmologic: Funduscopic (papilledema indicates increased intracranial pressure (mass lesions, pseudotumor cerebri)), pupils (Horner's syndrome can occur with cluster headache), signs of glaucoma (may present with eye pain—consider tonometry over age 40)

C. HEENT: Tympanic membrane, nares and sinus exams (for signs of infection/disease), TMJ exam (look for jaw tenderness, jaw click), temporal artery swelling and tenderness (especially over age 50), scalp exam (tenderness or trigger points), neck exam (nuchal rigidity, paraspinal tenderness or spasm, range of motion)

D. Neurologic: Visual fields, cranial nerves, motor, sensory, coordination, gait (looking for focal deficits) and mental status changes (which may indicate meningitis, mass lesions or increased intracranial pressure)

IV. DIFFERENTIAL DIAGNOSIS

A. Primary headaches (benign)

1. Tension-type headache (related to physical, mental and/or emotional stress): 47%
2. Migraine headache (with or without aura): 31%
3. Cluster headache: 7%
4. Mixed headache (usually migraine/tension)
5. Rebound headache: Watch especially for caffeine, Butalbital and narcotics
6. Neuralgias (trigeminal, occipital) characterized by brief electrical/lancating pains
7. Uncommon syndromes (chronic paroxysmal hemicrania, hemicrania continua, cough/exertional headache, coital headache)

   8. Miscellaneous: TMJ dysfunction, chronic sinus/allergies
B. Secondary headaches (not so benign)
   1. CNS mass lesions (tumor, abscess)
   2. Vascular (cerebral/subarachnoid hemorrhage, arteriovenous malformations, stroke/TIA)
      Note: sudden onset of worst headache of life is worrisome for subarachnoid hemorrhage
   3. Infectious (meningitis, sinusitis)
   4. Traumatic (epidural/subdural hematoma, subarachnoid/intracranial hemorrhage)
   5. Temporal arteritis: greater than age 50, increased sedimentation rate, jaw claudication, pain
      centered about one temple, visual symptoms
   6. Pseudotumor cerebri: headache with papilledema, visual loss and elevated CSF pressure
      (typically occurs in young, overweight females)
   7. Miscellaneous: Post lumbar puncture, sleep apnea (morning headaches), carbon monoxide
      poisoning, glaucoma, hypertensive
C. Red flags: worrisome features that indicate need for further workup
   1. First severe headache over 50 (temporal arteritis, mass lesion, stroke)
   2. Intense headache without prior history of headache (subarachnoid hemorrhage)
   3. Nuchal rigidity, Kernig's/Brudzinski's sign (meningitis)
   4. Papilledema
   5. Diplopia
   6. Fever
   7. New/persistent neurologic signs
   8. Elevated BP (diastolic > 110)
   9. Unexplained vomiting
   10. Exertional/cough headache (need MRI to rule out posterior fossa lesion)
   11. Sudden change in headache pattern (Note: prior history of benign headache does not rule
       out development of new cause for headache)
   12. History of head trauma, malignancy or coagulopathy

V. TESTING: Consider testing as appropriate when any of the "red flags" above are present
  A. Neuroimaging, including:
   1. Computed tomography (CT) scan: Best for detection of acute bleed (non-contrast)
   2. Magnetic resonance imaging (MRI) : Best for detection of posterior fossa disease, more
      sensitive than CT for most conditions, except acute bleed
   3. Magnetic resonance angiography (MRA): Aneurysm or other vascular lesion
  B. Lumbar puncture: Evaluating meningitis or subarachnoid hemorrhage, increased intracranial
     pressure (assuming neuroimaging shows no mass lesion)
  C. Electroencephalogram (EEG): Rarely helpful
  D. Other diagnostic tests including CBC, sed. rate, thyroid panel, drug levels (Lithium)

GEN

·DIAGNOSIS AND MANAGEMENT OF PRIMARY HEADACHES

Character	Tension-type headache	Migraine headache	Cluster Headache
Location	Bilateral intense about the neck	Usually unilateral	Strictly unilateral, retroorbital
Quality	Pressure, "vise-like"	Throbbing, aching	Sharp, stabbing
Severity	Mild to moderate	Moderate to severe	Extremely severe
Frequency	Variable, may be constant or intermittent	Intermittent (<15/month), not typically daily	Episodic, 1-4/day for weeks to months, same time each day, esp. night
Duration	Several hours/days, fluctuating	4-48 hours, gradual build-up and decline	15-120 minutes, rapid onset and decline
Aura	None	Occasional (16%), esp. visual(zig-zag scotoma,etc.)	None
Activity level	Variable	Passive, rest in dark room	Active, pacing
Precipitants	Stress	Numerous(foods, chocolate, menstrual cycle, etc.)	Alcohol
Associated symptoms	Muscular tenderness, mild photo/phonophobia	Photo/phonophobia, nausea/vomiting, diarrhea	Horner's syndrome, rhinorrhea, lacrimation

Therapy: Abortive	Acetaminophen
	NSAIDs
	ASA Muscle relaxants
	Relaxation, exercise
	Butalbital/narcotics*
	
	*Be careful with prolonged use (rebound, dependence)
		Acetaminophen
		NSAIDs
		Midrin 2 at onset,
		  repeat q 1 hr to max of 5
		Triptans (see below)
		DHE-45 1 mL IV/IM, may
		  repeat x 1 in 1 hr
		Intranasal
		  dihydriergotamine
			Sumatriptan 6mg SQ
			100% O₂ NRB mask
			  for 15 minutes
			DHE-45 1 mL IV/IM,
			  may repeat x 1 in 1 hr

Therapy: Prophylactic	Amitriptyline/Nortriptyline
	  10-100mg qhs
	SSRIs (less effective)
	Depakote 250mg bid
	Neurontin 100-600mg tid
	Biofeedback/relaxation
		Inderal 60-240mg qd (or
		  other Beta blockers)
		Depakote 250mg bid
		Amitriptyline/Nortriptyline
		  10-100mg qhs
		Verapamil 180-240mg qd
		Naproxen 500mg bid
		Neurontin 100-600mg tid
			Prednisone 60mg qd
			  and taper over 2-3
			  weeks for new/recur-
			  rent cluster
			Add prophylactic to
			  continue 2 wks after
			  headache controlled
			Verapamil 180-240mg qd
			Lithium 900mg qd
			Depakote 250mg bid

VI. TRIPTANS: Very effective for migraine, but contraindicated in coronary disease, uncontrolled hypertension, history of stroke and complicated migraine (hemiplegic, basilar)

Drug	mg	Speed of Onset	Efficacy	Rebound	Side Effects	Cost
Sumatriptan Imitrex/ IM	6	++++	++++	+++	++++	+++++
Sumatriptan Imitrex/ nas	10-20	+++	+++	+++	+++	++++
Sumatriptan Imitrex/ po	25-100	++	++	+++	++	++++
Zolmatriptan Zomig	2.5-5	++	++	++	+++	++++
Naratriptan Amerge	2.5	+	+	+	+	++++
Rizatriptan Maxalt	10 (5 w/ Inderal)	+++	+++	++	++	++++

Adapted from: National Headache Foundation. Standards of Care for Headache Diagnosis and Treatment. Chicago, Il: National Headache Foundation; 1996:6–7

CLINICAL PEARLS
- Myofascial pain, difficulty in concentration, emotional lability, divorce and job loss frequently accompany post-traumatic headache
- An epidural hematoma commonly presents with a history of trauma, seeming complete recovery (lucid interval), then worsening headache, vomiting, confusion, and focal neurologic signs
- Headaches typically worse in the morning are: pseudotumor cerebri, sleep apnea, carbon monoxide poisoning, and hypertensive
- Frequent use of Ergotamine, caffeine/Butalbital containing products, NSAIDs, and Excedrin can cause rebound headaches

References

Morgenstern LB, et al. Worst headache and subarachnoid hemorrhage: prospective, modern computed tomography and spinal fluid analysis. Ann Emerg Med September 1998;32:297–304.

National Headache Foundation. Standards of Care for Headache Diagnosis and Treatment. Chicago, IL: National Headache Foundation; 1996;6–7.

Smith R. Diagnosing headache. Hospital Medicine Jul 1997.

Evans RW. Diagnostic testing for the evaluation of headaches. Neurol Clin. 1996;14:1–26.

Davidoff RA. Migraine: manifestations, pathogenesis, and management. Philadelphia, PA: FA Davis Co; 1995.

Prager JM, Rosenblum J, Mikulis DJ, Diamond S, Freitag FG. Evaluation of headache patients by MRI. Headache Q 1991;2:192–195.

GEN

Michael B. Weinstock, MD
Geoffrey Eubank, MD

51. EVALUATION AND MANAGEMENT OF DIZZINESS

I. EVALUATION: The most important step is to define patient's type of dizziness

   A. Vertiginous dizziness: Illusion that either their body or the environment is moving (sensation of room spinning around the patient, sensation of standing on a ship) often associated with nausea. (See next table, Evaluation and Management of Vertiginous Dizziness)

     1. Peripheral lesions of the vestibular nerve and inner ear

       a. Benign positional vertigo (BPV): Calcium carbonate crystals which have fallen against the cupula of the posterior semicircular canal

       b. Ménière's disease (Endolymphatic hydrops)

       c. Vestibular neuronitis

       d. Labyrinthitis (serous or suppurative)

       e. Cerebellopontine angle tumors (acoustic schwannoma)

       f. Traumatic vertigo (labyrinthine concussion): Following head trauma

     2. Central lesions of the CNS

       a. Brain stem or cerebellar infarct: The 4 Ds—Dizziness, Diplopia, Dysarthria and Dysphagia. Also, change in motor and/or sensory function

       b. Vertebrobasilar insufficiency: Same symptoms as above, but occur transiently (seconds to minutes)

       c. Multiple sclerosis: Disease onset in young adulthood. MRI is abnormal in a majority of cases

       d. Vertebrobasilar migraines: Associated symptoms include visual changes, dysarthria, tinnitus, decreased hearing, ataxia, paresthesia, altered level of consciousness. Up to 25% of patients with migraines have symptoms consistent with basilar migraines

       e. Tumors of the posterior fossa or brainstem/cerebellar: Often have other signs of brainstem dysfunction

       f. Other

         i. CNS infection

         ii. Trauma: Intracranial bleed

iii. Temporal lobe epilepsy
  B. Presyncope/syncope: Lightheadedness, graying of vision with sitting/standing, diaphoresis
  1. Orthostatic hypotension: Sensation of light-headedness/vision going gray when standing or sitting up. Results from abnormal regulation of blood pressure
    a. Dehydration, blood loss
    b. Reflexive: Cough, valsalva, micturition
    c. Abnormal carotid baroreceptor response
  2. Cardiac: Valvular dysfunction, outflow obstruction, arrhythmia, ischemia
  3. Neuropathy (autonomic): Diabetic or alcoholic neuropathy, Guillain-Barre syndrome, nutritional
  4. Medications: Antihypertensives, vasodilators, anti-Parkinson drugs
  C. Imbalance and ataxia (disequilibrium): Imbalance, abnormal gait, lack of coordination
  1. Neuropathy (peripheral): Diabetes, B_{12} deficiency, tabes dorsalis
  2. Vascular: Carotid insufficiency, CVA, migraine, anemia
  3. Age related: Unfamiliar surroundings, poor lighting at night, sedative medications, cognitive defect
  4. Poor vision: Diplopia, decreased acuity
  5. Other
    a. Neoplastic
    b. Metabolic disorders: Hypoglycemia
    c. Trauma: Intracranial bleed, postconcussive syndrome
    d. Infectious: CNS infection
  D. Psychogenic dizziness: Symptoms are vague and imprecise (feeling apart from environment, fatigue, fullness in the head). Often associated with anxiety, panic disorders, hyperventilation syndrome. Diagnosis of exclusion. Reproduction of symptoms with hyperventilation strongly correlates with psychogenic dizziness

II. HISTORY
  A. Define the type of dizziness
  B. Provoking factors: Positional changes, changes in head positions
  C. Acuity of onset
  D. Aural symptoms: Hearing loss, tinnitus
  E. Focal neuro symptoms
  F. Visual symptoms: Diplopia, decreased acuity
  G. Cardiac symptoms: Palpitations, chest pain, shortness of breath
  H. Infectious symptoms
  I. Past medical history: Diabetes, alcohol, syphilis, migraine headaches, cardiac disease
  J. Medications
  K. Trauma

III. PHYSICAL EXAM
  A. Orthostatic BP and pulse
  B. Neuro exam: Cranial nerves, finger to nose, dysdiadochokinesia and Romberg—distinguish central from peripheral lesions
  C. Eye: Visual acuity, extra-ocular muscles, fundi and discs
  D. Ear: Tympanic membrane, external ear. Hearing test
  E. Neck: Nuchal rigidity or pain with movement. Reproduction of symptoms with movement. Carotid bruits
  F. Cardiac: Murmurs, signs of ischemia
  G. Gait
  H. Hallpike maneuver: Patient sits on bed while clinician supports head. Patient rapidly assumes supine position first with head straight, then turned 45° left then 45° right. With reproduction of symptoms, vertigo and nystagmus, benign positional vertigo is suggested. Also vertigo duration less than 1 minute, latency 2–20 seconds, unidirectional nystagmus, fatigability

IV. OTHER TESTS
  A. Caloric testing: Inject 5cc (then 10cc or 20cc if no response) of ice water over 5 seconds at posteroinferior quadrant of TM and observe for nystagmus, nausea and vertigo. If no response then vestibular apparatus is not functioning

B. Audiography: Low frequency loss in Ménière's disease
C. Electronystagmography (ENG): Most helpful in Ménière's disease and benign positional vertigo. Helpful in cases with medicolegal implications and psychogenic vertigo
D. Head CT or MRI
E. Lumbar puncture: Helpful when suspect multiple sclerosis, meningitis, or subarachnoid bleed
F. Cardiac evaluation if presyncope: Consider ECG, ECHO, EPS depending on symptoms

EVALUATION AND MANAGEMENT OF VERTIGINOUS DIZZINESS

Condition	Vertiginous symptoms	Nystagmus	Comments	Associated symptoms	Management
Benign positional vertigo	Vertigo: Positional, provoked by certain head positions.	Postional with latency, brief duration and fatigability. Horizontal.	Usually idiopathic, may result from head trauma, ear surgery, or sequelae of vestibular neuronitis.	None.	Postioning maneuvers to rid the posterior semicircular canal of debris.
Ménière's disease	Vertigo: Often with nausea and vomiting that lasts hours (not days or weeks).	Spontaneous during critical stage, postural in 25% of patients during first few weeks after an attack. Caloric testing reveals loss or impairment of thermally induced nystagmus on involved side.	Triad: Vertigo, tinnitus, hearing loss. Both ears affected in 30–50% of patients.	1. Tinnitus (louder during attacks). 2. Sensorineural hearing loss (low frequency). 3. Fullness in ear during attack.	Goal: To lower endolymphatic pressure. 1. Low salt diet (<2g Na$^+$/day). 2. Diuretics (HCTZ 50–100mg/day). 3. Surgical decompression.
Vestibular neuronitis	Vertigo accompanied by nausea and vomiting lasting days to weeks. Acute onset.	Increases when gaze is directed away from affected ear and is suppressed with visual fixation.	Auditory function *not* affected. BPV may develop as sequelae.	Antecedent or concomitant acute viral illness. Does not recur.	Symptomatic.
Labyrinthitis	Acute onset of vertigo *and* hearing loss which lasts 3–5 days. Rapid head movements may bring on vertigo.	Same as vestibular neuronitis.	Hearing loss may be total and permanent. Need to differentiate viral (serous) from bacterial (suppurative) labyrinthitis.	Antecedent or concomitant acute viral illness. Does not recur.	Tapered oral prednisone may be helpful. Suppurative labyrinthitis must be treated with antibiotics.
Acoustic schwannoma (acoustic neuroma)	Vertigo: Usually late, more often a progressive feeling of imbalance. Occasionally provoked by sudden head movements.	Spontaneous type frequently present.	Asymmetric sensorineural hearing loss. Usually unsteadiness and imbalance. Vertigo occurs in <20% of cases. Tinnitus is common. Diagnosed with MRI scanning.	1. Facial weakness. 2. Diplopia. 3. Headache. 4. Elevated CSF protein. 5. Hyperesthesia or hypoesthesia in distribution of eighth or fifth cranial nerve.	Surgery.
CNS vertigo	Vertigo: Nearly always positional — provoked by certain head positions.	Usually accompanies the vertigo.		1. Usually in the elderly. 2. Symptoms associated with arteriosclerosis, brainstem ischemia (visual symptoms), or cervical arthritis.	Directed to specific etiology.

V. SYMPTOMATIC MANAGEMENT OF TRUE VERTIGO

A. Acute vertigo: First few days
    1. Vestibular suppressants
        a. **Meclizine**: 12.5–25mg PO Q6hrs PRN
        b. **Valium**: 2–5mg PO Q6hrs PRN
    2. Antiemetics: **Compazine** or **Phenergan**. PO or rectal
    3. Bedrest
    4. Hospitalize if dehydrated or for other medical reasons
B. Subacute vertigo

GEN

1. Stop vestibular suppressants
2. Vestibular exercises

CLINICAL PEARLS
- Gait disturbance can be seen in central and peripheral vertigo
- In patients with multiple sclerosis, vertigo is the initial complaint in 5% and ultimately occurs in 50% of patients
- Symptoms of Ménière's disease may be mimicked in secondary and tertiary syphilis. Consider screening all patients with Ménière's disease with VDRL or RPR
- The average time from onset of symptoms to diagnosis of acoustic neuroma is 4 years with an incidence of 1 case in 100,000 persons

References
Lawson J, et al. Diagnosis of geriatric patients with severe dizziness. J Am Geriatr Soc Jan 1999;47:12–7.
Baloh RW. Vertigo. Lancet Dec 5, 1998;352: 1841–6.
Carroll L. Dizziness: easily diagnosed with good history-taking. Med Tribune 1995;36(14):6.
Spoelhof GD. When to suspect an acoustic neuroma. Am Fam Phys 1995;52:1768–74.

John A. Vaughn, MD

GEN

52. PREVENTION AND MANAGEMENT OF CVAs

I. INTRODUCTION
  A. There are an estimated 731,000 strokes annually
  B. There are 4 million stroke survivors
  C. The annual direct and indirect cost is $40 billion

II. ASYMPTOMATIC CAROTID ARTERY DISEASE
  A. An important risk factor for stroke
  B. The risk for cerebrovascular events increases with the degree of stenosis
  C. Screening
      1. There is insufficient evidence to recommend for or against screening for carotid artery stenosis using either physical examination or carotid ultrasound
          a. A carotid bruit only has a sensitivity of 63–76% and a specificity of 61–76% for clinically significant stenosis
          b. The positive predictive value of carotid duplex is 82–97%
      2. Men over 60 with risk factors for stroke and no contraindications to surgery are most likely to benefit from screening. A carotid bruit in these patients should be evaluated with vascular imaging
  D. Vascular imaging
      a. Venous Doppler Ultrasonography: It cannot distinguish between complete and near-complete occlusion but is non-invasive
      b. Cerebral angiography is the standard for the precise measurement of the degree of stenosis
  E. Management
      1. Surgical—**Carotid Endarterectomy (CEA):** Indicated for asymptomatic lesions *of at least 60% stenosis* with a local surgical risk of less than 3%
      2. Medical: Antithrombotic agent
          a. **Aspirin:** 50–325mg PO QD.
          b. For Aspirin intolerant chose one of the following:
              i. Clopidogrel (Plavix): 75mg PO QD
                  aa. Proven more effective than Aspirin for preventing vascular death (CVA, MI, peripheral vascular disease)
                  bb. Often used after aspirin failure
              ii. Ticlopidine (Ticlid): 250mg PO BID—Ticlid can cause hematologic abnormalities and a CBC should be obtained every 2 weeks for 3 months and then periodically thereafter

> iii. **Extended Release Dipyridamole (Persantine)** 200mg and **Aspirin** 25mg PO BID

III. SYMPTOMATIC CAROTID ARTERY DISEASE—TRANSIENT ISCHEMIC ATTACK (TIA) AND STROKE

A. Definition
  1. TIA: A neurologic deficit lasting *less than 24hrs* caused by reduced blood flow in a particular artery supplying the brain
  2. Stroke: A neurologic deficit lasting *greater than 24hrs*

B. Evaluation: Venous Doppler or Cerebral angiography (see II. D. a, b.)

C. Management
  1. Risk Factor Modification—National Stroke Association Recommendations:

Table 2. National Stroke Association Summary Recommendations for Prevention of a First Stroke

Condition	Recommendation
Hypertension	The Sixth Report of the Joint National Committee on Prevention, Detection, Evaluation, and Treatment of High Blood Pressure recommendations for lifestyle modification, initiation of specific therapy, and multidisciplinary management strategies
Myocardial infarction	Aspirin therapy if previous myocardial infarction (MI) or warfarin at an international normalized ration of 2-3 in patients with atrial fibrillation, left ventricular thrombus, or significant left ventricular dysfuntion, and statin agents after MI in patients with normal to high lipid levels
Atrial fibrillation*	Patients >75 years with or without risk factors should be treated with warfarin; patients aged 65-75 years with risk factors should be treated with warfarin and those without risk factors should be treated with warfarin or aspirin; patients <65 years with risk factors should be treated with warfarin, those without risk factors should be treated with aspirin
Diabetes mellitus	American Diabetes Association recommendations for control of diabetes to reduce microvascular complications (further studies are needed to determine if aggressive glycemic control lowers the risk of stroke)
Lipid levels	Statin agents in patients with high cholesterol and coronary heart disease and National Cholesterol Education Program guideline principles for dietary and pharmacologic management of patients with hyperlipidemia or atherosclerotic disease
Asymptomatic carotid artery disease†	Carotid endarterectomy for asymptomatic carotid stenosis ≥ 60% (but < 100%) When surgical morbidity and mortality is <3%
Lifestyle factors	Modification of smoking, alcohol consumption, physical activity, and diet according to published guidelines

* Adapted from Laupacis et al. Risk factors include previous transient ischemic attack, systemic embolism or stroke, hypertension, and left ventricular dysfunction. Efforts to improve patient and practitioner awareness regarding the benefits and risks of warfarin will serve as a first step toward increasing appropriate usage. The warfarin international normalized ratio goal is ranged 2.0 to 3.0 with a target value of 2.5.

† The at least 60% asymptomatic carotid artery stenosis cut point should be replicated in other studies.

Source: Gorelick PB, et al. Prevention of a first stroke. A review of guidelines and a multidisciplinary consensus statement from the National Stroke Association. JAMA Mar 24/31, 1999; 281:1115. Copyright 1999, American Medical Association. Used with permission.

  2. Medical: atherothrombotic TIA—see II. E. 2
  3. Medical: cardioembolic TIA (i.e., atrial fibrillation)
      a. Long term anti-coagulation with **Warfarin (Coumadin)** (goal INR 2.0–3.0)
      b. **Aspirin:** 50–325mg PO QD for patients with contraindications to Warfarin
  4. Surgical—CEA

a. 70–99% stenosis: Proven benefit in good surgical candidates who have had one TIA within the last 2 years. Three times as effective as medical therapy alone in reducing incidence of stroke

b. 50–69% stenosis: Absolute benefit is less than that for patients with higher degree of stenosis, retinal TIAs and women, *but patients with a recent TIA do have a reduced stroke rate with CEA*

c. < 50% stenosis: No benefit from CEA

IV. ACUTE ISCHEMIC STROKE

A. History
1. Assess for risk factors (above)
2. Establishment of the precise time of onset of clinical symptoms is very important in guiding therapy
3. Should emphasize the course of symptoms since onset to establish whether stroke is stable or unstable
4. Preceding TIA symptoms are more likely to be associated with an ischemic stroke
5. Headache more often occurs with hemorrhagic and embolic stroke

B. Differential diagnosis
1. Hemorrhagic stroke
2. Hypoglycemia
3. Migraine headaches
4. Seizures
5. Brain mass
6. Infectious: Meningitis vs. brain abscess

C. Physical exam
1. Neuro: May help to localize the lesion site
2. Cardiovascular: Assess heart rhythm, murmurs, blood pressure, carotid bruits
3. Ophthalmoscopy: Retinal cholesterol or platelet-fibrin emboli as well as evidence of chronic hypertensive or diabetic disease
4. Mental Status: Loss of consciousness or confusion should prompt consideration of other diagnoses

D. Laboratory evaluation
1. Complete blood count, platelet count, glucose, PT, PTT, lipid profile, and serum VDRL
2. Erythrocyte sedimentation rate (in the elderly) to exclude giant cell arteritis
3. Antiphospholipid antibodies (in the young) to identify immune-related disease processes predisposing to stroke
4. Protein C, protein S, and tests for platelet viscosity, function and collagen vascular diseases may also be indicated in younger patients
5. BUN, creatinine and serum electrolyte measurements help to establish systemic illnesses

E. Cardiac imaging
1. 12-lead EKG: To exclude MI, atrial fibrillation and other dysrhythmias
2. Cardiac Echo
   a. To evaluate for a cardiogenic source of emboli
   b. Yield is low in patients who have no history or physical evidence of cardiac disease

F. Vascular imaging
1. Ultrasonography: Cannot distinguish between complete and near-complete occlusion but is non-invasive and has a lower complication rate
2. Cerebral Angiography
   1. Most accurate method of assessing cerebrovascular system
   2. Complication rate is 0.5–3%
3. MR angiography
   1. Valuable for identifying lesions of extra-cranial carotid circulation
   2. Tends to overestimate degree of stenosis and, like ultrasonography, cannot distinguish between complete and near-complete occlusion
4. Ultrasonography combined with MR angiography
   1. May eliminate need for angiography
   2. Cheaper than angiography alone

GEN

G. Cerebral imaging
 1. CT scan (identifies acute bleeding better than MRI)
   a. Can identify or exclude hemorrhage as the cause of stroke
   b. Can identify other conditions that may mimic a stroke: neoplasm, abscess, extraparenchymal hemorrhage
   c. Infarct may not be reliably seen for 24–48hrs
   d. Posterior fossa and cortical infarcts may not be seen secondary to bone artifact
   e. Contrast enhancement allows greater detection of subacute infarcts
 2. MRI scan
   a. Reliably documents the extent and localization of infarct within 1 hour of onset
   b. Posterior fossa and cortical infarcts are clearly seen
   c. Identifies intracranial hemorrhage and other abnormalities

H. Management
 1. **Aspirin:** 160–325mg PO QD
   a. Recommended for patients not receiving tPA, IV Heparin or Warfarin
   b. Should be started within 48hrs of onset and may be used safely in combination with subcutaneous Heparin
 2. **Heparin**
   a. There is no conclusive evidence either for or against the use of Heparin in the treatment of acute stroke; it is a matter of individual clinical decision-making
   b. 3–5 days of IV Heparin is an option for cardioembolic stroke, large-artery atherosclerotic ischemic stroke and progressing thromboembolic stroke
   c. There is a small risk of cerebral hemorrhage
   d. If IV Heparin is used, a bolus is not recommended—a standardized sliding scale based on weight and PTT measurements should be used
   e. A brain CT should be done prior to initiation of IV Heparin to exclude hemorrhage and estimate the size of the infarction

V. POST-STROKE REHABILITATION
A. Acute care setting
 1. DVT prophylaxis in patients with restricted mobility
   a. Heparin 5000 U SQ Q12hr or low molecular weight Heparin
     i. Intermittent pneumatic compression devices for those with contraindications to anticoagulation
     ii. Swallowing assessment before starting oral intake
     iii. Maintenance of skin integrity
     iv. Continuous assessment of fall risk
     v. Minimizing use of chronic indwelling catheter for the treatment of urinary incontinence or retention
     vi. Mobilization as soon as medically possible

B. Rehabilitation facility
 1. Patients and caregivers should be educated about strokes in general as well as specific techniques needed to care for the patient
 2. Evaluation and treatment of persistent urinary incontinence
 3. Bowel management programs for patients with constipation or fecal incontinence
 4. Physical therapy directed at improving strength, motor control and functional performance
 5. Monitoring for signs and symptoms of depression and initiating appropriate therapy

C. Community residence
 1. Working with the patient and caregivers to avoid negative effects of caregiving on family functioning and caregiver health
 2. Facilitation of patient reintegration into family and social roles
 3. Fall prevention emphasizing reduction of patient, treatment and environmental risk factors
 4. Prevention of stroke recurrence and complications as well as health promotion
 5. Identifying valued activities and enabling participation

CLINICAL PEARLS
 • The use of Doppler ultrasonography instead of angiography for the evaluation of carotid

GEN

artery stenosis is currently being investigated
- All statin agents decrease the risk of stroke after MI, possibly through a separate mechanism from their lipid-lowering properties. The FDA has specifically approved Pravastatin (Pravachol) and Simvistatin (Zocor) for the prevention of stroke or TIA
- There is evidence that light to moderate drinking may have *beneficial* effects by increasing HDL and decreasing platelet aggregation and fibrinogen levels
- Angioplasty with stent placement and extracranial-intracranial bypass for the treatment of symptomatic carotid artery disease are both investigational and not recommended for general use
- Streptokinase and intra-arterial thrombolytic therapy for acute stroke are both investigational and not recommended for general use
- Tissue Plasminogen Activator (tPA) has been approved for the treatment of acute stroke if it is initiated within 3hrs of clearly defined symptom onset and the patient meets eligibility criteria

References

Barnett HJM, et al. Causes and severity of ischemic stroke in patients with internal carotid artery stenosis JAMA 2000;283:1429–1436.

Albers GW, et al. Supplement to the guidelines for the management of transient ischemic attacks—a statement from the Ad Hoc Committee on Guidelines for the Management of Transient Ischemic Attacks, Stroke Council, American Heart Association. Stroke 1999; 30: 2502–11.

Ascherio A, et al. Relation of consumption of vitamin E, vitamin C, and carotenoids to risk for stroke among men in the United States. Ann Intern Med Jun 15, 1999; 130:963–70.

Ezekowitz MD, Levine JA. Preventing stroke in patients with atrial fibrillation. JAMA May 19, 1999;281:1830–5.

Gorelick PB, et al. Prevention of a first stroke. A review of guidelines and a multidisciplinary consensus statement from the National Stroke Association. JAMA Mar 24/31, 1999; 281: 1112–20.

Albers GW, et al. Antithrombotic and thrombolytic therapy for ischemic stroke. Chest 1998;114:683–698.

Biller MD, et al. Guidelines for carotid endarterectomy: a statement for healthcare professionals from a special writing group of the Stroke Council, American Heart Association. Stroke 1998; 29:554–62.

Boult C, Brummel-Smith K. Post-stroke rehabilitation guidelines. The Clinical Practice Committee of the American Geriatrics Society. J Am Geriatr Soc Jul, 1997;45(7):881–3.

Lee TT, et al. Cost-effectiveness of screening for carotid stenosis in asymptomatic persons. Ann Intern Med 1997; 126(5): 337–46.

Daniel M. Neides, MD

53. LIVER FUNCTION TESTS

I. INTRODUCTION

- **A.** Liver function tests (LFTs) are often obtained on routine laboratory screenings; they are not a true measure of liver function. LFTs are actually enzymes present in the liver released into the blood when hepatocytes are injured, inflamed or destroyed
- **B.** It is important to repeat the test to confirm an abnormality (true positive) and assess whether the liver is actually the source
- **C.** Ultrasound is the most useful initial radiographic study of the liver (assesses size and presence of masses or ascites, and allows good visualization of the biliary tree and gallbladder)
- **D.** LFTs typically include ALT, AST, alkaline phosphatase, bilirubin, and GGT
- **E.** Protime and albumin are more accurate (but still indirect) measures of the liver's function

II. HISTORY AND PHYSICAL EXAMINATION

A. History

1. Alcohol and drugs
2. Medications (e.g., Acetaminophen, Isoniazid, Dilantin, barbiturates)

3. Previous medical history
4. Family history
5. Previous hepatitis (chronic hepatitis, hepatocellular cancer)
6. Sexual
7. Travel (amebiasis)
8. Transfusion
9. Pruritus (primary sclerosing cholangitis, primary biliary cirrhosis)
10. Arthritis (autoimmune hepatitis, hemochromatosis)
11. Weight loss, malaise, anorexia (hepatocellular cancer, pancreatic cancer, etc.)
12. COPD (α-1-antitrypsin), family history of emphysema at young age
13. Previous surgery (common bile duct stricture)

B. Physical Examination
1. Eyes: Scleral icterus or Kayser-Fleischer rings (Wilson's disease)
2. Skin: Spider angioma or palmar erythema
3. Face: Parotid enlargement
4. Signs of hypo-/hyperthyroidism
5. Musculoskeletal: Dupuytren's contracture
6. Abdomen: Tender right upper quadrant

III. LIVER ENZYMES
A. Aminotransferases (ALT/AST)
1. Useful in diagnosing *acute hepatocellular disease* such as hepatitis
2. ALT is present in high concentrations only in the liver
3. AST is found in the liver, cardiac and skeletal muscle, kidney, brain, pancreas, lung, WBCs, and RBCs
4. Increases in both ALT and AST indicate hepatocellular necrosis or inflammation
5. In liver disease secondary to alcohol, the transaminase values rarely exceed 300 U/L. Levels that are markedly increased in an alcoholic patient suggest another etiology such as viral hepatitis, drug-induced disease, or ischemia
6. AST/ALT > 2 is suggestive of alcohol-induced liver disease
7. Viral hepatitis may show an increase in ALT and AST about 1 week preceding the onset of jaundice (See Chapter 55, Diagnosis and Management of Hepatitis B)

B. Alkaline phosphatase (Alk Phos)
1. Elevation usually indicates *cholestatic liver disease* (defined as intra- or extrahepatic biliary obstruction)
2. Primarily found in liver, bone, intestines, kidney, WBCs, and placenta
3. If the Alk Phos is the only abnormality on the laboratory screen, consider a GGT to help differentiate liver vs. bone as the source
4. Patients with infiltrative disease of the liver (metastatic disease, fatty liver, amyloid, granulomatous hepatitis) may present with a markedly increased Alk Phos

C. Gamma-glutamyl transpeptidase (GGT)
1. Elevated GGT is often seen in *cholestatic liver disease* (along with a concurrent increased Alk Phos). May be elevated secondary to *drugs* (alcohol, Dilantin, barbiturates)
2. GGT may be increased in thyrotoxicosis, renal failure, status post myocardial infarction, pancreatitis, diabetes, and prostate cancer
3. Found in liver, kidney, pancreas, heart and brain
4. A GGT level which is disproportionately higher than the AST, ALT, or Alk Phos in a patient not taking Dilantin or barbiturates suggests alcohol as the etiology

D. Bilirubin (Bili)
1. Bilirubin is an end-product of hemoglobin metabolism. The unconjugated Bili is bound to albumin in serum and transported to the liver. It is conjugated in the liver, becomes water soluble and is excreted in the bile. Elevated direct (conjugated) or indirect (unconjugated) Bili is useful in diagnosing liver disease
2. Direct (conjugated) hyperbilirubinemia is almost always due to *hepatobiliary disease*
3. Indirect (unconjugated) hyperbilirubinemia
   a. Gilbert's disease is the most common. This is a benign disease caused by abnormal

GEN

hepatic metabolism of unconjugated Bili. The Bili level is usually < 3mg/dL. Patients with Gilbert's disease have no evidence of hemolysis and the other LFTs are normal. May be present in 7–10% of the population

    b. Hemolysis. The work-up includes checking H/H, reticulocyte count, Coombs test, haptoglobin (increased with hemolysis), G6PD level, and abnormal peripheral smear

E. Albumin

    1. Is a good indicator (along with the Protime) of the liver's ability to function properly and make proteins

    2. Decreased dietary protein and increased alcohol consumption can affect albumin synthesis

    3. Trauma, sepsis, or severe burns may rapidly lower the albumin level due to fluid shifts

    4. The albumin to total protein ratio should be > 1:2. If not, it may indicate presence of other proteins (multiple myeloma, monoclonal gammopathy of undetermined significance)

F. Prothrombin time (Protime)

    1. Reflects hepatic synthesis of Factors I, II, V, VII, and X; elevated Protime may be due to a deficiency of at least 1 of these factors

    2. An elevated Protime may also be caused by hepatocellular disease or vitamin K deficiency (Factors II, VII, IX, and X are dependent on vitamin K for normal functioning)

    3. To determine the etiology of an increased Protime in patients with cholestasis, give the patient vitamin K 10mg IM and recheck the Protime in 24hrs. Hepatocellular function is satisfactory if the Protime improves by at least 30%

    4. Consider a Factor VIII level in difficult cases. A low level indicates a primary hematologic problem

G. Bile salts

    1. A component of bile (formed by the metabolism of cholesterol in the liver). Bile salts help with the absorption of dietary fat

    2. May be *elevated in cholestatic or obstructive liver disease* but use of serum bile salt levels are limited since many conditions can yield an abnormal level

IV. ETIOLOGY OF LIVER DISEASE: LFT PATTERN AND DIAGNOSING DISEASE

    A. Inflammatory: Elevated ALT and/or AST

        1. Hepatitis A, B, C, D (antibody titers)

        2. CMV hepatitis (antibody titers)

        3. EBV hepatitis (antibody titers)

        4. Alcoholic hepatitis

        5. α-1-antitrypsin deficiency (α-1-antitrypsin level)

        6. Drug toxicity (Acetaminophen, INH, CCl_4)

        7. Hemochromatosis (iron studies, CAT scan)

    B. Chronic active: May see low grade elevation of LFTs

        1. Autoimmune hepatitis (anti-smooth muscle antibody: SMA, ANA)

        2. Viral hepatitis (antibody titers)

        3. Wilson's disease (ceruloplasmin level)

        4. Glycogen storage disease Type I (decreased activity of glucose-6-phosphatase)

        5. α-1-antitrypsin deficiency

    C. Cholestasis: Elevated Alk Phos and GGT; elevated Bili and/or jaundice may or may not be present

        1. Extrahepatic obstruction:

            a. Cholelithiasis (ultrasound)

            b. Pancreatic cancer (CT or ultrasound)

            c. Choledochal cyst (CT, ultrasound, or ERCP)

            d. Common bile duct stricture (ERCP)

            e. Cholangiocarcinoma (CT)

        2. Intrahepatic obstruction:

            a. Primary biliary cirrhosis (anti-mitochondrial antibody)

            b. Alcoholic hepatitis

GEN

      c. Drugs (barbiturates and Dilantin)

      d. Primary or metastatic liver cancer (CT)

  D. Impaired excretion: Increased direct Bili and normal bile salts

    1. Dubin-Johnson syndrome (increased urinary coproporphyrin I)

    2. Rotor's syndrome (increased total urinary coproporphyrin)

  E. Impaired conjugation: Increased indirect Bili

    1. Gilbert's disease (increased indirect Bili, other LFTs normal)

    2. Crigler-Najjar syndrome (glucuronyl transferase)

    3. Hypothyroidism (TSH, T_4)

V. HEPATITIS B SEROLOGY—See Chapter 55, Diagnosis and Management of Hepatitis B

CLINICAL PEARLS

- Abnormalities associated with drug-induced liver injury should resolve once the drug has been stopped. The presence of jaundice suggests more severe injury
- An alcohol user/abuser with elevated transaminases who stops drinking for 2–4 weeks should significantly lower those levels. Abstinence improves the prognosis in many stages of alcohol-induced liver disease
- If an unexpected result occurs on routine screening labs repeat the test, obtain an ALT if the AST is abnormal, a GGT if the Alk Phos is abnormal, or a fractionated Bili if the total Bili is abnormal
- The most common causes of asymptomatic liver enzyme elevation in the population are obesity and alcohol
- In an asymptomatic middle aged female with elevated liver enzymes, consider primary biliary cirrhosis and obtain a serum anti-mitochondrial antibody (AMA)
- In evaluating cholestasis, consider ultrasound early in the work-up to rule out bile duct enlargement

References

Herlong F. Approach to the patient with abnormal liver enzymes. Hosp Practice 1994;29(11):32–8.

Herrera JL. Abnormal liver enzyme levels. Postgrad Med 1993;93(2):113–30.

Interpretation of laboratory tests for the detection of hepatitis B virus infection. Minnesota Dept of Health Disease Control Newsletter 1992;20(1):6.

McKenna JP, Moskovitz M, Cox JL. Abnormal liver function tests in asymptomatic patients. Am Fam Phys 1989;39:117–26.

Michael B. Weinstock, MD

---

54. DIAGNOSIS AND MANAGEMENT OF THYROID DISEASE

I. INTRODUCTION/BACKGROUND: The following recommendations are for non-pregnant patients

  A. Thyroid-stimulating hormone (TSH): Secreted by the pituitary. Stimulates the steps of thyroid hormone production

  B. The thyroid gland: Secretes mostly T_4 and a small amount of T_3

  C. The most active thyroid hormone is T_3. About 90% of circulating T_3 is derived from peripheral deiodination of T_4

  D. Over 99% of circulating thyroid hormones are bound to proteins, mostly thyroid-binding globulin (TBG)

II. DIFFERENTIAL DIAGNOSIS

  A. Hyperthyroidism

    1. Toxic diffuse goiter (Graves' disease)

    2. Toxic adenoma

    3. Toxic multinodular goiter

    4. Painful subacute thyroiditis

    5. Silent thyroiditis including lymphocytic and postpartum variations

6. Iodine-induced hyperthyroidism
7. Excessive pituitary TSH (TSH secreting pituitary adenoma) or trophoblastic disease
8. Excessive ingestion of thyroid hormone (Thyrotoxicosis factitia)

B. Hypothyroidism
1. Primary hypothyroidism
   a. Autoimmune thyroiditis (Hashimoto's thyroiditis/Chronic lymphocytic thyroiditis): Most common cause in the US
   b. Surgical removal of the thyroid gland
   c. Radioactive iodine thyroid gland ablation
   d. External irradiation
   e. Thyroid gland iodine organification defect
   f. Idiopathic
2. Secondary (central) hypothyroidism
   a. Pituitary disease
   b. Hypothalamic disease

III. SIGNS AND SYMPTOMS AND LAB ABNORMALITIES

A. Hyperthyroidism: Severity of symptoms may vary (age of patient, duration of illness, magnitude of hormone excess)
1. General: Weight loss, poor sleep, alterations in appetite, fatigue, heat intolerance, increased sweating, mental disturbances
2. Eye: Vision change, photophobia, diplopia, exophthalmos
3. Neck: Possibly thyroid enlargement
4. Cardio: Palpitations and tachycardia, exertional intolerance/dyspnea on exertion
5. Neuro: Tremor, sudden paralysis
6. GYN: Menstrual disturbance (decreased flow), impaired fertility
7. Extremities: Pretibial myxedema (Graves' disease)

B. Hypothyroidism
1. General: Weight gain, poor sleep, alterations in appetite, fatigue, cold intolerance, hypothermia, dry skin, yellow skin, loss of hair, constipation
2. ENT: Thick tongue
3. Neck: Possibly thyroid enlargement (goiter)
4. Cardio: Bradycardia, cardiomyopathy
5. Neuro: Reflex delay, ataxia, memory and mental impairment, decreased concentration, depression, myalgias
6. GYN: Menstrual disturbance (increased flow), impaired fertility
7. Extremities: Myxedema
8. Lab abnormalities: In addition to abnormal thyroid tests (see below), increased cholesterol, increased liver enzymes and CPK, increased prolactin, hyponatremia, hypoglycemia, anemia (normal or increased MCV)

IV. TECHNIQUE FOR PHYSICAL EXAMINATION OF THE THYROID GLAND

A. Inspection: Located below the cricoid cartilage, observe while patient is swallowing water
B. Palpation
1. Examine from behind the patient
2. Palpate with 3 fingers on either side of the lower trachea (index fingers just below the cricoid) for size, shape, consistency, tenderness or nodularity
C. Examination during swallowing: The thyroid gland moves upward with swallowing and may be more easily palpated

V. INTERPRETATION OF LAB TESTS

A. Introduction
1. The primary screening test for thyroid abnormalities is TSH (ultrasensitive)
2. FTI (free thyroxine index) is a more precise way of measuring *active* (unbound) thyroxine than T_4. The T_4 level may not be a true indication of a patient's thyroid status because it is affected by altered states of protein binding
3. Free T_4 can also be measured directly, but is expensive and FTI is usually adequate
4. Causes of abnormal T_4 levels when free (active) thyroxine is normal

GEN

    a. Causes of increased T_4 secondary to increased thyroid binding proteins
        i. High estrogen states including pregnancy, oral contraceptives, estrogen replacement therapy, neonates
        ii. Acute illness including acute infectious hepatitis, AIDS, primary biliary cirrhosis
        iii. Drugs including Fluorouracil, Heroin, Methadone, Amiodarone, T_4 replacement therapy
        iv. Familial thyroid hormone binding abnormalities
        v. Hyperemesis gravidarum
    b. Causes of decreased T_4 secondary to decreased thyroid binding proteins
        i. Chronic debilitating illness including malnutrition, chronic renal failure, hypoproteinemia, cirrhosis
        ii. Nephrotic syndrome
        iii. Drugs including glucocorticoids, androgens, phenytoin, Phenobarbital, Carbamazepine, large doses of salicylates
        iv. Heredity TBG deficiency

B. Definition of commonly obtained thyroid tests:
    1. TSH: (High—hypothyroid; low—hyperthyroid) May be artificially elevated by severe illness, Metoclopramide, Haloperidol and artificially decreased by dopamine, steroids, or pregnancy (with morning-sickness). If abnormal, then check FTI or free T_4
    2. T_4: Measures thyroxine by radioimmunoassay and is affected by states of altered thyroxine binding (see above). It measures both circulating thyroxine bound to protein and active (unbound) thyroxine
    3. T_3RU: Does not measure T_3. It measures the *percentage* of T_4 *not bound* to protein. If this test is normal you know that thyroid binding proteins are not significantly altering the T_4 measurement, and T_4 will usually be an accurate estimation of *free T_4*. If T_3RU is abnormal, then look at FTI
    4. FTI: The FTI = T_4 × T_3RU/100. The FTI *usually* corrects for abnormalities of thyroxine binding and is a good approximation of the amount of active (unbound) thyroxine
    5. Free T_4: Measures the actual free T_4. Limitations are cost. May be falsely elevated in patients receiving Heparin (especially with dialysis) or depressed with severe nonthyroid illness
    6. T_3: For diagnosis of T_3 thyrotoxicosis (thyrotoxicosis with normal T_4 values). Like T_4, only measures *bound* T_3. Not useful in hypothyroidism. Obtain when suspect thyrotoxicosis in patients with low TSH and normal or low T_4 (T_3 toxicosis)
    7. Reverse T_3 (RT_3): RT_3 is an inactive isomer of T_3. Level is increased in hyperthyroidism, by drugs that block conversion of T_4 to T_3 (Amiodarone, Propranolol), and in nonthyroid illnesses that decrease the T_3 concentration
    8. Serum thyroglobulin: Storage site for thyroid hormones. Elevated in hyperthyroidism and thyroiditis. Reduced or undetectable in thyrotoxicosis factitia (exogenous thyroid hormone suppresses endogenous production)
    9. Thyroid antibodies: Found in 5–10% of normal subjects
        a. Antimicrosomal antibodies: Elevated in Hashimoto's thyroiditis. Can be elevated in Graves' disease
        b. Antithyroglobulin antibodies: Elevated in Hashimoto's thyroiditis or Graves' disease

VI. OTHER TESTS
    A. Radioiodine (^{123}I) Uptake and scan of thyroid gland: Provides a picture of thyroid uptake
        1. Elevated: *Graves' disease, toxic nodular goiter, toxic adenoma,* dietary iodine deficiency, pregnancy, early Hashimoto's thyroiditis, nephrotic syndrome, recovery from thyroid hormone suppression, recovery from subacute thyroiditis, some thyroid enzyme deficiencies
        2. Decreased: Administration of iodine (including drugs, contrast dyes, etc.), antithyroid drugs, subacute thyroiditis, thyroid hormone administration, severe (high turnover) Graves' disease, thyroid gland damage (thyroiditis, surgery, radioiodine), ectopic functioning thyroid tissue
    B. Ultrasound: To differentiate solid from cystic nodules. Purely cystic are usually not cancer
    C. Fine-needle aspiration (FNA) thyroid biopsy: See X. below
    D. Calcitonin assay: Useful serum marker in medullary thyroid carcinoma

VII. ALGORITHM FOR EVALUATION OF THYROID STATUS IN AMBULATORY PATIENTS

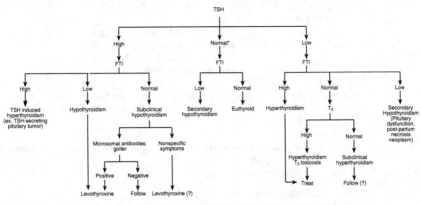

* — Serum TSH may be in normal range in patients with hyperthyroidism secondary to hypothalamic or pituitary disease

Source: Pittman JG. Evaluation of patients with mildly abnormal thyroid function tests. Am Fam Phys 1996;54:962. Used with permission.

VIII. MANAGEMENT OF HYPERTHYROIDISM (OR DECREASED TSH)

A. Graves' disease
1. Diagnosis: Symptoms of hyperthyroidism, low TSH, high FTI/free T$_4$, elevated antithyroglobulin and antimicrosomal antibodies, diffusely enlarged thyroid gland
2. ß-blockers (**Propranolol**)
   a. Symptomatic relief. No effect on thyroid hormone secretion
   b. Dose: Begin with 10mg PO QD and increase. Usual dose is 20mg PO QID
   c. Caution with nursing mothers as it is secreted in breast milk
3. **Radioactive iodine**: Treatment of choice
   a. May be given in an ablative dose (with life-long thyroid replacement therapy necessary) or in a smaller dose to attempt to induce a euthyroid state
   b. Elderly or patients with cardiac history may benefit from treatment with antithyroid drugs before radioactive iodine therapy (to deplete the gland of stored hormone)
   c. Contraindicated in pregnancy
   d. Patients usually become hypothyroid by 3 months. May require partial thyroid replacement 2 months after radioactive iodine treatment. Note: TSH may not be a good indicator of thyroid status for the first several months after treatment
   e. Frequency of follow-up: 3 months, 6 months, 1 year, then, if thyroid status has normalized (with replacement therapy), every 1–2 years
4. Antithyroid drugs
   a. Indications inc. hyperthyroidism in pregnancy, "pretreatment" in elderly or cardiac patients
   b. **Propylthiouracil (PTU)**
      i. Drug of choice in breast-feeding or pregnancy
      ii. Blocks peripheral conversion of T$_4$ to T$_3$
      iii. Dose 300–600mg PO QD in 4 divided doses
   c. **Methimazole (Tapazole)**
   d. Side effects: Minor skin rashes, rarely agranulocytosis, hepatitis
5. Surgery
   a. Uncommonly performed in the US, but may be appropriate with pregnant women intolerant of antithyroid drugs or non-pregnant patients who desire definitive therapy but who refuse radioactive iodine. Consider in pediatric patients
   b. Complications include hypoparathyroidism and vocal cord paralysis

B. Toxic solitary thyroid nodules
1. **Definition:** A single hyperfunctioning thyroid nodule causing hyperthyroidism
2. Symptomatic: **Propranolol**
3. Definitive treatment
   a. **Radioactive iodine**: Permanent hypothyroidism occurs in less than 10% of patients

          b. Surgery: Recommended if radioactive iodine is contraindicated

C. Toxic multinodular goiter
1. General: Usually affects older patients
2. Symptomatic: **Propranolol**
3. Antithyroid medications: 95% recurrence rate after thioureas are stopped
4. Definitive treatment
    a. **Radioactive iodine**: Thiourea treatment before iodine. Requires high doses of radioactive iodine. Recurrences are common—patients need close follow-up
    b. Surgery: Reserved for cosmetic purposes or pressure symptoms

D. Subacute thyroiditis
1. General: Painless inflammation of the thyroid gland lasting weeks to months causing transient hypo or hyperthyroidism. Subsides spontaneously after several weeks to months
2. Symptomatic hyperthyroidism: **Propranolol** is treatment of choice, 10–40mg PO QID
3. Treat transient hypothyroidism with **Levothyroxine** 0.05–0.1mg PO QD if symptomatic
4. Antithyroid medication: Ineffective as thyroid hormone production is low
5. **Radioactive iodine**: Ineffective since thyroid iodine uptake is low
6. Pain management with NSAIDs

E. Suppurative (bacterial) thyroiditis
1. Often occurs during course of systemic infection
2. Antibiotics: Empiric
3. Surgical drainage if fluctuant

F. Thyrotoxicosis factitia
1. Occurs from exogenous ingestion of thyroid hormone
2. If it is suspected, then check serum thyroglobulin. The thyroglobulin level is reduced or undetectable in thyrotoxicosis factitia (exogenous thyroid hormone suppresses endogenous production)
3. Manage with patient education or psychiatric referral

G. Subclinical hyperthyroidism
1. Definiton: Low TSH and normal T_4 and T_3
2. These patients have a 3 fold higher risk of developing atrial fibrillation within 10 years and some may be at risk of developing thyroid induced osteoporosis
3. Should be treated if associated with toxic goiter, toxic adenoma or toxic multinodular goiter
4. If asymptomatic, should probably not be treated, but followed closely for development of hyperthyroidism

IX. MANAGEMENT OF HYPOTHYROIDISM (OR INCREASED TSH)

A. Autoimmune thyroiditis (Hashimoto's thyroiditis): Chronic lymphocytic thyroiditis
1. Thyroid autoantibodies are positive 95% of the time
2. Management
    a. Elderly or patients with coronary disease: Start with **Levothyroxine (Synthroid, Levothyroid)** 0.025–0.05mg PO QD for 1 week, then increase by 0.025mg every week to a total dose of 0.075–0.15mg QD
    b. Young patients/healthy patients: Start with **Levothyroxine (Synthroid)** 0.05–0.1mg PO QD for 1 week, then increase by 0.025mg every week until TSH normalizes (usually 0.1–0.2mg QD)
    c. Note: Older patients generally require ²/₃ the amount as younger patients
3. Follow-up: Once TSH normalizes and patient is asymptomatic, then check TSH every 1–2 years
4. The half-life of T_4 is about 7 days. Check TSH level 6–8 weeks after a change in dosage of thyroid replacement. Early testing may lead to over-treatment
5. Drugs which increase the rate of thyroxine clearance: Phenytoin, Lovastatin, Carbamazepine, Amiodarone

B. Surgical removal of the thyroid gland
1. Hypothyroidism develops in 25% at 8–12 years post-op in patients with subtotal thyroidectomy
2. Management as above

C. Radioactive iodine thyroid gland ablation
1. Hypothyroidism develops at rate of 2–5% per year (30–70% at 10–15 years after treatment)
2. Management as above

D. Subclinical hypothyroidism
1. Normal T_4 (FTI) and high TSH
2. Longitudinal progression to hypothyroidism of 5–8% per year in patients with high TSH and significant titer of antimicrosomal antibodies. The incidence of hypothyroidism in patients over 65 years of age is 80% over 4 years
3. Indications for Levothyroid replacement therapy
   a. All patients with elevated TSH and a significant titer of antimicrosomal antibodies
   b. Elderly patients with TSH greater than 20 µU/mL (20mU/L) and a negative antimicrosomal antibody test
   c. Patients with elevated TSH and goiter (+/- antimicrosomal antibodies)
   d. History of radioiodine treatment for thyrotoxicosis and elevated TSH
   e. Consider in symptomatic patients with elevated TSH: Start at sub-therapeutic dose of 0.05–0.075mg PO QD
4. If treatment is not initiated, then follow closely

X. DIAGNOSIS AND MANAGEMENT OF SOLITARY THYROID NODULES
A. May occur in up to 50% of the population with sensitive imaging techniques. Most are benign, less than 5% are malignant. If an incidental nodule > 1 cm is found, then consider fine needle aspiration. Solitary nodules are associated with higher incidence of malignancy
B. Risk factors for thyroid cancer
1. History
   a. Age < 20 or > age 45
   b. Male
   c. Exposure to ionizing radiation (especially in childhood)
   d. Family history
2. Physical exam
   a. Cervical lymphadenopathy
   b. Vocal cord paralysis
   c. Very firm nodule
   d. Rapid tumor growth
   e. Fixation to adjacent structures
C. Factors which *do not* differentiate benign from malignant nodules:
1. History and physical exam
2. Thyroid function tests
3. Antithyroglobulin and antimicrosomal antibodies
4. Ultrasound: May be able to differentiate solid from cystic, but either type may be malignant
5. Thyroid radioiodine uptake and scan: May differentiate between a "cold" (nonfunctioning) nodule which is more likely to be malignant, and a "hot" (functioning nodule) which is less likely to be malignant, but does not *reliably* distinguish between benign and malignant nodules
D. Fine needle aspiration (FNA): Test of choice
1. Safe, reliable, inexpensive
2. Performed as an outpatient
3. Technique
   a. No anesthesia necessary
   b. Aspiration with 25 gauge needle
   c. Place material on slide and place second slide over the first, then draw the slides apart to obtain a thin smear. The first slide is air dried and the second slide is preserved in 95% alcohol and both are submitted to pathology
E. Results
1. If positive (suspicious or malignant), then referral for definitive therapy (surgery)
2. If indeterminate, then consider:
   a. Repeat FNA—*or*—
   b. Radionuclide scanning: If "hot" then follow and if "cold" then surgery—*or*—
   c. Trial of suppression therapy with monthly follow-up over 6 months

GEN

　　　　i. If size increases, then surgery
　　　　ii. If size decreases, then follow
　　　　iii. If size does not change, then consider surgery or repeat FNA
　　3. If inadequate, then consider referral for surgical excision in patients with one or more risk factors
　　4. If benign, then trial of suppression therapy with monthly follow-up over 6 months

XI. EVALUATION OF GOITER

A. Differential diagnosis
　　1. Hashimoto's thyroiditis
　　2. Iodide deficiency
　　3. Genetic thyroid hormone defects
　　4. Drug goitrogens: Lithium, iodide, PTU, Methimazole, Phenylbutazone, sulfonamides, Amiodarone
　　5. Infiltrating diseases: Cancer, sarcoidosis

B. Evaluation
　　1. History and physical exam as above
　　2. Obtain TSH, FTI (T_4 and T_3RU)
　　3. Consider thyroid radioiodine uptake and scan
　　4. Consider ultrasound and FNA if nodules are present

C. Management: Per specific diagnosis

CLINICAL PEARLS

- Free T_4 represents about 0.025% of total T_4 (bound and unbound)
- Amiodarone causes clinically significant hypothyroidism in about 8% of patients and asymptomatic hypothyroidism in another 17% of patients due to the high iodine concentration. (TSH high and T_4 low or normal)
- Use caution with diagnosis of hospitalized patients. Up to 70% of moderately ill hospitalized patients will have thyroid function abnormalities
- Symptoms of thyrotoxicosis vary with age and may be atypical, especially in the elderly

GEN

References

Bartalena L, et al. Relation between therapy for hyperthyroidism and the course of Graves' Ophthalmopathy. N Engl J Med 1998;338:73–8.

Hennessey JV. Diagnosis and management of thyrotoxocisis. Am Fam Phys 1996;54:1315.

Pittman JG. Evaluation of patients with mildly abnormal thyroid function tests. Am Fam Phys 1996;54:961.

Garcia M, et al. AACE treatment guidelines for hyperthyroidism and hypothyroidism. Endocr Practice 1995;1:54–62.

Costa AJ. Interpreting thyroid tests. Am Fam Phys 1995;52:2325.

Rifat SF. Management of thyroid nodules. Am Fam Phys 1994;50:785.

Mazzaferri EL, et al. Management of a solitary thyroid nodule. N Engl J Med 1993;328:553–9.

Michael B. Weinstock, MD

55. DIAGNOSIS AND MANAGEMENT
OF HEPATITIS B

I. BACKGROUND
A. Transmission of hepatitis B is by infected blood or blood products or by vertical transmission
B. Incubation period is 6 weeks to 6 months (may be prolonged with administration of HB immune globulin)
C. Fulminant hepatitis occurs in less than 1% of infected patients, but has a mortality rate of ~60%
D. Of all patients infected with hepatitis B, 5–10% develop chronic hepatitis or a chronic carrier state
E. In patients with chronic HBV, 20% develop cirrhosis within 20 years
F. Chronic hepatitis is caused by HBV (and HDV), and HCV and is defined as elevated serum aminotransferase levels for more than 6 months
G. If a patient has acute or chronic hepatitis B, then they should be checked for HCV and HDV

II. INTERPRETATION OF LAB TESTS
A. Overview: First look at HBsAg and HBsAb (see table, below)
  1. *If the HBsAg is positive*, then the patient usually has either acute hepatitis B or chronic infection
  2. *If the HBsAb is positive*, then the patient usually has either had past infection (and is noninfectious and protected from hepatitis B) or they have received the HBV vaccine
  3. If both are negative (rare), then the patient may be in the "window phase" (see below)
  4. If both are positive (rare), then see below
B. Tests
  1. **HBsAg:** First manifestation of HBV infection and persists throughout clinical illness. Persistence associated with chronic hepatitis and implies infectivity
  2. **HBsAb:** Occurs in most patients after clearance of HBsAg and implies noninfectivity and protection from recurrent HBV infection. (Occasionally, the appearance of HBsAb is delayed until clearance of HBsAg and during this "window phase," both HBsAb and HBsAg may be negative—see below)
  3. **HBcAb IgM:** Appears during acute hepatitis B and indicates a diagnosis of acute hepatitis B
  4. **HBcAb IgG:** Appears during acute hepatitis B and persists indefinitely
  5. **HBeAg:** Indicates viral replication and infectivity
  6. **HBeAb:** Follows HBeAg and signifies diminished viral replication
  7. **HBV DNA:** Usually parallels the presence of HBeAg, but is a more precise marker of viral replication and infectivity

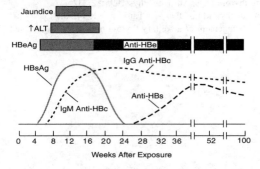

Source: Harrison's principles of internal medicine, 13th ed. New York, NY: McGraw-Hill, 1994:1458–83. Used with permission.

C. Result of HBV serologic tests and interpretation: (see below for management of patients diagnosed with active hepatitis B, chronic hepatitis B, and immunity)
  1. If HBsAg is positive and ...

     a. HBcAb IgM is positive and HBeAg is positive,
       the patient has *active hepatitis B*
     b. HBcAb IgG is positive and HBeAg is positive,
       the patient has *chronic hepatitis B* with active viral replication
     c. HBcAb IgG is positive and HBeAb is positive,
       the patient has *chronic hepatitis B* with low viral replication
     d. HBcAb IgG is positive and HBsAb is positive (HBeAg and HBeAb may be positive or negative)
       the patient has *chronic hepatitis B* with heterotypic HBsAb (~10% of cases)

2. If HBsAb is positive and ...
     a. All other tests are negative,
       the patient has received a vaccine and is *immune*
     b. HBcAb IgG is positive (HBeAb may be positive or negative),
       the patient has recovered from hepatitis B and is *immune*

3. If HBsAg and HBsAb are both negative and ...
     a. HBcAb IgM is positive (HBeAg positive or negative),
       the patient has acute hepatitis B and is in the "window phase"
     b. HBcAb IgG is positive and all other tests are negative,
       this is usually a false positive

COMMON SEROLOGIC PATTERNS IN HEPATITIS B INFECTION AND THEIR INTERPRETATION

HBsAg	HBsAb	HBcAb	HBeAg	HBeAb	Interpretation
+	-	IgM	+	-	Acute hepatitis B
+	-	IgG	+	-	Chronic hepatitis B with active viral replication
+	-	IgC	-	+	Chronic hepatitis B with low viral replication
+	+	IgC	+ or -	+ or -	Chronic hepatitis with heterotypic HBsAb (~10% of cases)
-	-	IgM	+ or -	-	Acute hepatitis B
-	+	IgG	-	+ or -	Recovery from hepatitis B (immunity)
-	+	-	-	-	Vaccination (immunity)
-	-	IgG	-	-	False positive; less commonly, infection in remote past

Source: Tierney LM, et al. current medical diagnosis and treatment. 36th ed. Norwalk, CT: Appleton & Lange, 1997: 611. Used with permission.

III. ACTION

A. Patient has active hepatitis B
  1. The acute illness usually subsides over 2–3 weeks and lab values are normalized within 16 weeks unless the patient develops chronic hepatitis (see below)
  2. Clinical picture: Variable clinical picture with symptoms ranging from asymptomatic to general malaise, myalgia, arthralgia, easy fatigability, anorexia, nausea/vomiting, diarrhea, fever/chills, jaundice (occurs after 5–10days)
  3. Physical exam: Hepatomegaly (over 50% of the time), splenomegaly (15%), lymphadenopathy
  4. Lab: Low WBC, elevated ALT or AST, elevated bilirubin and alkaline phosphatase, elevated prothrombin time (in severe hepatitis), mild proteinuria and bilirubinuria
  5. Management
     a. Acute disease—Symptomatic: Rest, good diet, avoidance of hepatotoxins (alcohol). Avoidance of behaviors which may transmit hepatitis B (blood donation, unprotected sex, etc.)
     b. Long-term management: Follow LFT's and HBsAg every month until disappearance of HBsAg. When this occurs, then check for appearance of HBsAb. If HBsAg is still positive after 6 months, then the patient has **chronic hepatitis** (see III.B.)
  6. Indications for hospital admission
     a. Encephalopathy
     b. Prothrombin time (PT) prolonged > 3 seconds

GEN

      c. Intractable vomiting

      d. Hypoglycemia

      e. Bilirubin > 20mg/dL

      f. Age > 45 years

      g. Immunosupression

B. Patient has chronic hepatitis B

  1. Definition: Persistent HBsAg > 6 months, chronic liver inflammation and characteristic histologic findings

    a. Chronic active hepatitis (replicative phase)

      i. Persistent HBsAg > 6 months

      ii. Persistent presence of HBV DNA or HBeAg

      iii. Liver injury (Persistent elevation of LFTs > 6 months)

    b. Chronic persistent hepatitis (nonreplicative phase)

      i. Persistent HBsAg > 6 months

      ii. Absence of HBV DNA and HBeAg (possibly presence of HBeAb)

      iii. Minimal liver injury (Modest LFT elevation)

    ** Remissions are characterized by the disappearance of HBV DNA and HBeAg (HBsAg persists). This means that the virus is in a non-replicative phase, and the patient is classified as having chronic persistent hepatitis—an important distinction from chronic active hepatitis, which is characterized by higher infectivity and greater risk of progression to cirrhosis. The likelihood of converting from replicative to nonreplicative disease is approx. 10–15% per year

  2. Clinical picture

    a. Chronic persistent hepatitis: Range from asymptomatic to mild symptoms; fatigue, anorexia, nausea

    b. Chronic active hepatitis: Asymptomatic to mild or severe constitutional symptoms, especially fatigue. Possibly jaundice, arthralgias, anorexia. End-stage: ascites, edema, bleeding varices, hepatic encephalopathy, coagulopathy

  3. Physical exam

    a. Chronic persistent hepatitis: Minimal findings—occasionally hepatomegaly

    b. Chronic active hepatitis: Symptoms associated with chronic liver disease

  4. Lab: Aminotransferase elevations (usually 100–1000 units), minimally elevated alkaline phosphatase, hyperbilirubinemia, hypoalbuminemia, prolongation of prothrombin time

  5. Management with interferon

    a. Indications for treatment of chronic hepatitis B with interferon—all must be present (Patients with normal aminotransferase values should not be treated)

      i. Persistent elevations in serum aminotransferase concentrations (greater than 6 months)

      ii. Detectable levels of HBsAg, HBeAg, and HBV DNA in serum

      iii. Chronic hepatitis on liver biopsy

      iv. Compensated liver disease

    b. Dose: Recommended regimen is 5 million units daily or 10 million units 3 times per week, subcutaneously for 4–6 months (Induces remission in 25–40% of patients compared to 12% of controls)

    c. Response to interferon: Patient is considered to be in remission if the HBeAg (and HBV DNA) disappears

  C. Patient has recovered from hepatitis B or has been vaccinated and is immune: No further action required

IV. INDICATIONS FOR HB IMMUNE GLOBULIN (Must be given within 7 days of exposure)

  A. Sexual contacts of persons with HBV infection

  B. Individuals exposed to HBsAg containing material via mucous membranes or breaks in the skin

  C. Newborn infants of HBsAg positive mothers (followed by the vaccine series)

CLINICAL PEARLS

    • The risk of chronic infection in a neonate is 90% (when transmitted at the time of delivery by HBsAg positive mothers). They must receive the HB immune globulin, followed by the vaccine series

    • Up to 50% of cases of HCV are attributable to IV drug use. HCV is responsible for over 90%

GEN

of cases of post-transfusion hepatitis
- HDV is a defective virus that only causes hepatitis in the presence of HBV infection. In the USA, infection is primarily with IV drug users
- There has been a 60% reduction in occupationally acquired hepatitis B infection due to immunization programs
- The hepatitis B vaccine series induces protective antibodies in 95% of healthy volunteers 20–39 y/o
- In patients with chronic HCV, 50% develop cirrhosis within 40 years
- The incidence of hepatocellular carcinoma increases 200–300 fold in patients with chronic hepatitis B

References

Hoofnagle JH, DiBisceglie AM. The treatment of chronic viral hepatitis. N Engl J Med 1997; 336:347–55.

Molloy PJ, et al. Treatment of chronic hepatitis B and hepatitis C with interferon Alfa-2b. Am Fam Phys 1996;54:1598–1602.

Tintinalli JE, ed. Emergency medicine, a comprehensive study guide. 5th ed. New York: McGraw-Hill, 2000; 499–503.

Isselbacher KJ, et al. Harrison's principles of internal medicine. 13th ed. New York; 1994:1458–83.

Daniel M. Neides, MD

GEN

56. ANEMIA

DEFINITION: A decrease in the number of red blood cells or a decrease in the concentration of hemoglobin. Anemia should be divided into microcytic (MCV < 83 mcm^3), normocytic (MCV 83–100 mcm^3), or macrocytic (MCV > 100 mcm^3)

—PART ONE: MICROCYTIC ANEMIA (MCV <83 mcm^3)—

I. INTRODUCTION
   A. **Microcytosis** is the presence of small red blood cells (RBCs) and characterized by a mean corpuscular volume (MCV) < 83 mcm^3
   B. Differential diagnosis
      1. Iron deficiency anemia (the most common cause of microcytosis)
      2. (Anemia of) chronic disease
      3. Thalassemia
      4. Sideroblastic anemia
      5. Lead toxicity

II. IRON DEFICIENCY ANEMIA
   A. Physiology of normal iron metabolism
      1. Most iron absorption takes place in the small intestine with the duodenum being the most active site of absorption
      2. Mucosal iron is stored as ferritin; the mucosal transport protein is transferrin
      3. Iron storage (as ferritin) is primarily found in the bone marrow, spleen, liver and skeletal muscle
      4. Iron is required for hemoglobin and DNA synthesis
      5. The daily dietary intake of iron in the US is approximately 10–20mg/day. The USRDA is 10mg/day
   B. Etiology of iron deficiency anemia
      1. Blood loss: PUD, colon cancer (or any malignancy), menstruation, trauma, drugs, pulmonary hemosiderosis, polycythemia, inflammatory bowel disease (IBD)
      2. Decreased ingestion: Infants and children
      3. Increased requirements: Pregnancy
      4. Decreased absorption: Malabsorption syndromes (IBD), partial gastrectomy
   C. History and physical examination

1. Many patients with mild anemia will be asymptomatic
2. History: Fatigue, weakness, headache, increased irritability, palpitations, paresthesias, sore tongue, brittle nails, or PICA (the desire to eat dirt, ice, paint)
3. Physical examination may be normal. Abnormal findings may include tachycardia, murmur, CHF, papillary atrophy of the tongue, retinal hemorrhages, glossitis, brittle nails, or splenomegaly

D. An algorithmic approach to microcytic anemia

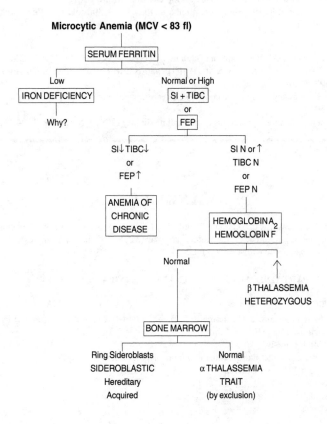

FEP = Free Erythrocyte Protoporphyrin; **N** = Normal; **SI** = serum iron; **TIBC** = total iron binding capacity.

Source: Wheby MS. Anemia: classification, mechanisms, diagnosis and physiologic effects. In Thorup OA, et al., eds. Leavell and Thorup's fundamentals of clinical hematology. Philadelphia: W.B. Saunders, 1987:171. Used with permission.

ETIOLOGY	SERUM Fe	TIBC	FERRITIN	BONE MARROW Fe STORES	HgbA$_2$ AND F (FETAL)
Iron Deficiency	Decreased	Increased	Decreased	NONE	Normal
Chronic Disease	Decreased	Normal or Decreased	Normal or *Increased*	Normal or Increased	Normal
Thalassemia	Normal	Normal	Normal or Increased	Normal	Increased in b-thal; Normal in a-thal
Sideroblastic anemia	Normal or Increased	Normal or Increased	Normal or Increased	Increased	Normal

E. Laboratory data in iron deficiency anemia (and other causes of microcytosis)

F. Management of iron deficiency anemia
    1. Evaluating the gastrointestinal tract in iron deficiency anemia
        a. Idiopathic iron deficiency anemia in adults most often occurs from blood loss somewhere in the GI tract
        b. Patients with unexplained iron deficiency anemia should be questioned regarding symptoms associated with upper and/or lower GI tract disease. A fecal occult blood test should be obtained
        c. An endoscopic evaluation should be considered (either EGD or colonoscopy depending on patient's symptoms)
        d. For asymptomatic adults, a colonoscopy should be obtained first, followed by an EGD if the colonoscopic examination is negative
    2. Replacement therapy with either oral or parenteral iron should be initiated once the diagnosis of iron deficiency is made
        a. Adults: **FeSO$_4$** 325mg PO BID–TID
        b. Children: 3–6mg elemental **Fe**/kg/day PO divided TID (e.g., Fer-in-sol)
        c. Side effects: Cramping, nausea, constipation and/or diarrhea (if these develop, decrease the dose to either QD or BID)

— PART TWO: MACROCYTIC ANEMIA (MCV > 100 mcm^3)—

I. DIFFERENTIAL DIAGNOSIS
    A. Alcohol abuse
    B. B$_{12}$ or folate deficiency (see section III for etiologies)
    C. Hemolysis or bleeding
    D. Liver disease
    E. Hypothyroidism
    F. Myelodysplasia
    G. Chemotherapeutic agents or other drugs

II. HISTORY AND PHYSICAL EXAMINATION
    A. History
        1. Determine number of alcoholic beverages patient drinks per *day.* (Ask *CAGE* questions if appropriate.) Ask about blackouts, missed work, recent DUI convictions
        2. Diet: Strict vegetarians are susceptible to developing B$_{12}$ deficiency. Patients with a high carbohydrate diet (and nothing else) are susceptible to folate deficiency
        3. Past medical history (including malabsorption syndromes, inflammatory bowel disease)
        4. Past surgical history: Partial or total gastrectomy predisposes the patient to B$_{12}$ deficiency (pernicious anemia)
        5. Neurologic symptoms: Paresthesias or gait disturbances
        6. Symptoms of hypothyroidism: Anorexia, constipation, dysphagia, alopecia, brittle hair, dry skin, depression, vertigo, or fatigue

GEN

7. History of chemical or radiation exposure (myelodysplasia)
8. Medications including Zidovudine (AZT), Stavudine (d4t), Dilantin, Phenobarbital, OCPs, Sulfa, Trimethoprim, Colchicine, Neomycin

B. Physical examination: Will often be normal
1. Spider angiomata, sore tongue, tremor, ataxia, weight loss (alcohol abuse)
2. Weakness, gait disturbance, or decreased sensation (B_{12} deficiency)
3. Jaundice, ascites or hepatosplenomegaly (liver disease)

C. An algorithmic approach to macrocytic anemia

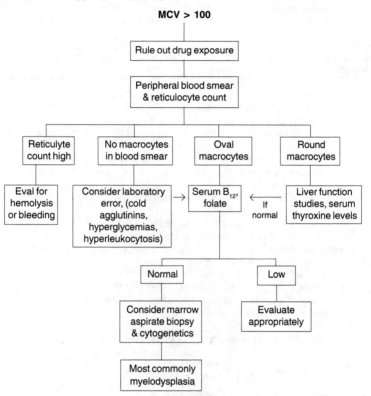

Source: Colon-Otero G, Menke D, Hook CC. A practical approach to the differential diagnosis and evaluation of the adult patient with macrocytic anemia. In Wheby MS, ed. Medical Clinics N Am. Philadelphia: W.B. Saunders, 1992: 590. Used with permission.

D. Laboratory evaluation
1. Peripheral blood smear: Look for target cells (liver disease), hyposegmented neutrophils (myelodysplasia) and hypersegmented neutrophils (B_{12} or folate deficiency)
2. Labs: B_{12} and folate levels, TSH, reticulocyte count, and liver function tests
3. Bone marrow aspirate: Should be considered on an individualized basis (patients with normal B_{12} and folate levels, not on chemotherapy)
4. Schilling test and/or anti-intrinsic factor antibiotics: B_{12} malabsorption

III. ETIOLOGIES OF B_{12} AND FOLATE DEFICIENCIES AND TREATMENTS
A. B_{12} deficiency
1. Decreased intake: Strict vegetarian
2. Decreased absorption: Pernicious anemia, abnormal (or deficient) intrinsic factor, gastrectomy, gastric atrophy, Crohn's disease, ileal resection, celiac disease, tropical sprue, chronic

pancreatitis, bacterial overgrowth
3. Decreased utilization: Nitrous oxide inhalation, inborn errors of metabolism
4. **Treatment of B$_{12}$ deficiency:** B$_{12}$ injection (**Cyanocobalamin**) 1mg IM Q month—*or*—**vitamin B$_{12}$** 25–250mcg PO QD (if secondary to decreased intake)—*or*—**Cyanocobalamin** intranasal spray (**Nascobal**) 500mcg once weekly following injectable B$_{12}$ therapy (maintenance)

B. Folate
1. Decreased intake
2. Decreased absorption: Tropical sprue, celiac disease, short gut syndrome
3. Drugs: Dilantin, Phenobarbital, alcohol, OCs, Trimethoprim, Sulfa
4. Increased demands: Pregnancy, infancy, hemolytic anemia
5. Treatment of folate deficiency
   a. Children: 0.5–1.0mg PO QD
   b. Adults: 1mg PO QD
   c. Note: May also give IM, IV, or subcutaneously

—PART THREE: NORMOCYTIC ANEMIA (MCV 83–100 mcm^3)—

I. DIFFERENTIAL DIAGNOSIS
 A. Early iron deficiency anemia
 B. Anemia of chronic disease (can be normocytic or microcytic)
 C. Chronic renal insufficiency
 D. Endocrine disorders: Thyroid disease, hyperparathyroidism, adrenal insufficiency
 E. Bone marrow failure: Radiation, drugs (chemotherapy), viruses (HIV, hepatitis B)
 F. Bone marrow replacement: Metastatic cancer, myelofibrosis, leukemia
 G. Acute blood loss
 H. Drugs

GEN

CLINICAL PEARLS
 • A patient with neurologic symptoms secondary to a B$_{12}$ deficiency who is treated with folic acid may develop worsening symptoms
 • Anemia is the most common hematologic abnormality in pregnancy
 • Hgb > 12g/dL should be considered normal in elderly men and women. Observation alone may be reasonable in an elderly patient whose Hgb is 11–12g/dL with normal reticulocyte count, normocytic and normochromic indices, normal WBC and platelet count, negative fecal occult blood, and normal serum ferritin. Further work-up would be indicated if the anemia worsened or the indices changed

References
Little DR. Ambulatory management of common Forms of anemia. Am Fam Phys 1999;59:1598.
Rockey DC, Cello JP. Evaluation of the gastrointestinal tract in patients with iron deficiency anemia. N Engl J Med 1993;329:1691–5.
Massey AC. Microcytic anemia: differential diagnosis and management of iron deficiency anemia. In: Wheby MS, ed. Medical Clinics N Am. Philadelphia: W.B. Saunders, 1992:549–66.
Colon-Otero G, Menke D, Hook CC. A practical approach to the differential diagnosis and evaluation of the adult patient with macrocytic anemia. In: Wheby MS, ed. Medical Clinics N Am. Philadelphia: W.B. Saunders, 1992:581–97.
Mansouri A, Lipschitz DA. Anemia in the elderly patient. In: Wheby MS, ed. Medical Clinics N Am. Philadelphia: W.B. Saunders, 1992:622–3.
Wheby MS. Anemia: classification, mechanisms, diagnosis and physiologic effects. In: Thorup OA, et al., eds. Leavell and Thorup's fundamentals of clinical hematology. Philadelphia: W.B. Saunders, 1987:171.

57. EVALUATION OF DIARRHEA IN ADULTS

DEFINITION: A change in bowel habits, including increased stool volume, looseness, or frequency

I. DIFFERENTIAL DIAGNOSIS OF DIARRHEA
A. **Viral:** Rotavirus, Norwalk, Adenovirus, Enterovirus, HIV
B. **Bacterial**: *Salmonella, Shigella, Yersinia, Campylobacter, E. coli, Vibrio cholerae, Vibrio parahaemolyticus, Staphylococcus aureus, Clostridium perfringens*
C. **Parasitic:** *Giardia lamblia, Entamoeba histolytica, Cryptosporidium*
D. **Drugs:** Laxatives, Antibiotics, Caffeine, Alcohol, Digitalis
E. **Inflammatory:** Ulcerative colitis, Crohn's disease, Ischemic colitis, Pseudomembranous colitis (*C. difficile*)
F. **Malabsorption:** Sprue, Lymphoma, Whipple's disease, Pancreatic insufficiency, Lactose intolerance
G. **Tumors:** Intestinal carcinoma, Carcinoid, Islet-cell tumors, Medullary carcinoma of the thyroid, Villous adenoma
H. **Functional:** Irritable bowel syndrome, Diverticulosis
I. **Postsurgical:** Postgastrectomy dumping syndrome, Parasympathetic denervation, Short bowel syndrome, enteroenteric fistulas
J. **Other:** Cirrhosis, Diabetes mellitus, Hyperthyroidism, Addison's disease, Scleroderma, Amyloidosis, Radiation enteritis

II. HISTORY
A. **Bowel Movements:** Frequency, consistency, and volume; determine presence of blood, pus, or mucus
B. **Abdominal Pain:** Periumbilical or RLQ pain and large stool volume likely have a small bowel etiology; LLQ pain and frequent, small volume stools likely have a colonic etiology
C. **Fever**
D. **Travel History:** Camping (infected water supply or well water exposure), other countries
E. **Food exposure:** Onset of symptoms within hours of eating contaminated food
F. **Drug history:** Recent antibiotics, laxative use, antacids, excessive alcohol, caffeinated beverages, sorbitol (sugar-free gum or candy)
G. **Sexual history:** Anal intercourse may result in a polymicrobial etiology

III. PHYSICAL EXAMINATION
A. **Vital signs:** Blood pressure (postural hypotension) and heart rate (tachycardia)—may reflect dehydration; temperature; weight
B. **Abdomen:** Guarding, rebound tenderness, hypo- or hyperactive bowel sounds, hepatomegaly, ascites, or masses
C. **Rectal**: Guaiac stool, note any fistulas
D. **Skin**: Rash (may be viral or bacterial etiology) or jaundice

IV. LABORATORY—If indicated:
A. **Stool specimen:** Blood, fecal leukocytes, culture and sensitivity (typically will test for *Salmonella, Shigella, Yersinia, and Campylobacter*), ova and parasites, and *C. difficile*   (recent antibiotic use)
B. **Complete blood count:** Decreased H/H (anemia from chronic blood loss) or elevated WBC's with left shift (infectious etiology)
C. **Serum chemistry:** Hypernatremia and/or elevated BUN/creatinine (dehydration); hypokalemia, metabolic acidosis due to bicarbonate loss; lactic acidosis due to dehydration

V. OTHER STUDIES
A. **Abdominal x-rays:** Patients with severe pain or any evidence on exam that indicates intestinal obstruction, mass, or perforation
B. **Colonoscopy** or **Sigmoidoscopy:** Patients with bloody diarrhea (IBD) or if *C. difficile* is suspected

VI. MANAGEMENT

A. Rehydration: Replace fluid loss and electrolytes (oral rehydration solution)

B. Diet: Try to avoid fruits or fruit juices that may promote diarrhea (apples or prunes); otherwise may advance diet as tolerated

C. Anti-diarrheal agents: Contraindicated in patients with an infectious etiology to their diarrhea or bloody stool

   1. **Imodium:** 4mg PO initially, then 2mg after each unformed stool (max: 16mg/day)

   2. **Pepto-Bismol**

D. Antibiotics: Useful when identification of a parasite or bacteria is determined; may be used empirically when diarrhea persists despite negative stool cultures

   1. *Salmonella*—Adults: **Ciprofloxacin** 500mg PO BID for 3–5 days

      Children: **TMP/SMX DS** 1 tablet PO bid for 3–5 days; **TMP/SMX** 8mg/40mg/kg/day in 2 divided doses

   2. *Shigella*—Adults: **Ciprofloxacin** 500mg PO BID for 3–5 days

      Children: **TMP/SMX DS** 1 tablet PO BID for 3–5 days; **TMP/SMX** 8mg/40mg/kg/day in 2 divided doses

   3. *Yersinia*—Adults: **Ciprofloxacin** 500mg PO BID for 3–5 days

      Children: **TMP/SMX DS** 1 tablet PO BID for 3–5 days; **TMP/SMX** 8mg/40mg/kg/day in 2 divided doses

   4. *Campylobacter*—Adults: **Ciprofloxacin** 500mg PO BID for 5 days

      Children: **Erythromycin** 500mg PO BID for 5 days; 20mg/kg/day in 2 divided doses

   5. *C. difficile*—**Flagyl** 250mg PO TID for 7–14 days

   6. *E. coli*—Adults: **Ciprofloxacin** 500mg PO BID for 3–5 days

      Children: **TMP/SMX DS** 1 tablet PO BID for 3–5 days; **TMP/SMX** 8mg/40mg/kg/day in 2 divided doses

   7. *Vibrio cholera*—Adults: **Ciprofloxacin** 1g PO × 1 dose

      Children: **Tetracycline** or **TMP/SMX** (if under age 9)

   8. *Giardia*—**Flagyl** 250mg PO TID for 5 days

   9. *Entamoeba histolytica*—**Flagyl** 750mg PO TID for 10 days

   10. *Cryptosporidium*—No agent with proven efficacy

GEN

CLINICAL PEARLS

- Traveller's diarrhea can occur from contaminated ice cubes or water used to wash fruits or vegetables
- Patients taking Flagyl for an infectious diarrhea should avoid alcohol (may cause an antabuse-like reaction)
- Test for HIV in patients diagnosed with *Cryptosporidium*

References
Lipsky MS. Chronic diarrhea: Evaluation and treatment. Am Fam Phys 1993;48:1461.
Heck JE. Traveler's diarrhea. Am Fam Phys 1993;48:793.

Ken Griffiths, MD
Beth Weinstock, MD
Frank Weinstock, MD, FACS

58. SCREENING, DIAGNOSIS, AND MANAGEMENT OF OCULAR DISORDERS

I. INDICATIONS FOR REFERRAL TO OPHTHALMOLOGIST
A. Immediate referral
1. **Penetrating trauma:** History of missile type injury, high velocity, metal on metal, irregular pupil
2. **Acute glaucoma:** Red and painful eye, pupil semi-dilated and fixed, hazy cornea decreased vision. May have nausea and abdominal pain. Family history
3. **Corneal ulcer:** Red and painful eye, photophobia, fluorescein staining on cornea. Usually associated with trauma, poor lid apposition, or contact lens wear
4. **Postoperative infection/endophthalmitis:** Pain, decreased vision, white cell level in anterior chamber, purulent drainage. Can result from any invasive ophthalmologic procedure
5. **Iritis:** Limbal flush, photophobia, small pupil, sore eye. Usually post-traumatic
6. **Floaters, flashes, or sudden decreased vision:** Differential includes retinal detachment or hole, occlusion of the retinal vein or artery, trauma, or stroke
7. **Corneal foreign body or rust ring that cannot be removed**
8. **Orbital cellulitis**
9. **Chemical exposure,** especially alkali/lye solutions
B. Referral within several days: Poor healing of corneal abrasion, unresponsive conjunctivitis, double vision or any visual problem that does not improve with treatment

II. HISTORY
A. Onset of vision loss, pain, redness,etc
B. Length of symptoms
C. Change in vision: floaters, halos, scotoma (zigzags), photopsia (flashing lights), specific visual field defects
D. Photophobia
E. Pain, with or without eye movement
F. Diplopia
G. Itching, burning, crusting
H. Contact lens wear
I. Vision decrease or difficulty seeing at night
J. Recent eye surgery or trauma (if so, was the patient wearing safety glasses)
K. Systemic symptoms: CVA/TIA symptoms, nausea, vomiting, abdominal pain, fever, temporal pain, jaw claudication (c/w temporal arteritis), etc.

III. PHYSICAL EXAMINATION
A. Check visual acuity of each eye with correction. If corrective lenses not available, use:
Pinhole—Patient reads visual acuity chart through a pinhole; should compensate for any uncorrected refractive errors if patient does not have corrective lenses available (i.e., in a trauma situation). If no eye chart available, use newspapers, fingers etc. If not corrected through pinhole, then should suspect disease
OD (oculus dexter) = right eye
OS (oculus sinister) = left eye
OU (oculus uterque) = both eyes
B. Check pupils
1. Size: May be unequal in size (anisocoria) but should still be reactive. Patient can usually tell you if this is a new finding
2. Reactivity: reactive vs. nonreactive
3. Swinging flashlight test: checks consensual response in opposite pupil
C. Inspect lids: May need to evert lid to check for foreign body. This is easily done if the patient is looking down while upper lid is everted with pressure from a cotton swab. Check for lid

eversion (ectropion), lid inversion (entropion), lash growth toward the cornea (trichiasis), chalazion (see below). Also check for lash loss or crusting

D. Extraocular muscle function: Motility and position
  1. Cranial N. III—medial, inferior, and superior rectus and inf. oblique as well as levator muscle of lid
  2. Cranial N. IV—superior oblique
  3. Cranial N. VI—innervates lateral rectus
  Strabismus—misalignment of the eyes; important to recognize early in pediatric patients
E. Fluorescein staining: Will stain areas of denuded epithelium
F. Tonometry: If glaucoma is suspected. Normal intraocular pressure is 20 mmHg or below
G. Funduscopic Exam: Eyes may be dilated with **Neo-Synephrine 2.5%** or **1% Mydriacyl** (effects will reverse in 4–6hrs, maximum effect in about 20 minutes). Atropine drops should not be used because mydriasis will last up to 1–2 weeks. Dilation causing an attack of acute angle closure glaucoma is extremely uncommon; do not dilate if anterior chamber appears shallow
  1. Check red reflex bilaterally; should be equal
  2. Hemorrhages
  3. Retinal detachments
  4. Cotton wool spots—infarctions of nerve fibers
  5. Cherry red spot in macula—central retinal artery occlusion
  6. Also check for papilledema, A-V nicking, optic pallor
  7. Cup to disk rate (normal is ≤0.3)
H. Confrontation Visual field: Examiner should be at least 3 feet in front of patient. Used to detect gross hemianopic and other visual field defects
I. Slit lamp exam, if available: Used to examine anterior segment of eye. Helpful if attempting to diagnose and remove foreign bodies. Use cobalt blue filter to highlight fluorescein-stained areas of denuded epithelium. Check for inflammatory cells in anterior chamber:
  Hyphema—blood in anterior chamber
  Hypopyon—purulence in anterior chamber (seen in iritis or infection)
  Flare—light scatter caused by inflammatory cells in the aqueous fluid

IV. MANAGEMENT
A. Conjunctivitis:
  1. Bacterial: Purulent drainage, red eye, minimal pain, no change in vision
    a. Three most common pathogens are: *Strep pneumoniae, H. Influenzae,* and *S. aureus*
    b. Drops are given every 1–2hrs while awake for the first 1–2 days, then QID. 1 drop is sufficient. Encourage frequent hand washing
    c. **Tobramycin (Tobrex)** or **Gentamicin (Garamycin):** Good broad spectrum ATB
    d. **Trimethoprim–Polymyxin B (Polytrim):** Good in adults and children
    e. **Sulfacetamide 10% (Bleph-10):** Less effective but inexpensive
    f. **Ofloxacin (Ocuflox)** and **Norfloxacin (Chibroxin):** Broad spectrum, expensive
  2. Allergic: Bilateral itchy, red eyes without matting/purulence
    a. **Note:** *Levocabastine, Ketorolac and Lodoxamide should not be used with soft contact lenses*
    b. **Cromolyn Sodium (Crolom):** Mast cell stabilizer: 1–2 gtts OU 4–6 ×/day
    c. **Lodoxamide (Alomide):** Mast cell stabilizer: 1–2 gtts OU 4–6 ×/ day
    d. **Olopatadine (Patanol):** Mast cell stabilizer: 1–2 gtts OU BID
    e. **Levocabastine (Livostin):** Antihistamine: 1 gtt OU QID for up to 2 weeks
    f. **NaphConA (vasoconstrictor/ antihistamine):** 1 gtt OU Q 3–4hrs PRN; should not be used for a prolonged time due to rebound
    f. **Ketorolac (Acular):** Anti-inflammatory 1 gtt QID for 7 days
    h. **Note:** A weak steroid drop may be used for severe cases, but this is usually prescribed only by an ophthalmologist
B. Corneal abrasion:
Must distinguish from corneal foreign body, herpes simplex (dendritic appearance to corneal stain) or corneal ulcer (will see an infiltrate around corneal defect in the case of corneal ulcer). Symptoms include a history of mild trauma (i.e., fingernail scratch, tree branch, contact lens), photophobia, conjunctival injection, involuntary lid closure, increased tearing

GEN

1. Examine eye as outlined above. Slit lamp used to facilitate exam. Visual acuity may be decreased if abrasion is in central cornea (20/80 to 20/200). If no slip lamp is available, the ophthalmoscope is important for direct observation or by localizing the abrasion or FB against the red reflex
2. Topical anesthetic (to relieve discomfort and facilitate examination): 1 drop of **Tetracaine** or **Proparcaine**. Will lead to immediate relief of pain. *Do not* send patient home with anesthetic drops as they may inhibit corneal healing
3. Prophylactic antibiotics may be prescribed. Can also give cycloplegic drops (**1% Cyclogyl** or **Homatropine 2%** TID) which will make patient more comfortable (only give in cases of severe discomfort)
4. If patient is uncomfortable, may patch the eye tightly overnight. Does not speed healing. Make sure lid is closed under patch
5. Tell patients that they may feel as if something is in their eye for several days
6. Patient should follow-up in 1–4 days if not healed

C. Corneal foreign body: Consider referral
1. Examine and use topical anesthetic as used in corneal abrasion
2. Remove corneal foreign body with blunt instrument, cotton swab, or forceps. Avoid needles
3. Patient may return to normal activities immediately. No need to patch eye
4. Prophylactic antibiotic drops
5. If a rust ring remains or foreign body cannot be removed, then refer

D. Conjunctival foreign body
1. No anesthetic necessary
2. Evert upper eyelid and remove foreign body with a cotton swab—pain should be essentially relieved
3. May see linear, vertical corneal abrasions (ice-skate track abrasions) indicating retained foreign bodies in the superior tarsal conjunctiva

E. Blepharitis: Look for erythema of lid margin, dandruff-like deposits on lashes, fibrinous scales around individual lashes (collarettes), lash loss, recurrent mild conjunctivitis. Patient will complain of irritation, burning, excessive tearing (epiphora), foreign body sensation
1. Caused by seborrhea, staph infection, and/or meibomian gland dysfunction
2. Wash hands after touching eyes
3. Antibacterial eye drops, treat 7–10 days. If recurs, then:
4. Wash lids every day with baby shampoo (eyes closed)
5. Warm compresses to eye TID

F. Sudden onset double vision (diplopia)
Distinguish monocular or binocular double vision: binocular will resolve when either eye is covered. Monocular is secondary to uncorrected refractive error, dry eye, corneal scar, or cataract, etc. Binocular diplopia may be secondary to nerve palsies (III, IV, or VI), decompensated strabismus, myasthenia gravis, thyroid eye disease, blow-out fracture
1. Patch either eye for symptomatic relief while awaiting definitive diagnosis
2. Evaluate for diabetes, hypertension, hyper-/hypothyroidism, myasthenia gravis, trauma, multiple sclerosis, CNS lesion
3. Refer to ophthalmologist

G. Stye (hordeolum)
1. Painful, erythematous, often pointed nodule on surface of skin (external stye) or on conjunctival surface (internal stye)
2. Usually caused by a staph infection of a sebaceous gland of the lid
3. Treatment: Warm compresses, topical antibiotic drops
4. No systemic antibiotics necessary

H. Chalazion
1. Firm well-demarcated nodule just below lid margin; may have grayish discoloration on conjunctival surface
2. Secondary to a lipogranulomatous inflammation of meibomian gland
3. May be symptom-free, or nodule may be tender and erythematous
4. Treatment includes frequent warm compresses and antibiotic drops initially, then after 1 month ophthalmologist may lance or excise the chalazion
5. No systemic antibiotics necessary

I. Open-angle glaucoma: More prevalent. Tends to be more severe in African-Americans. Increased incidence if positive family history

    1. Refers to a group of diseases with progressive optic nerve damage and visual field loss, usually with associated elevations in intraocular pressure

    2. Normal intraocular pressure is 10–21mmHg

    3. Damage from glaucoma is manifested by optic nerve "cupping" (caused by loss of neurons and glial tissue). Cup-to-disc of 0.6 or greater, or asymmetry is one sign of glaucoma

    4. Visual field loss over time (usually spares the central visual field)

    5. Prevalence—0.5% of population

J. Angle-closure glaucoma: May have acute severe eye pain, red eye and blurry vision, with associated nausea, vomiting, diaphoresis, abdominal pain. May see halos around light fixtures. *Ophthalmologic emergency*

V. PRIMARY/PREVENTIVE OPHTHALMOLOGY SCHEDULE

A. Neonates

    1. Ophthalmologic screen for retinopathy of prematurity if birth weight <1500g, <33 weeks gestation, or received O_2 therapy for > 48hrs at birth; should be done within 1 month

    2. In all other neonates red reflexes should be checked at birth and every visit thereafter to screen for congenital cataracts, retinoblastoma, congenital glaucoma. Cataracts should be treated before the age of 3 months to prevent amblyopia, so this exam is important! In more darkly pigmented individuals, the red reflex may look dull orange or whitish orange—make sure this is symmetric and uniform across entire reflex. Refer if eyes are not straight

B. Preschool

    1. Screen for strabismus (exotropia and esotropia) with cover-uncover test and pupillary light reflex test (normally both light reflexes should be centered in each pupil). Begin screening at birth—prior to 4 months of age infants may show variable crossing or drifting out of the eyes due to underdevelopment of the macula. If strabismus not picked up early, it may lead to amblyopia (decreased vision in 1 eye). Refer for ophthalmololgic evaluation

    2. Vision screening is feasible at around age 3½ years; will initially use the Allen test (pictures) until child is able to read numbers or letters

C. School-aged children: Should have vision screen at least every 2–3 years if asymptomatic

D. Adults

    1. Routine glaucoma exam (Funduscopic exam and IOP) at age 35 then every 2 years (yearly if family history of glaucoma)

    2. Funduscopic exam at least yearly in patients at increased risk—diabetes mellitus, family history of retinal detachments, or glaucoma corticosteroid therapy, Plaquenil, Mellaril

    3. Age > 65 years; full eye exam every 1–2 years regardless of risk factors

    4. African-American (Recommendation of the Comprehensive Adult Eye Evaluation)—Comprehensive eye evaluation by an ophthalmologist:

        a. Age 20–39: Every 3–5 years

        b. Age 40–64: Every 2–4 years

        c. Age 65 or older: Every 1–2 years

E. Diabetes: Ophthalmologic exam every year

VI. SPECIFIC PEDIATRIC OPHTHALMOLOGIC DISORDERS

A. Conjunctivitis

    1. In neonates, may be toxic conjunctivitis from routine perinatal prophylaxis

    2. Infectious conjunctivitis may be caused by *staph, chlamydia*, herpes virus, gonorrhea. If discharge is purulent and excessive, gonorrhea is probable; blindness can result in 24–48hrs, should be immediately referred for evaluation and treatment

B. Nasolacrimal duct obstruction (congenital)

    1. Obstruction is usually unilateral

    2. Origin is usually congenital due to lack of patency of the inferior ostium of the nasolacrimal duct; very common

    3. Tear lake is elevated, and lashes appear wet

    4. May get bacterial superinfection: Eyelids will be adherent with purulent matter on awakening. Lids are red with tearing of the eye

GEN

    5. Infection will recur in spite of topical antibiotics, unless duct opens or is opened with probing

    6. Can put pressure on nasolacrimal sac with a Q-tip or finger; if expression of mucopurulent material is seen from the puncta, then nasolacrimal duct obstruction is the diagnosis

    7. Approximately 75% spontaneously open within first 6 months of life. Should be referred for duct probing after 6 months if no resolution. If persistent purulent drainage, refer earlier

    8. Parent should massage over the duct 3–4 ×/day; this will relieve most obstructions

C. Preseptal Cellulitis

    1. Eyelids are erythematous and edematous; may be sharply circumscribed or diffuse

    2. Conjunctival injection may be present as well as mucopurulent discharge from the nasolacrimal duct, if this is the source of infection

    3. **Orbital cellulitis** should be suspected if proptosis, sluggish pupil, vision change, or extraocular motility disturbance is present; should obtain immediate CAT scan to evaluate for orbital involvement

    4. If child < 2 years, then should be hospitalized for IV antibiotics regardless if cellulitis preseptal or orbital

    5. If child > 2 years, may try oral antibiotics, but if no improvement in 48hrs, should be admitted for IV antibiotics

D. Strabismus (See Preventive schedule)

    1. Inward, outward, or upward deviation of 1 or both eyes; pupils are misaligned

    2. Any patient with constant deviation, or deviation that develops after the first 3 to 4 months of life, should be referred immediately to ophthalmologist

    4. Therapy usually involves patching of good eye and/or corrective lenses (after evaluation to rule-out tumor, cataract, etc.)

    5. Ideally, eyes should be straightened before age 2 to increase chance of stereopsis (normal depth perception)

CLINICAL PEARLS

- It is not always necessary to patch the eye or to use dilating drops for corneal abrasions or after removing corneal foreign bodies or rust rings
- Vertically oriented, linear corneal abrasions may indicate a conjunctival foreign body under the upper lid. Evert the upper lid with a cotton swab
- Never send anesthetic eye drops home with patients with corneal abrasions; they delay healing by preventing re-epithelialization of the cornea, and may damage the cornea, resulting in blindness
- Always check vision before examination and treatment
- Be alert for herpes simplex; dendritic appearance under fluorescein staining
- Patients with diabetes should have an ophthalmological examination by an ophthalmologist every year starting at the time of diagnosis for adult onset diabetes and within 5 years after diagnosis of juvenile diabetes
- Neomycin can cause allergic reaction in up to 10% of patients

References

American Diabetes Association: Diabetic retinopathy (Position Statement). Diabetes Care 23 (Suppl. 1):S73–S76, 2000.

Quilen D. Common causes of vision loss in elderly patients. Am Fam Phys 1999;60:99–108.

Weinstock FJ, Weinstock MB. Common eye disorders: six patients to refer. Postgrad Med Apr 1996; 99(4):107–10, 113–6.

American Diabetes Association: Clinical Practice Recommendations 1998. Position Statement, Jan 1998. Diabetic Retinopathy. Diabetes Care 21(s1):47–9, 1998.

Morrow GL, Abbott RL. Conjunctivitis. Am Fam Phys 1998;57:735.

Weinstock FJ; Assaad MH. Recurrent corneal erosions. Management by the primary care physician. Postgrad Med Nov 1995; 98(5):155, 159–60.

Weinstock FJ, Weinstock MB. Common eye disorders: six patients to treat, pitfalls to avoid. Postgrad Med Apr 1996(4):119–23.

Coston CC, Craven RA. Reading the red eye: conjunctivitis and its mimics. Emergency Med Sep 1994:15–29.

Bienfang DC, et al. Ophthalmology. N Engl J Med 1990; 323(14):956–66.

Ryan Hanson, MD
Michael Weinstock, MD

59. ALLERGIC RHINITIS/
SEASONAL ALLERGIES

I. DEFINITION:

Allergic rhinitis is an immunologically mediated disease. It is initiated by a type I antigen-antibody reaction. Inhaled allergens interact with T and B cell lymphocytes to produce IgE antibodies which then attach to mast cells and basophils resulting in the release of histamine and chemotactic factors and allergic rhinitis symptoms. Seasonal allergies are one of the most common primary care problems and affect 10–20% of the population. The most recent guidelines from the Joint Task Force on Practice Parameters in Allergy, Asthma and Immunology defines rhinitis ". . . as inflammation of the membranes lining the nose, and is characterized by nasal congestion, rhinorrhea, sneezing, itching of the nose and/or postnasal drainage."

II. HISTORY

   A. Seasonal prevalence
   B. Paroxysmal sneezing, rhinitis, dry, watery or pruritic eyes, pharyngeal itch, cough
   C. Triggering exposures
   D. Anosmia (decreased sense of smell)
   E. Age at onset
   F. Medication use (inquire specifically about intranasal decongestants, also see list below)
   G. History of nasal trauma
   H. History of atopy
   I. Family history of allergies
   J. Nasal polyps: Often unilateral and associated with asthma and aspirin sensitivity. May mimic allergic rhinitis

III. PHYSICAL EXAM

   A. Rhinorrhea
   B. Nasal congestion
   C. Pale, boggy, blue-gray, edematous nasal turbinates
   D. Nasal crease ("allergic salute")
   E. Dark circles under eyes
   F. Skin folds under eyes (Denies lines)
   G. Cobblestoning of posterior pharynx

IV. LABS/TESTING:

Allergy testing is useful if the patient requires proof of cause, the diagnosis is puzzling or if you are considering immunotherapy. Before skin testing, discontinue all anti-histamines for 1 week

   A. Prick testing: Small amount of antigen is pricked into the skin, can easily be done in the office if one has a supply of antigens
   B. Intradermal testing: Antigen is injected into the dermis
   C. RAST (radioallergosorbent testing): Blood is analyzed for specific anti-IgE antibodies to known antigens, useful for patients with extensive eczema, dermatographism or prior anaphylaxis, young, or cannot discontinue antihistamines
   D. Nasal smears: Eosinophilia can be supportive but is not diagnostic

V. DIFFERENTIAL DIAGNOSIS: May mimic symptoms of allergic rhinitis

   A. Vasomotor rhinitis: Related to autonomic dysfunction and more common in women
   B. Infectious rhinitis: Viral URI, bacterial sinusitis
   C. Rhinitis medicamentosa: Tachyphylaxis after use of nasal decongestant. Nasal mucosa bright red and swollen

GEN

D. Nonallergic rhinitis with eosinophilia syndrome (NARES): Nasal eosinophils in patients who have perennial symptoms and occasionally loss of sense of smell

E. Hormonal rhinitis: Pregnancy (usually second trimester to term, resolving after delivery) and hypothyroidism

F. Drug-induced rhinitis: Aspirin, Clonidine, Hydralazine, Labetolol, Propranolol, Methyldopa, Prazosin, Terazosin, Reserpine, oral contraceptives

G. Gustatory rhinitis: Exposure to hot, spicy foods

H. Nasal polyps: May be associated with asthma and aspirin sensitivity

I. Other: Alcoholism, cocaine abuse, nasal septal deviation, tumors, adenoidal hypertrophy, hypertrophy of the nasal turbinates

VI. MANAGEMENT

A. Environmental controls

1. Indoor: Avoid active and passive tobacco smoke, remove bedroom carpet, foam pillows, enclose mattress and box springs in plastic, use air conditioning in the summer
2. Outdoor: Masks, long-sleeve clothing, filter air from outside
3. Dust mites: Control bedroom: wash bedding weekly, impermeable covers on pillows and mattresses, keep humidity below 50%, HEPA (high density particulate air) filter
4. Molds: Remove any visible mold/mildew, treat with a retardant, frost-free refrigerator, keep firewood outside, avoid house-plants, clean heating and cooling systems, remove old books
5. Animals: Avoid furry animals and birds or eliminate carpeting and keep floors polished and upholstery frequently cleaned, HEPA vacuum. Animals should stay out of the bedroom

B. Pharmocotherapy

1. Non-sedating antihistamines: Slower onset of action than sedating antihistamines
   a. **Fexofenadine (Allegra)**
      i. 12 years and older: 60mg PO BID or 180mg PO QD
      ii. Children 6–11 years: 30mg PO BID
      iii. Onset of action: 60 minutes
      iv. Also available as Allegra D (with 120mg Pseudoephedrine) PO BID
   b. **Cetirizine (Zyrtec)**
      i. Dose: 5–10mg PO QD (slightly sedating in some patients)
      ii. Approved for children 2–5 years old with seasonal and perennial allergic rhinitis and chronic idiopathic urticaria at 5mg QD (available 5mg/5cc). Dose for 6–11 years old is 5–10mg QD
      iii. Onset of action 15–30 minutes
   c. **Loratadine (Claritin)**
      i. Dose: 10mg PO QD
      ii. Approved for children ≥ 6 years with seasonal allergic rhinitis and chronic idiopathic urticaria at 10mg QD (available 5mg/5cc)
      iii. Onset of action: 3hrs
      iv. Also available as Claritin D 12hr (5mg Loratadine/120mg Pseudoephedrine) and Claritin D 24hr (10mg Loratadine/240mg Pseudoephedrine)
2. **Sedating antihistamines:** Caution in patients with BPH and in the elderly secondary to urinary retention and risk of glaucoma
   a. **Diphenhydramine (Benadryl)**
      i. Adults: 25–50mg PO TID–QID
      ii. Children>9 kg: 5mg/kg/24 hrs. divided QID PRN
   b. **Chlorpheniramine (Chlor-trimeton):** 4mg PO QID PRN
   c. **Hydroxyzine (Atarax, Vistaril):** 25mg PO QID PRN
3. **Oral decongestants:** Stimulatory CNS effects may offset sedative effects of sedating antihistamines (see Chapter 116, Symptomatic Medications)
   a. **Phenylephrine**
   b. **Pseudoephedrine**—e.g., **Sudafed**
   c. **Phenylpropanolamine**—e.g., **Entex LA** (also contains Guaifenesin)
4. **Local Medications:** Often helpful in conjunction with oral antihistamines
   a. **Steroid nasal inhalers:** Consider glaucoma screening within 3 months of starting in patients over 60 years old. If results are negative at that time, then continue intranasal steroid use

i. **Beclamethasone Diproprionate (Vancenase/Beconase)** 1 spray in each nostril BID to QID. May decrease to QD once therapeutic. Also Vancenase DS for QD dosing

ii. **Fluticasone Propionate (Flonase):** 2 sprays in each nostril QD or 1 spray in each BID

iii. **Triamcinolone (Nasacort):** 2 sprays per nostril QD

iv. **Flunisolide (Nasalide):** 2 sprays in each nostril BID

v. **Budesonide (Rhinocort):** 2 sprays in each nostril BID

vi. **Mometasone (Nasonex):** 2 sprays in each nostril QD

  b. Mast cell stabilizers—**Cromolyn Sodium (Nasalcrom):** 1 spray in each nostril 3–6 ×/day

  c. Saline nasal spray—Safe, inexpensive, helps thin mucous, use 3–6 ×/day, e.g., **SalineX, Ocean Nasal Mist, NaSal**

  d. Nasal vasoconstrictors—Should not use more than 3–4 days or rebound vasodilitation and worsening of symptoms (Rhinitis medicamentosa). May be helpful in acute sinusitis or for airplane flights

    i. **Neo-Synephrine (Phenylephrine):** 0.25, 0.5 or 1.0%: 2–3 sprays in each nostril q4hrs PRN

    ii. **Oxymethazoline (Afrin)**

  e. Ophthalmic solutions—See Chapter 58, Screening, Diagnosis, and Management of Ocular Disorders, IV.A.2.a-h

5. Systemic steroids: Rarely necessary, but may be helpful in severe cases of complete nasal obstruction. Short course of prednisone for 1 week or less

C. Immunotherapy

1. Indications

  a. Unable to manage symptoms with environmental modification or medications

  b. Patients who require medications for greater than 6 months of the year

  c. Intolerable side effects to medications

2. Perform RAST testing or skin testing to identify the offending allergen

3. Weekly injections are initiated with a small amount of antigen, which is gradually increased. The length of time between injections is also gradually increased to once every 3–4 weeks

4. Side effects: Local reaction at injection site, anaphylaxis (rare)

5. Often able to discontinue after 3–5 seasons

CLINICAL PEARLS

- Environmental control is often the key for many patients
- It can often be helpful with copious rhinitis to give an oral decongestant (Pseudoephedrine, Phenylephrine) along with an antihistamine and intranasal medication
- Intranasal medications are much more effective if the patient blows nose before using
- Onset of allergic rhinitis is before age 30 in 70% of patients
- Pharmacotherapy is much more effective when used prophylactically
- Therapy for rhinitis medicamentosa involves weaning the intranasal decongestant over 1 week and combining with oral steroids (0.5–1.0mg/kg/day) tapered over 7–10 days
- Cystic fibrosis should be considered in the differential diagnosis in children with nasal polyps

References

Lee NP, Arriola ER. How to treat allergic rhinitis. West J Med Jul 1999;171:31–4.

Dykewicz MS, Fineman S, Skoner DP, et al. Diagnosis and management of rhinitis: complete guidelines of Joint Task Force on Practice Parameters in Allergy, Asthma and Immunology. Ann Allergy, Asthma, Immunol Nov 1998; 81(5):478–518.

Titi MJ, Sloan, RW. A critical look at ocular allergy drugs. Am Fam Phys 1996;53(8).

Ferguson BJ. Allergic rhinitis—Recognizing signs, symptoms, and triggering allergens. Postgraduate Medicine 1997;101:110–6.

Ferguson BJ. Allergic rhinitis—Options for pharmacotherapy and immunotherapy. Postgraduate Medicine 1997;101:117–131.

GEN

Daniel M. Neides, MD

60. SINUSITIS

DEFINITION: Inflammation of the mucosa of 1 or more of the paranasal sinuses

I. ETIOLOGY
    A. Bacterial pathogens: *S. pneumoniæ, H. influenzæ, S. aureus, M. catarrhalis, S. pyogenes*
    B. Viral

II. HISTORY
The classic complaint from patients is a "cold that won't go away." Related symptoms include fever, nasal congestion, rhinorrhea, headache, nasal irritation, fatigue, and malaise
    A. Facial pain may occur above and below the eyes
    B. Nasal secretions may turn from clear to a yellow/green
    C. Productive cough secondary to secretions draining posteriorly into the throat (post-nasal drip)
    D. Sense of taste and smell may be reduced
    E. Halitosis

III. PHYSICAL EXAMINATION
    A. Purulence in the nares or nasopharynx (not always visible)
    B. Irritation of the nasal mucosa: Leads to inflammation with a bright red, irregular appearance
    C. Nasal polyps: Prolonged nasal inflammation may lead to polypoid degeneration of nasal mucosa and formation of polyps
    D. Facial tenderness to palpation or percussion
        1. Maxillary: Subzygomatic over cheek and upper teeth
        2. Ethmoid: Periorbital
        3. Frontal: Forehead above eyebrow
        4. Sphenoid
            a. Usually retrobulbar, often not well localized
            b. Infection in the sphenoid sinus may lead to pain and tenderness over the vertex of the skull, the mastoid bones, and the occipital portion of the head
    E. Periorbital tissue swelling or erythema of the skin overlying the affected sinus may be seen

IV. DIAGNOSTIC PROCEDURES
    A. Radiography: Not necessary to obtain in an uncomplicated acute sinusitis. Should be reserved for evaluating recurrent or chronic sinus infections
        1. Plain films (conventional sinus x-rays)
            a. The basic studies consist of 3 views
                i. Waters': Useful for evaluating maxillary and frontal sinuses
                ii. Caldwell: Evaluates ethmoid sinuses
                iii. Lateral: Evaluates sphenoid sinus and any nasopharyngeal masses
            b. Positive findings include diffuse opacification, mucosal thickening of at least 4mm, or an air-fluid level
            c. Neither sensitive or specific. Many clinicians proceed directly to CT
        2. CT scan
            a. Many institutions will perform a "screening CT of the sinuses" which limits the number of slices but specifically targets the sinuses
            b. The cost is higher than plain films, but the sensitivity is much greater
        3. MRI
            a. Offers the best soft tissue contrast. Valuable in evaluating neoplasms and complicated infections; no radiation involved
            b. Limitations include high cost, long imaging times, and the inability to directly display bony landmarks
    B. Rhinoscopy (flexible): Allows a detailed examination of the upper nasal cavities and posterior

GEN

nasopharynx. This technique is also valuable in identifying polyps, high nasal vault, and structural abnormalities

C. Nasal cytology: > 5 neutrophils or eosinophils per high power field usually indicates sinus films will be positive. Not commonly performed

D. Maxillary sinus aspiration: Indicated when precise microbial identification is required; the specimen should be cultured for anaerobes, aerobes, and fungi

E. Transillumination: Its use is limited to adults with suspected acute maxillary or frontal sinusitis. This technique has been unreliable in diagnosing acute sinusitis

V. MEDICAL TREATMENT OF ACUTE UNCOMPLICATED SINUSITIS

A. Initial therapy (use any *ONE* of these)
1. **Amoxicillin**
   a. Adults: 500mg PO TID for 14–21 days
   b. Children: 40mg/kg/day in 3 divided doses Q8hrs for 14–21 days
2. **Trimethoprim-Sulfamethoxazole (Bactrim/Septra)**
   a. Adults: 1 double-strength tablet Q12hrs for 14–21 days
   b. Children: (pediatric suspension) 8mg/kg/day **TMP** and 40mg/kg/day **SMX** in 2 divided doses Q12hrs for 14–21 days
3. **Doxycycline (Vibramycin)**
   Adults: 100mg PO BID for 14–21 days

B. Treatment failure (treat for 3–4 weeks)
1. Antibiotics
   a. Consider trying different first-line antibiotic (i.e., **TMP/SMZ** if **Amoxicillin** was used initially)
   b. **Cefuroxime Axetil (Ceftin)**
   c. **Amoxicillin-Clavulanate (Augmentin)**
   d. **Loracarbef (Lorabid)**
   e. **Erythromycin-Sulfisoxazole (Pediazole)**
2. Nasal steroid inhaler
3. Antihistamines and decongestants
   a. Limited studies of decongestants show that they decrease nasal-airway resistance; however, their overall effect on the clinical course of acute sinusitis is not well known
   b. Antihistamines should be reserved for patients with known allergies
4. Nasal irrigation
   a. May be used for patients with increased mucus drainage
   b. A bulb syringe is used to irrigate the nasal passage with saline. This is performed 3–4 × /day as needed

C. Failure despite above approaches
1. Radiologic studies to obtain definitive diagnosis
2. Antibiotics: Consider using a different second line agent for 4–6 weeks in conjunction with nasal steroids and a decongestant
3. Referral to an allergist or ENT

VI. RECURRENT OR CHRONIC SINUSITIS

A. In children the most common cause of recurrent sinusitis is recurrent viral upper respiratory infection

B. Other conditions predisposing patients to chronic sinusitis include allergic inflammation, cystic fibrosis, immunodeficiency disorders (insufficient or dysfunctional immunoglobulins), ciliary dyskinesia (immotile cilia syndrome, Kartagener's syndrome), nasal polyps, or an anatomical problem

C. The evaluation of children with recurrent or chronic sinusitis may include consulting an allergist, a sweat test, measurement of immunoglobulins and their subclasses, and possibly a mucosal biopsy (to assess ciliary function and structure)

VII. COMPLICATIONS OF ACUTE SINUSITIS (AND THEIR TREATMENT)

A. Subperiosteal abscess of the orbit: Manifested by eye swelling, exophthalmos, and impaired extraocular eye movements

B. Intracranial abscess: Manifested by signs of increased intracranial pressure, meningeal

GEN

irritation, and focal neurologic deficits
C. Treatment
1. A CT scan is necessary for diagnosis
2. IV antibiotics and surgical drainage are usually required for successful treatment

VIII. INDICATIONS FOR SURGERY OR REFERRAL

A. Patients with chronic or recurrent sinusitis who have failed an extended course of antibiotics, nasal steroids and allergy management
B. Patients with chronic sinusitis and worsening pulmonary disease
C. Patients with severe asthma which is exacerbated by recurrent sinus symptoms

CLINICAL PEARLS

- *Pseudomonas* is a common pathogen causing acute sinusitis in patients with cystic fibrosis
- Patients with HIV can present with recurrent sinusitis
- Sinusitis is an overly diagnosed condition. Before committing a patient to the diagnosis of *chronic* sinusitis, consider radiologic studies
- The 3 most common causes of chronic cough (90–95%) are post-nasal drip (often secondary to sinusitis), asthma and gastroesophageal reflux disease (GERD)

References

de Ferranti S, et al. Are amoxicillin and folate inhibitors as effective as other antibiotics for acute sinusitis? A meta-analysis. BMJ Sep 5, 1998;317:632–7.
Diagnosis and treatment of acute bacterial rhinosinusitis. Summary (AHCPR Publication No. 99–E016).
Wald ER. Sinusitis in children. N Engl J Med 1992;326:319–23.
Diament MJ. The diagnosis of sinusitis in infants and children: x-ray, computed tomography, and magnetic resonance imaging. J Allergy Clin Immunol 1992;90:442–4.
Druce HM. Diagnosis of sinusitis in adults: history, physical examination, nasal cytology, echo, and rhinoscope. J Allergy Clin Immunol 1992;90:436–41.
Fireman P. Diagnosis of sinusitis in children: emphasis on the history and physical examination. J Allergy Clin Immunol 1992;90:433–6.

GEN

Daniel M. Neides, MD
Deb Frankowski, MD

61. GASTROESOPHAGEAL REFLUX DISEASE AND PEPTIC ULCER DISEASE

— PART ONE: GASTROESOPHAGEAL REFLUX DISEASE (GERD) —

I. SYMPTOMS OF REFLUX of gastric, biliary, pancreatic secretions into the esophagus:
   A. Heartburn
   B. Regurgitation
   C. Dyspepsia
   D. Chest pain

II. ETIOLOGY
   A. **Incompetent lower esophageal sphincter (LES):** Exacerbating factors include foods such as onion, fats, mint, ETOH, chocolate, caffeine as well as medications such as anticholinergics, ß-blockers, progesterone containing oral contraceptives, NSAIDs, Prednisone
   B. **Impaired esophageal peristalsis:** Associated diseases include CREST, scleroderma, Raynaud's, relfux-induced injury
   C. **Decreased salivation:** Associated conditions include Sjogren's, cigarette use, and anticholinergic medications
   D. **Delayed gastric emptying:** Associated conditions include gastroparesis, hiatal hernia, gastric outlet obstruction
   E. **Increased secretion of gastric acid:** Associated conditions include gastrinoma, Zollinger-Ellison syndrome
   F. **Direct irritants:** Citrus, tomato, cola, coffee

III. EVALUATION
   A. **Empiric treatment** may be attempted in patients with typical "uncomplicated" symptoms (see Table 1)
   B. **Further evaluation,** as below, is required in patients with:
      1. Atypical symptoms (early satiety, anorexia, dysphagia, odynophagia, cough, chest pain, asthma, laryngitis)
      2. Patients over age 50 with new onset symptoms
      3. Patients whose symptoms persist after 8 weeks of treatment
      4. Patients presenting with complications (anemia, guaiac positive stool, weight loss, stricture)
   C. **Patients treated empirically who do not respond** in 2 weeks or whose symptoms recur after 6 weeks of treatment should undergo further evaluation
   D. **Evaluations** include:
      1. Upper endoscopy with biopsy: Best assessment of extent of mucosal damage, Barrett's esophagus, stricture
      2. Esophageal pH monitoring: The "gold standard" for diagnosing reflux and especially useful in patients with atypical symptoms of chronic cough, chest pain, asthma, laryngitis
      3. Upper GI: May identify ulcers or stricture, but is insensitive for reflux
      4. Esophageal motility: Useful assessment of motor function of the esophagus, especially preoperatively
      5. Gastroesophageal scintigraphy: Noninvasive evaluation of esophageal emptying, especially useful in pediatric population

IV. MANAGEMENT
   A. **Behavior modification**
      1. Avoid foods that are direct irritants or decrease LES pressure (see above)
      2. Weight loss
      3. Avoid tight fitting clothes
      4. Remain upright for 3hrs after eating

GEN

    5. 4–8 inch blocks under head of mattress

B. Antacids provide symptom relief but do not heal esophagitis

C. H₂ blockers: See Table 1

D. Proton pump inhibitors: See Table 1

E. Prokinetic agents aid in the competence of LES. They are approximately equivalent to H₂ blockers for mild GERD and maintenance

    1. **Metoclopramide (Reglan):** 10mg PO QID, significant side effects

F. Mucosal protective agents: See PUD, IV.A.2

G. Combinations: Prilosec plus **Reglan** is more effective than **Prilosec** alone

H. Surgery: Nissen fundoplication is the therapy of choice for patients with strictures requiring repeated dilation or for patients who fail medical therapy. Surgery has a 90% efficacy and is especially effective in patients with atypical symptoms such as chronic cough, asthma, etc. Laparoscopic methods have lower morbidity than the standard open technique

V. COMPLICATIONS

A. Degree of injury is poorly correlated with degree of symptoms

B. Specific complications include:

    1. **Barrett's Esophagus:** In 10% of patients with chronic reflux, esophageal squamous cells may undergo metaplasia to columnar cells. Esophageal adenocarcinoma may develop in up to 10% of patients with metaplasia. If multiple foci of high grade dysplasia are found on EGD, elective esophagectomy versus Q6 month EGDs with biopsy must be considered. For Barrett's esophagus metaplasia without dysplasia, EGD with biopsy must be performed Q1–2 years

    2. **Stricture:** EGD should confirm the stricture (usually at the GE junction) and dilation may be performed at the same time. Long term proton pump therapy should follow dilation

    3. **Extra-esophageal complications** include asthma (aspiration versus vagal), laryngitis, chronic cough, sleep apnea

Table 1—Common Medications Used in GERD/PUD

	Famotidine (Pepcid) H₂ blocker	Ranitidine (Zantac) H₂ blocker	Cimetidine (Tagamet) H₂ blocker	Nizatidine (Axid) H₂ blocker	Omeprazole (Prilosec) Proton pump inhibitor	Lansoprazole (Prevacid) Proton pump inhibitor	Rabeprazole (AcipHex) Proton pump inhibitor
Acute duodenal ulcer	20mg BID or 40mg hs × 6–8 wks	150mg BID or 300mg hs × 6–8 wks	800mg hs × 6–8 wks or 400mg BID	150mg BID or 300mg hs × 6–8 wks	20mg QD × 4–8 wks	15mg QD × 4–8 wks	20mg QD × 4 wks
Maintenance duodenal ulcer	20mg hs	150mg hs	400mg hs	150mg hs	20mg QD	15mg QD	20mg QD
Acute gastric ulcer	40mg hs × 6–8 wks	150mg BID or 300mg hs × 6–8 wks	800mg hs × 6–8 wks	300mg hs × 6–8 wks	40mg QD ×4–8 wks	30mg QD × 4–8 wks	20mg QD × 4-8 wks
GERD symptoms	20mg BID	150mg BID	400mg BID	150mg BID	20mg QD	15mg QD	20mg QD
Esophageal lesions	40mg BID	150mg BID	800mg BID or 400mg QID	200mg BID	20mg QD	30mg QD	20mg QD
Maintenance esophageal ulcers / severe GERD		150mg BID			20mg QD	15mg QD	20mg QD

— PART TWO: PEPTIC ULCER DISEASE (PUD) —

I. SYMPTOMS

A. Duodenal ulcers frequently present with burning epigastric pain relieved by antacids. Symptoms may awaken the patient

B. Gastric ulcers often present with nausea, vomiting, pain made worse by food, early satiety

C. Nonspecific symptoms include dyspepsia, bloating, gas

II. ETIOLOGY

A. *Helicobacter Pylori:* This bacteria is a cofactor in 95% of duodenal ulcers and 80% of gastric ulcers. Almost 100% of patients with *H. pylori* have chronic antral gastritis although only 15–20% develop ulcers

B. NSAID use: Clinical ulcers (usually gastric) develop in 1% per patient per year of NSAID use. Risk of complications include increased age, prior GI disease, concomitant steroid or antico-agulant use, female sex, increased dose, older agents (especially aspirin). Newer NSAIDs are probably safer (Relafen, Lodine, Daypro, Ibuprofen). Cytotec (Misoprostol) provides some protection

C. Hypersecretory state: Zollinger Ellison Syndrome, gastrinoma

D. Exacerbating factors
1. Tobacco: One study showed that the risk of duodenal ulcer, failure to heal, and recurrence was directly proportional to number of cigarettes
2. Alcohol is a strong stimulant of acid secretion
3. Corticosteroids
4. Diet (controversial)

III. EVALUATION

A. For ulcers: As in GERD (see GERD III.B.), upper GI may be useful for screening symptomatic patients but EGD with biopsies must follow if abnormal (especially if gastric ulcer). A CBC and stool guaiac should also be done

B. For *H. pylori*:
1. CLO test: Performed on biopsy tissue, it detects urea positive organisms
2. Histology: Not sensitive
3. Culture: Not sensitive
4. Serology (IgG and IgA): Test has similar sensitivity and specificity to EGD but does not evaluate for gastric carcinoma. Titers remain elevated months after eradication
5. Breath test for urea: Though not widely available, the test is sensitive and specific before and 4 weeks after eradication

IV. TREATMENT

A. Healing acute ulcers (duodenal or gastric)
1. Antisecretory drugs (see Table 1, above)
   a. Proton pump inhibitors include Omeprazole (Prilosec), Lansoprazole (Prevacid), and Rabeprazole (AcipHex)
   b. H$_2$ blockers include Ranitidine (Zantac), Cimetidine (Tagamet), Famotidine (Pepcid), and Nizatidine (Axid)
2. Mucosal protective agents:
   a. **Sucralfate (Carafate)**
      i. Forms a barrier at the ulcer base and stimulates production of mucous, HCO$_3$, and prostaglandins
      ii. Comparable to H$_2$ blockers in healing duodenal ulcers and in GERD
      iii. Dose: 1g PO QID × 6–8 weeks
   b. Antacids
      i. Help relieve symptoms and are comparable to H$_2$ blockers in healing duodenal ul-cers and in GERD
      ii. Example: Mylanta
   c. Bismuth (Pepto-Bismol) stimulates production of HCO$_3$ and prostaglandins

B. Maintenance therapy
1. Duodenal ulcers: H$_2$ blockers (or proton pump inhibitors) given at HS at half treatment dose (full dose in smokers or complicated disease)—*or*—**Carafate** 1g PO BID
2. Gastric ulcers: No approved maintenance therapy
3. NSAID ulcers: **Misoprostol (Cytotec)** acts as a prostaglandin analog and stimulates HCO$_3$ and mucous production. It is dosed at 200mcg PO QID with meals. Diarrhea and miscar-riage induction limit its use

GEN

V. ERADICATION OF *H. pylori*

   A. In nontreated *H. pylori*, there is an 85% recurrence rate of PUD. All patients with ulcers with *H. pylori* should be treated. Patients with GERD without ulcers who are *H. pylori* positive should probably be treated

   B. Eradication requires a multiple-drug regimen (see Table 2)

Table 2: *H. pylori* Treatment Regimens from JAMA Consensus Statement (Feb 1996)

KEY:	Meds	Comments	Adverse Effects
	Bismuth (Pepto-Bismol)	2 tabs or 1tsp QAC+HS, works topically	black stools
	Metronidazole (Flagyl)	*H. pylori* easily develops resistance	nausea, metallic taste
	Tetracycline	500mg QAC+HS, works topically	metallic taste
	Omeprazole (Prilosec)		
	Clarithromycin (Biaxin)		
	Amoxicillin (Amoxil)	works topically, can't use Ampicillin IV	allergic reactions

Regimen #	Regimen	Length of treatment	Cure rate
1	B 2 tabs QAC+HS M 250mg QAC+HS T 500mg QAC+HS	1–2 weeks	88%
2	Add O 20mg BID with meals to Regimen 1	1 week	94–98%
3	B 2 tabs QAC+HS M 250mg QAC+HS A 500mg QAC+HS	1 week 2 weeks	75–81% 80–86%
4	M 500mg BID with meals O 20mg BID with meals C 500mg BID with meals	1 week 2 weeks	87–91% slightly increased
5	A 1000mg BID with meals O 20mg BID with meals C 500mg BID with meals	1 week 2 weeks	86–91% slightly increased
6	M 500mg BID with meals O 20mg BID with meals A 1000mg BID with meals	2 weeks	77–83%

VI. COMPLICATIONS OF PUD

   A. Hemorrhage: Symptoms include coffee ground emesis, hematemesis, melena, or hematochezia. Up to 20% of patients with PUD may develop bleeding

   B. Perforation: Seen in up to 5% of ulcer patients. Usually occurs from ulcers on the anterior wall of the stomach or duodenum. Patients will usually have absent bowel sounds, rebound tenderness, and a very rigid abdomen. Upright or decubitus plain abdominal films will aid in diagnosis (free intraperitoneal air)

   C. Gastric outlet obstruction: Occurs in 2% of ulcer patients due to edema or scarring of the pylorus or duodenal bulb. Upper endoscopy is necessary to define the extent of obstruction and to rule out carcinoma

CLINICAL PEARLS

   • Patient education regarding Aspirin and NSAID use is important. Patients should be made aware of common signs and symptoms of PUD and instructed to inform the physician if they should develop (bleeding may be the first sign of PUD in patients taking NSAIDs)

   • Smoking cessation is imperative in patients with PUD. Physician assistance will greatly increase the likelihood of quitting

   • If patients need to continue NSAIDs despite being diagnosed with PUD, consider cox-2 inhibitors (Celebrex, Vioxx) or shorter acting NSAIDs (so that dosage can be titrated) rather than the potent once-a-day NSAIDs

   • Consider Cytotec for prevention of PUD in chronic NSAID users

GEN

References

Ahuja V. Head and neck manifestations of gastroesophageal reflux disease. Am Fam Phys 1999;60:873–86.

Bardhan KD, et al. Symptomatic gastro-oesophageal reflux disease: double blind controlled study of intermittent treatment with omeprazole or rantidine. BMJ Feb 20, 1999;318:502–7.

Chey WD, et al. The ^{13}C-urea blood test accurately detects active *Helicobacter pylori* infection: a United States, multicenter trial. Am J Gastroenterol Jun 1999;94:1522–4.

Trus TL, et al. Improvement in quality of life measures after laparoscopic antireflux surgery. Ann Surg March 1999;229:331–6.

Ing AJ, Ngu MC. Cough and gastro-oesophageal reflux. Lancet Mar 20, 1999;353:944–6.

Hawkey CJ, et al. Omeprazole compared with misoprostol for ulcers associated with nonsteroidal antiinflammatory drugs. N Engl J Med 1998;338:727–34.

Fisher RS, Parkman HP. Management of nonulcer dyspepsia. N Engl J Med 1998;339:1376–81.

Talley NJ, Silverstein MD, Agreus L, Nyren O, Sonnenberg A, Holtmann G. AGA technical review: evaluation of dyspepsia. Gastroenterology 1998; 114:582–95.

Yeomans ND, et al. A comparison of omeprazole with ranitidine for ulcers associated with nonsteroidal antiinflammatory drugs. N Engl J Med 1998;338:719–26.

Fass R, et al. Contemporary medical therapy for gastroesophageal reflux disease. Am Fam Phys 1997(55);1:205–11.

Ofman JJ, et al. Management strategies for Helicobacter pylori-seropositive patients with dyspepsia: clinical and economic consequences. Ann Intern Med 1997;126:280–91.

Roth SH. NSAID gastropathy: a new understanding. Arch Intern Med 1996;156:1623–7.

Soll AH. Medical treatment of peptic ulcer disease: practice guidelines. JAMA 1996(275);8:622–9.

Walsh JH, Peterson WL. The treatment of Helicobacter Pylori infection in the management of peptic ulcer disease. N Engl J Med 1995 (333);15:984–9.

Daniel M. Neides, MD
Steve Markovich, MD
Miriam Chan, PharmD

62. SEIZURE DISORDERS

I. CLASSIFICATION OF SEIZURES

A. Generalized seizures

1. Absence (*petit mal*): Brief lapses in awareness sometimes accompanied by staring, rhythmic eye blinking, or head dropping; no postictal period
2. Tonic-clonic (*grand mal*): Tonic movements appear as sustained muscle contraction that results in limb and trunk rigidity. Clonic movement is rhythmic jerking and flexor spasms of the extremities. Up to 30 seconds of apnea is common. Often accompanied by *incontinence of urine/stool, tongue or lip biting, increased salivation and postictal period*
3. Myoclonic: Brief muscle contractions that occur unilaterally or bilaterally. Often occurs in healthy people as they fall asleep
4. Atonic: Usually begins in childhood. Loss of muscle tone can cause eyes to close, head to droop or even a complete collapse

B. Partial seizures

1. Simple partial: Seizures with motor, somatosensory, autonomic, or psychic symptoms; no loss of consciousness is observed
2. Complex partial: Cognitive, affective, or psychosensory symptoms may occur (behavioral automatisms or alterations in perception, hallucinations, or memory); a change in consciousness or an aura may occur

C. Other epileptic syndromes

1. Infantile spasms
   a. Occur at age 4–7 months and generally cease by age 4 years
   b. Associated with flexor, extensor or mixed spasm
   c. EEG shows hyperarrhythmic patterns
2. Febrile seizures
   a. The most common seizure of childhood

b. Diagnosis: Tonic-clonic movements associated with temperature > 100.4° F (38.0° C)
    i. Generally in children between 6 months and 5 years
    ii. Duration of seizure activity < 15 minutes
    iii. Seizure activity within 24hrs of onset of fever
    iv. Normal development and neurologic exam
    v. No family history of epilepsy
    vi. *Diagnosis of febrile seizure is a diagnosis of exclusion*
c. Appropriate laboratory tests, including lumbar puncture, should always be considered in any child with a seizure, especially if age < 18 months
d. Overall risk of a second febrile seizure is 25–30% and increases with height of fever, younger age and family history of febrile seizures

II. ETIOLOGY

A. Infection: Meningitis, encephalitis, intracranial abscess, subacute bacterial endocarditis, rabies, pertussis, tetanus, syphilis

B. Trauma: Concussion, subdural or epidural hemorrhage, subarachnoid hemorrhage

C. Metabolic: Hyper- or hypoglycemia, hyponatremia, hypernatremia, hypocalcemia, hypomagnesemia, kernicterus, inborn errors of metabolism (phenylketonuria, amino and organic acidemias), uremia, or hypoxemia

D. Intoxication (partial list): Aspirin, amphetamine, anticholinergics (tricyclics, phenothiazines, organophosphates), Theophylline, carbon monoxide, PCP, Cocaine, Propoxyphene, lead, alcohol or sedative toxicity or withdrawal, Romazicon administration

E. Degenerative/Deficiency: Pyridoxine deficiency, Tay-Sachs, Huntington's chorea, metachromic leukodystrophy

F. Neoplasms: Primary or metastatic disease

G. Vascular: Intracranial hematoma, hypertensive encephalopathy, stroke, or cerebral hypoperfusion, subarachnoid bleeding

H. Epilepsy: Idiopathic

III. DIAGNOSIS

Question the patient and any witnesses to determine if a seizure actually occurred

A. Initial assessment (patient's history)
1. Inquire about characteristics of the seizure, frequency, associated sensory and autonomic function, and behavioral changes
2. Determine if fever, intoxications, perinatal asphyxia, trauma, or preexisting abnormalities in growth and development have occurred
3. Inquire about bowel or bladder incontinence, tongue biting, or muscle fatigue during the episode

B. Physical examination: Perform a complete exam with emphasis on the neurologic exam including a careful assessment of asymmetry, head circumference (infants), increased intracranial pressure, infection, or petechial skin rash

C. Laboratory (if indicated)
1. Chemistries: Glucose (chemstrip) level should be obtained on all patients; obtain electrolytes, Ca^{++}, Mg^{++}, and PO_4 as indicated. ABG and EKG if indicated
2. Hematology: A complete blood count and blood cultures are indicated for febrile patients
3. Lumbar puncture: Consider in the febrile patient; send fluid for gram stain, culture and sensitivity, cell count, and glucose and protein levels
4. Drug levels: Evaluate for possible ingestion as indicated; obtain anticonvulsant drug levels for patients receiving chronic therapy

D. Radiographic studies
1. Head CT
    a. Should be done with first seizure
    b. Useful emergently to rule out mass effect or acute intracranial bleed
2. MRI: Most sensitive for anatomic detail, vascular malformations and demyelinating disorders
3. PET and SPECT scans: Measure brain metabolism and regional cerebral blood flow respectively. May be useful for surgical evaluation in patients with refractory seizures. Not used routinely

E. Electroencephalogram (EEG): Indicated to assess electrical seizure activity. The routine

GEN

EEG lasts approximately 1hr and is taken to be a representative sample of electrical activity. Since the test may occur when no epileptiform activity is present, a sleep-deprived EEG or repeat routine EEG (at a later date) may be necessary

IV. TREATMENT OPTIONS
A. Initial management: Stabilize the patient—ABCs
    1. Correct possible metabolic derangement: Glucose, oxygen, IV fluids
    2. Treat possible opioid overdose: Narcan
    3. **Diazepam (Valium)** is drug of choice for status epilepticus
B. Maintenance medication (See tables)
    1. Generally indicated if:
        a. More than one unprovoked seizure within one year with or without an abnormal EEG
        b. Two or more unprovoked seizures within a 6–12 month period
        c. Identification of risk factors (abnormal EEG, trauma, central lesion)
    2. Choose medication based on type of seizure
    3. No medication is without side-effect
C. Surgery
    1. Severe, refractory patients may benefit from surgical intervention
    2. Requires identification of the "epileptogenic zone"

GEN

GUIDELINES FOR ANTIEPILEPTIC DRUGS IN CHILDREN

Drug	Indication	Starting Dose (mg/kg/day)	Maintenance Dose (mg/kg/day)	Doses/Day	Target Plasma Concentration (mcg/mL)	Side Effects
Phenobarbitol	Generalized Complex partial Status epilepticus	4	4-8	1-2	10–40	Alters mood, aggression insomnia, Dupuytren's contracture
Phenytoin (Dilantin)	Generalized Complex partial Status epilepticus	5	5-15	1–2	10–20	Gum hypertrophy, acne, ataxia, tremor, nystagmus
Diazepam (Valium)	Status epilepticus	0.2-0.5mg/kg/dose IV Q 15-30 min Max total dose <5 yr - 5mg >5 yr - 10mg Rectal doses: 0.5mg/kg dose, repeat 0.25mg/kg/dose in 10 min PRN	NA	NA	NA	Sedation
Lorazepam (Ativan)	Status epilepticus	0.05-0.1mg/kg/ dose IV over 2-5 min max 4mg/dose	NA	NA	NA	Sedation
Carbamazepine (Tegretol)	Generalized Complex partial	5 (not to exceed 100mg/day)	10–25	2–4	6–12	Morbilloform rash, lethargy, agranulocytosis
Ethosuximide (Zarontin)	Absence (petit mal)	10	15-30	1-2	40–100	Nausea, vomiting, lethargy, dizziness, ataxia
Valproic acid (Depakene)	Generalized Partial Absence	10	15–40	1–3	50–100	Hepatotoxicity, pancreatitis, thrombocytopenia, tremor, weight gain
Felbamate (Felbatol)	NOT FIRST LINE Generalized Complex partial	15	15-45	3-4	NA	Life threatening aplastic anemia and liver toxicity. Requires weekly blood tests
Primidone (Mysoline)	Generalized Complex partial Myoclonic	10	20-30	1-2	5–12	Fatigue, rash, aganulocytosis, lupus-like syndrome
Clonazepam (Klonopin)	Myoclonic Infantile spasm Status epilepticus	0.025	0.025-0.1	2-3	NA	Aggression, hyperkinesia
Lamotrigine (Lamictal)	Adjunct for Generalized Partial Complex	2 (no valproic acid) 0.2 (with valproic acid)	5-15	2	NA	Life threatening skin rash, tremor, headache, nausea

GUIDELINES FOR ANTIEPILEPTIC DRUGS IN ADULTS

Drug	Indication	Starting Dose (mg/day)	Maintenance Dose (mg/day)	Doses/Day	Target Plasma Concentration (mcg/mL)	Side Effects
Phenobarbitol	Generalized Complex partial Status epilepticus	60	60-240	1-2	10–40	Alters mood, aggression insomnia, Dupuytren's syndrome
Phenytoin (Dilantin)	Generalized Complex partial Status epilepticus	200 PO 3–5mg/kg 10-15mg/kg IV for status	200–600	1-3	10–20	Gum hypertrophy, acne, ataxia, tremor, nystagmus
Diazepam (Valium)	Status epilepticus	5-10mg IV	NA	NA	NA	Sedation
Lorazepam (Ativan)	Status epilepticus	4-8mg IV	NA	NA	NA	Sedation
Carbamazepine (Tegretol)	Generalized Complex partial	200	400–1200	2–4	6–12	Morbilloform rash, agranulocytosis
Ethosuximide (Zarontin)	Absence (Petit mal)	500	500-2000	1-2	40–100	Nausea, vomiting, lethargy, dizziness, ataxia
Valproic acid (Depakene)	Generalized Partial Absence	500	500–3000	1-2	50–100	Hepatotoxicity, pancreatitis, thrombocytopenia, tremor, weight gain
Felbamate (Felbatol)	NOT FIRST LINE Generalized Complex partial	1200	1200-3600	3-4	NA	Life-threatening aplastic anemia and liver toxicity. Requires weekly blood tests
Lamotrigine (Lamictal)	Generalized Partial complex	50	300-500	2	NA	Life threatening skin rash, tremor, headache, nausea
Gabapentin (Neurontin)	Generalized Partial complex	300	900-1800	3	NA	Somnolence, ataxia, fatigue
Primidone (Mysoline)	Generalized Complex partial Myoclonic	250	250-1500	1-2	5–12	Fatigue, rash, agranulocytosis, lupus-like syndrome
Clonazepam (Klonopin)	Myoclonic Status epilepticus	1	2-8	1-2	NA	Aggression, hyperkinesia
Tiagabine (Gabitril)	Complex Partial	4	32-56	2-4	NA	Impaired concentration, speech problems, somnolence
Oxcarbazepine (Trileptal)	Partial	600mg	600-2400	2	NA	Somnolence, dizziness, diplopia, fatigue, hyponatremia

GEN

CLINICAL PEARLS

- In 50% of children with seizures, the etiology will be undetermined despite an appropriate work-up
- Breath-holding spells, benign paroxysmal vertigo, and syncope are often confused with seizures and should be considered in differential diagnosis
- If a child with a febrile seizure meets all of the criteria listed above (Section I.C.2) *and* the child appears fine, an antipyretic may be given and no further studies or treatment are necessary. The risk of recurrence is 25–30% with simple febrile seizures
- 75% of epileptics have their first seizure during childhood
- Unprovoked seizures have a 31–71% recurrence rate
- Many antiepileptic drugs decrease oral contraceptive effectiveness
- Carbamazepine and Valproic Acid are associated with increased risk of neural tube defect in pregnancy
- Non-compliance is the most common reason for incomplete seizure control

References

Montouris GD, Moser RP. Management of epilepsy. Am Fam Phys monograph 1997;1:4–20.
Brodie MJ, Dichter MA. Antiepileptic drugs. N Engl J Med 1996;334:168–75.
Brodie MJ, Dichter MA. New antiepileptic drugs. N Engl J Med 1996;334:1583–90.
Freeman JM, Vining EPG. Febrile seizures: a decision making analysis. Am Fam Phys 1995;52:1401–8.
Devinsky O. Seizure disorders. Clinical symposia 1994;46:2–20.

63. SEXUAL DYSFUNCTION

— PART ONE: MALE —

I. INTRODUCTION
    A. Definition: Consistent inability to achieve and/or maintain an erect penis which is adequate for satisfactory sexual performance
    B. Affects 15–25% males greater than 65 years. About 80% of cases are secondary to organic disease. Overall, this affects 10–18 million men

II. DIFFERENTIAL DIAGNOSIS
    A. Hormonal
    B. Neurologic
    C. Vascular
    D. Medications
    E. Psychogenic

III. HISTORY
    A. Distinguish loss of libido vs. loss of erections: If libido and erections are intact, the cause is usually psychogenic
    B. Onset and duration of impotence: Gradual loss of erections over time suggests organic cause
    C. Erections: Difficulty in obtaining or maintaining erections and presence of nocturnal erections. If normal erections do occur, then the cause is usually psychogenic
    D. Past medical history: Diabetes mellitus, coronary artery disease, peripheral vascular disease, hypertension, hyperlipidemia, hypogonadism, multiple sclerosis, neurologic disease, thyroid disorders, renal failure, adrenal disorders
    E. Medications: Antidepressants, antihypertensives, anxiolytics, antipsychotics, hormonal preparations, 5-α reductase inhibitors, histamine H_2 blockers, Metoclopramide, Digoxin
    F. Drugs: Alcohol, nicotine, illicit drug use
    G. Past surgical history: Pelvic surgery or spinal cord injury

IV. PHYSICAL
    A. Vascular disease: Check blood pressure, auscultate vessels for bruits (aorta, femoral)
    B. Secondary sexual characteristics: Masculinization
    C. Neurological exam: Check rectal tone, bulbocavernosus reflex, peripheral sensory exam
    D. Genital: Penile scarring or plaque formation (Peyronie's disease). Testicular abnormalities, tunics and erectile tissue
    E. Rectal: Prostate exam (DRE)
    F. Consider psychological evaluation: Especially if young or psychogenic cause is suspected

V. LABORATORY AND DIAGNOSTIC TESTS (If necessary after history and physical exam)
    A. Labs: CBC, SMA-12, glucose, HgbA1C, lipid profile, PSA, testosterone, thyroid function tests, urinalysis
    B. If testosterone is abnormal: Check FSH, LH, prolactin
    C. Nocturnal penile tumescence testing: If erections are obtained, this suggests psychogenic etiology. This test is not necessary if the history indicates that a patient has erections
    D. Injection of vasoactive substance into penis: If this results in erection, then a vascular cause is excluded; this is also done to determine therapeutic options
    E. Color Doppler ultrasonography: If there is a suggestion of vascular disease

VI. TREATMENT OF ORGANIC IMPOTENCE: (Listed in increasing order of invasiveness)
For treatment of psychogenic impotence, refer to other sources
    A. Minimize medications with side effects of sexual dysfunction, or change to a different class of agents
      1. Agents that may cause erectile dysfunction:
        a. Anticonvulsants
        b. Antihistamines

GEN

    c. Antihypertensives
      i. ß-blockers
      ii. Calcium channel blockers
      iii. Centrally acting α-agonists
      iv. Diuretics
    d. Antipsychotics
    e. Anxiolytics
    f. Drugs of abuse
      i. Alcohol
      ii. Anabolic steroids
      iii. Heroin
      iv. Marijuana
    g. Miscellaneous
      i. Cimetidine (Tagamet)
      ii. Corticosteroids
      iii. Finasteride (Proscar)
      iv. Gemfibrozil (Lopid)

B. Smoking cessation, alcohol in moderation, healthy diet, regular exercise

C. Sildenafil (Viagra)
1. Dose: 50mg PO taken 30 minutes to 4hrs before sexual activity. May increase to 100mg if not effective. If > age 65 or with hepatic or renal impairment, then start with 25mg
2. Side effects: Headache (16%), flushing (10%), dyspepsia (7%), nasal congestion (4%)
3. Interactions: Cytochrome P450 3A inhibitors: Erythromycin, Ketoconazole, Itraconazole, Cisapride. Contraindicated in patients on nitrates
4. Trials: 21 randomized, double blind trials up to 6 months in duration with 3000 patients aged 19–89 showed improvement in 63% (25mg), 74% (50mg), and 82% (100mg) compared to 24% with placebo. Men with DM or radical prostrate surgery did not do as well
5. Available: Tabs 25, 50, 100mg
6. Cost: ~ $7 wholesale for all strengths

D. Testosterone supplementation: Use only for men who are hypogonadal and do not have prostate cancer after adequate evaluation. This may speed up BPH in older men, follow-up every 6 months with DRE and PSA. Can be given intramuscularly or transdermal:
1. **Depo-Testosterone**: 200mg every 3 weeks of **Testosterone Cypionate**. Follow every 6 weeks with testosterone levels and liver function tests
2. Transdermal patches include **Testoderm** or **Androderm** and should be changed daily; however absorption is erratic and higher risk of hepatotoxicity

E. Yohimbine
1. α₂ adrenergic receptor antagonist
2. Dose: 5.4mg PO TID

F. Urethral suppository
1. **Muse (Alprostadil):** Supervise initial application
2. Initially 125 or 250mcg suppository is inserted into urethra after urination. May adjust dose in stepwise increments on separate occasion. Maximum 2 suppositories/day

G. Vacuum constriction devices: Consist of a hollow cylinder placed over the penis, a vacuum is generated and a rubber ring is rolled onto the erect penis to the base to trap blood maintaining the erection. Often the choice of older men
1. Low cost
2. Disadvantages include: Use can be uncomfortable, may be associated with ecchymoses
3. Use for 30 minutes only

H. Penile self-injection of vasoactive agents into corpora cavernosa, may use single agent or mixture
1. **Caverject (Alprostadil):** Self-injection into dorso-lateral aspect of proximal third of penis. Effective dose should be determined initially in the office. Initially, start at 1.25 or 2.5mcg. If no response, may give second dose after 1hr. Increase dose in increments of 2.5 to 5mcg until desired response. If partial erection occurs, wait 24hrs before next dose. Maximum dose is 60mcg and 3 injections/week. Reduce the dose if erection lasts longer than 1hr. Must counsel patient on potential for priapism and to seek medical attention if erection lasts longer than 3–4hrs

2. Contraindications include sickle cell anemia, schizophrenia, psychoses, severe venous incompetence, poor manual dexterity (for injections)
3. Complications: Mild penile pain, hypotension and dizziness, syncope, infection, and priapism (must counsel patient on risks of priapism and need to seek immediate medical attention if erection lasts longer than 3–4hrs)

I. Surgical options
1. Penile prosthesis: Either malleable or inflatable
2. Vascular reconstruction

— PART TWO: FEMALE —

I. INTRODUCTION: Sexual dysfunction in women is common and should be brought up by the physician during the history

II. DIFFERENTIAL DIAGNOSIS
A. Inhibited sexual desire
B. Orgasmic dysfunction
C. Decreased satisfaction
D. Dyspareunia

III. HISTORY
A. **Family background:** Repressive background/upbringing
B. **Onset and duration:** Primary vs. secondary
C. **Trauma:** Rape, abusive relationship, sexual abuse or incest (childhood or adult)
D. **Sexual orientation**
E. **Life changes in the past year:** Losses, pregnancy, stresses
F. **Relationship with sexual partner(s)**
G. **Menarche/menopause**
H. **Past medical history:** Chronic illness, sexually transmitted diseases, HIV/AIDS, cancer (breast)
I. **Drugs:** Alcohol, nicotine, illicit injection of drugs, sedatives/hypnotics, ß-blockers
J. **Past surgical history:** Pelvic surgery (number and type) or spinal cord injury
K. **Hormonal changes:** Postpartum, breast-feeding

IV. PHYSICAL
A. **Genital:** Infections, mass, lesions, discharge. Surgical changes (female circumcision, episiotomy)
B. **Pelvic exam:** Important looking for adnexal tenderness and signs of endometriosis such as uterosacral nodularity and decreased pelvic organ mobility

V. MANAGEMENT
A. **Orgasmic problems**
1. Primary anorgasmia (never experienced orgasm in any situation)
   a. Causes: May be due to fear of pregnancy, satisfaction, losing control. Anxiety is often a factor
   b. Treatment
      i. Extinguish the woman's subconscious overcontrol and enhance sensory stimulation
      ii. Focus on erotic thoughts and fantasies
      iii. Self-stimulation
      iv. Heighten arousal and lubrication before penetration
2. Secondary anorgasmia
   a. In depth exploration of differences in life situation now and in the past (when she was able to obtain an orgasm)
   b. Use the above techniques
B. **Dyspareunia**
1. Secondary to inadequate vaginal lubrication
   a. Lubricants such as K-Y jelly, Lubrin, Replens
   b. Vaginal creams containing estrogen can reverse vaginal atrophy in perimenopausal women
   c. Low dose oral contraceptive therapy; or hormone replacement therapy can alleviate vaginal dryness
2. Vaginismus
   a. Painful reflex spasm of the perivaginal muscles due to fear of sex (young and

GEN

inexperienced, often from strict homes) or prior rape or incest
  b. Gradual vaginal dilation with woman's finger, partner's finger or dilator
  c. Psychotherapy
 3. Other causes: Endometriosis, ovarian cysts, etc and may require further work-up to determine if change in pain relates to menstrual cycle

C. Decreased libido
 1. The short term addition of androgens has been helpful in some women in restoring sexual desire
 2. **Estratest (Estrogen and Methyltestosterone)** comes in 0.625 or 1.25mg of **Estrogen** and 1.25 or 2.5mg **Methyltestosterone** PO QD and is given cyclically
 3. If secondary to relationship or marital strife, then address these problems or refer for psychotherapy

CLINICAL PEARLS
 • Premature ejaculation is usually psychogenic (performance anxiety)
 • 8–10% of adult women in the US have never had an orgasm. 10% may achieve orgasm with fantasy alone
 • At age 60, men have an average of one erection per week

References
Miller T. Diagnostic evaluation of erectile dysfunction. Am Fam Phys 2000;61:95–104, 109–10.
Goldstein I, et al. Oral sildenafil in the treatment of erectile dysfunction. N Engl J Med 1998;338:13.
Dewire DM. Evaluation and treatment of erectile dysfunction. Am Fam Phys 1996;53:2101.
NIH Consensus Conference: Impotence. JAMA 1993;270:83.

Michael B. Weinstock, MD

64. DIFFERENTIAL DIAGNOSIS OF ARTHRITIS

I. DIFFERENTIAL DIAGNOSIS: HISTORY AND PHYSICAL
 A. History: Inquire about the location and number of joints involved, onset of pain, exacerbating and relieving factors, morning stiffness, prior injury, prior diagnosis and medications which helped, prior illness, extra-articular symptoms (fever, rash, neuropathy)
 B. Physical examination
  1. Presence of swelling, heat, tenderness, pain with motion, range of motion, joint distribution
  2. Heberden's nodes: Affect distal interphalangeal joints (DIP) in degenerative joint disease (DJD)
  3. Bouchard's nodes: Affect proximal interphalangeal joints (PIP) in DJD
  4. Extra-articular manifestations including rash, subcutaneous nodules, lymphadenopathy, splenomegaly

II. DIFFERENTIAL DIAGNOSIS BY JOINT PATTERN *
 A. Inflammation of joints
  1. **Present:** Rheumatoid arthritis (RA), systemic lupus erythematosus (SLE), gout, osteoarthritis (OA)
  2. **Absent:** OA
 B. Number of joints involved
  1. **Monoarticular** (1 joint): Gout, trauma, septic arthritis, Lyme disease, OA
  2. **Oligoarticular** (2–4 joints): Reiter's disease, psoriatic arthritis, inflammatory bowel disease (IBD), OA
  3. **Polyarticular** (>5 joints): RA, SLE
 C. Location of joint involvement
  1. **Distal interphalangeal joints** (DIP): OA, psoriatic arthritis
  2. **Metacarpal phalangeal joints** (MCP), **PIP joints, wrists**: RA, SLE
  3. **First metatarsal phalangeal joint** (MTP): Gout, OA
*Adapted from Hellman DB. Arthritis and musculoskeletal disorders. In: Tierney LM, et al. Current medical diagnosis and treatment. 34th ed. Norwalk, CT: Appleton & Lange, 1995:695. Used with permission.

III. DIFFERENTIAL DIAGNOSIS BY EXAMINATION OF JOINT FLUID

	Normal	Noninflammatory	Inflammatory	Septic
Clarity	Transparent	Transparent	Transparent-opaque	Opaque
Color	Clear	Yellow	Yellow/opalescent	Yellow/green
WBC (per uL)	< 200	200–3000	3000–50,000	> 50,000†
PMNs(%)	< 25%	< 25%	≥ 50%	≥ 75% †
Culture	Negative	Negative	Negative	Usually positive
Glucose (mg/dL)	Nearly equal to serum	Nearly equal to serum	> 25mg/dL but lower than serum	< 25 (much lower than serum)
DIFFERENTIAL DIAGNOSIS:	Consider "non-inflam-matory" causes	1. Osteoarthritis 2. Trauma 3. Osteochond-ritis dissecans 4. Osteochond-romatosis 5. Neuropathic arthropathy 6. Rheumatic fever 7. SLE 8. Scleroderma	1. Rheumatoid arthritis 2. Gout and pseudogout 3. Reiter's syndrome 4. Ankylosing spondylitis 5. Psoriatic arthritis 6. Arthritis accompanying IBD 7. Rheumatic fever 8. SLE 9. Scleroderma 10. Tuberculosis 11. Mycotic infections	Pyogenic bacterial infections † The total cell count may be lower if the infection has been partially treated or if organisms have a low virulence

Adapted from Hellman DB. Arthritis and musculoskeletal disorders. In: Tierney LM, et al. Current medical diagnosis and treatment. 34th ed. Norwalk, CT: Appleton & Lange, 1995:696, and Rodan GP, ed. Primer on the rheumatic diseases. 7th ed. JAMA 1973;224(supp):662. Copyright 1973, American Medical Association. Used with permission.

IV. DIFFERENTIAL DIAGNOSIS BETWEEN OA AND RA

	OSTEOARTHRITIS	RHEUMATOID ARTHRITIS
Morning stiffness	Absent or brief	Present
Systemic manifestations*	Absent	Present
Joint involvement	DIP joints, less commonly MCP, hip, knees, cervical and lumbar spine. May affect any joint with previous trauma.	PIP and MCP joints, wrists, knees ankles, toes
Onset	Insidious	Insidious
Lab — RF, ANA, ESR	Usually normal	RF positive >75%, ANA positive ~ 20%, ESR usually increased
X-ray findings	Narrowed joint space, osteophytes, bony cysts, increased density of subchondral bone	Juxta-articular osteoporosis, joint erosions, narrowed joint space

* Systemic manifestations of RA may include malaise, fever, weight loss, morning stiffness, pleural effusion, pericarditis, lymphadenopathy, splenomegaly, and vasculitis

References

Litman K. A rational approach to the diagnosis of arthritis. Am Fam Phys 1996;53:1295.

Hellman DB. Arthritis and musculoskeletal disorders. In: Tierney LM, et al. Current medical diagnosis and treatment. 34th ed. Norwalk, CT: Appleton & Lange, 1995:695–6.

Smith CA, Arnett Jr. FC. Diagnosing rheumatoid arthritis. Am Fam Phys 1991;44:863–70.

Rodan GP, ed. Primer on the rheumatic diseases. 7th ed. JAMA 1973;224(supp):662.

Linda Stone, MD
Michael B. Weinstock, MD

65. OSTEOARTHRITIS

I. INTRODUCTION

Synonymous with degenerative joint disease (DJD). Osteoarthritis (OA) is the most common form of joint disease. Affects 20 millions adults in the USA. Marked by *loss of cartilage and joint margin changes*. Its cause is unknown, but it is more common in the presence of other disorders such as RA, gout, Paget's and trauma

II. SYMPTOMS AND SIGNS

A. Joint use will increase symptoms
B. Joint pain develops over time
C. Disuse (sleeping, sitting) will increase stiffness
D. Decreased range of motion
E. Joints will enlarge over time
F. Appearance of nodes: Heberden's nodes (DIP joints) and Bouchard's nodes (PIP joints)

III. PATIENTS AT INCREASED RISK

A. Increasing age
B. History of injury
C. Obesity
D. Occupations with repetitive motion

IV. LABORATORY

See Chapter 64, Differential Diagnosis of Arthritis, IV. Chart. Usually negative

V. X-RAY

See Chapter 64, Differential Diagnosis of Arthritis, IV. Chart. Usually normal in early stages

VI. DIFFERENTIAL DIAGNOSIS BETWEEN OA AND RA

See Chapter 64, Differential Diagnosis of Arthritis, IV. Chart

VII. MANAGEMENT

A. **Weight reduction:** Extremely important!
B. **Maintaining range of motion:** Stretching, use of joint
C. **Muscle strengthening exercises:** Consider involving physical therapy
D. **Use of ambulatory aids:** Walker, cane
E. **Heat**
F. **NSAIDs, Acetaminophen:** Acetaminophen has the same efficacy as Ibuprofen in the treatment of OA of the knee. Selective COX-2 inhibitors should be considered in patients who need NSAID, but are at risk of NSAID's GI side effects
G. **Capsaicin (Zostrix):** Topical analgesic 0.025%, 0.075%. Apply 3–4 × QD. Wash hands after use. May not notice effect for 4–6 weeks
   Intra-articular glucocorticoid provides immediate pain relief. Limit to not >3 month for any given joint
   Intra-articular hyaluronic acid (Hyalgan, Synvisc) improves visco elasticity of synovial fluid. Given in series of doses and are expensive
   Glucosamine and **Chondroitin** have been used to relieve pain. Their efficiency has yet to be established
H. **Surgical correction** of developmental anomalies, deformities, unequal leg length, severe OA of hip and knee (consider hip or knee replacement)
I. **Educate patients** and involve them in community support groups (e.g., Arthritis Foundation)

CLINICAL PEARLS

- Watch for side effects of NSAIDs, especially in the elderly patient: Inquire about signs of GI bleed and renal compromise. Monitor renal labs
- Discuss prognosis so that patient can have realistic expectations of future

References

Manek NJ, et al. Osteoarthritis: Current concepts in diagnosis and management. Am Fam Phys 2000;61:1795–804.

Langman MJ, et al. Adverse upper gastrointestinal effects of rofecoxib compared with NSAIDs. JAMA 1999;282:1929–33.

Simon LS, Weaver AL, Graham DY, et al. Anti-inflammatory and upper gastrointestinal effects of celecoxib in rheumatoid arthritis: a randomized controlled trial. JAMA. 1999;282:1921–28.

Altman RD, Lozada CJ. Practice guidelines in the management of osteoarthritis. Osteoarthritis Cartilage 1998;6(suppl A):22–4.

Creamer P, Flores R, Hochberg MC. Management of osteoarthritis in older adults. Clin Geriatr Med 1998;14:435–54.

Frizziero L, Govoni E, Bacchini P. Intra-articular hyaluronic acid in the treatment of osteoarthritis of the knee: clinical and morphological study. Clin Exp Rheumatol 1998;16;441–9.

Lane NE, Thompson JM. Management of osteoarthritis in the primary-care setting: an evidence-based approach to treatment. Am J Med 1997;103:25S–30S.

Towheed TE, Hochberg MC. A systematic review of randomized controlled trials of pharmacological therapy in osteoarthritis of the knee, with an emphasis on trial methodology. Semin Arthritis Rheum 1997;26:755–70.

Hochberg MC, Altman RD, Brandt KD, et al. Guidelines for the medical management of osteoarthritis, I: osteoarthritis of the hip. Arthritis Rheum 1995;38:1535–40.

Hochberg MC, Altman RD, Brandt KD, et al. Guidelines for the medical management of osteoarthritis, II: osteoarthritis of the knee. Arthritis Rheum 1995;38:1541–6.

GEN

Laurie Dangler, MD
Miriam Chan, PharmD

66. RHEUMATOID ARTHRITIS

I. DEFINITION: A chronic, systemic inflammatory connective tissue disease characterized by symmetric, erosive synovitis and sometimes multisystem involvement. Etiology is unknown

II. EPIDEMIOLOGY
- **A.** Estimated prevalence of 1–2% of adult population worldwide
- **B.** Prevalence increases with age (> 10% in persons over age 65)
- **C.** Women 2.5 times as often as men
- **D.** Much higher concordance in monozygotic twins compared to dizygotic twins, suggesting genetic predisposition; also higher incidence with certain HLA subtypes (DR4 and DR 1)

III. DIFFERENTIAL DIAGNOSIS OF POLYARTHRITIDES
- **A. Connective tissue diseases:** Systemic lupus erythematosus (SLE), primary Sjogren's syndrome, scleroderma, polymyositis/dermatomyositis
- **B. Vasculitic syndromes:** Polyarteritis nodosa, giant cell arteritis, cryoglobulinemia, Bechet's syndrome, Wegener's granulomatosis
- **C. Seronegative spondyloarthropathies:** Ankylosing spondylitis, Reiter's disease, reactive arthritis, psoriatic arthritis, inflammatory bowel disease, Whipple's disease
- **D. Crystalline disorders:** Gout, pseudogout
- **E. Infectious arthritides:** Human immunodeficiency virus (HIV), viral, bacterial, tuberculous, fungal, subacute bacterial endocarditis (SBE), rheumatic fever, Lyme disease
- **F. Metabolic disorders:** Hypothyroidism, hyperparathyroidism, hemochromatosis
- **G. Paraneoplastic syndromes:** Lymphoproliferative disorders, hypertrophic osterarthropathy, carcinomatous polyarthritis
- **H. Miscellaneous arthritides:** Hemoglobinopathies, pancreatic disease, hyperlipoproteinemia, multicentric reticulohistiocytosis

IV. SIGNS AND SYMPTOMS
- **A.** Insidious development of symptoms over several weeks
- **B.** Symmetric inflammation of smaller joints, esp. MCP, PIP, and MTP joints, but may also affect large joints, particularly later in the disease (involvement of DIP joints is more typical of

osteoarthritis and psoriatic arthritis)

C. Morning stiffness often lasting over 1hr

D. Joint deformity: Caused by laxity of ligaments and tendons around the joints

1. Swan-neck: flexion of PIP and hyperextension at DIP joints
2. Ulnar deviation of MCP joints
3. Atlantoaxial subluxation of cervical spine: May cause myelopathy or even death (esp. if in car accident or other trauma with subluxation)

E. Joint destruction: Often not apparent on x-ray until one year after onset of disease; initially osteopenia followed by erosion of bone and decalcification

F. Rheumatoid nodules: Occur over pressure points and may be confused with tophi

G. Sjogren's syndrome: May occur secondarily, esp. in older patients with long-standing disease

H. Anemia: Often have mild normochromic, normocytic anemia; must rule out chronic blood loss

I. Other: May also have vasculitis, pulmonary manifestations, nerve entrapment syndromes (e.g., carpal tunnel), low-grade fever, malaise, fatigue, and weight loss

V. DIAGNOSIS

A. Rheumatoid Factor: Nonspecific but present in up to 90% of patients with RA, usually associated with more severe, erosive disease

B. Inflammatory markers: ESR and C-reactive protein elevated but very nonspecific, however, may be used to clinically follow disease with changes in treatment

C. Synovial fluid analysis: WBC count typically 10,000–20,000 with 60–75% PMN's

D. Diagnosis: Based on American College of Rheumatology Criteria

The 1987 American College of Rheumatology Revised Criteria for Classification of Rheumatoid Arthritis (Traditional Format)

CRITERION	DEFINITION
1. Morning stiffness	Morning stiffness in and around the joints lasting at least one hour before maximal improvement
2. Arthritis of three or more joint areas	At least three joint areas with simultaneous soft tissue swelling or fluid (not bony overgrowth alone) observed by a physician. The 14 possible joint areas are right or left PIP, MCP, wrist, elbow, knee, ankle and MTP joints
3. Arthritis of hand joints	At least one joint area swollen as above in a wrist, MCP or PIP
4. Symmetric arthritis	Simultaneous involvement of the same joint areas on both sides of the body; bilateral involvement of PIP, MCP or MTP joints is acceptable without absolute symmetry
5. Rheumatoid nodules	Subcutaneous nodules, over bony prominences, or extensor surfaces, or juxta-articular regions, observed by a physician
6. Serum rheumatoid factor	Demonstration of abnormal amounts of rheumatoid factor by any method that has been positive in less than 5% of normal control subjects
7. Radiologic changes	Radiologic changes typical of rheumatoid arthritis on postanterior hand and wrist roentgenograms, which must include erosions or unequivocal bony decalcification localized to or most marked adjacent to the involved joints (osteoarthritis changes alone do not qualify)

NOTE: For classification purposes, a patient shall be said to have rheumatoid arthritis if at least four of the seven criteria are present. Criteria 1 through 4 must have been present for at least six weeks. Patients with two clinical diagnoses are not excluded. Designation as "classic," "definite" or "probable" rheumatoid arthritis is not made

PIP = proximal interphalangeal joint; MCP = metacarpophalangeal joint; MTP = metatarsophalangeal joint

Source: Arnett FC. Revised criteria for the classification of rheumatoid arthritis. Bull Rheum Dis 1989;38(5):1–6. Used with permission.

VI. MANAGEMENT

A. Goals

1. Relief of symptoms
2. Preservation of function
3. Prevention of structural damage and deformity

4. Maintenance of a normal life-style
B. Education: Explain goals of therapy and chronic disease course to patients, enroll help of family members and other support groups
C. Physical and occupational therapy
D. Systemic rest: Depends on the severity of disease (e.g., mild disease may require only 2hrs of rest per day)
E. Articular rest: Relaxation and stretching of the hip and knee muscles to prevent contractures
F. Exercise: To preserve joint motion, and enhance muscular strength and endurance
G. Assistive devices: Raised toilet seat, gripping bar, cane, crutches, etc. (See Chapter 105, Falls in the Elderly)
H. Weight loss: Will aid with arthritis of the lower extremities
I. Local therapies
1. Heat and cold: For analgesic effects (heat or cold) and muscle-relaxing effects (prior to exercising or stretching (local moist heat or warm tub baths). Note: Heat may exacerbate joint inflammation
2. Injections of corticosteroids: See Chapter 86, Corticosteroid Injection of Joints
3. Splints: To provide joint rest, reduce pain, prevent contracture. Should be applied for the shortest period of time possible and should be removed at least twice per day for stretching and range of motion exercises. May coordinate with physical or occupational therapist
   a. Night splints to the wrist and/or hand in position of function
   b. Knee splint in full extension
   c. Ankle splint at 90° angle
J. Medications
1. **Non-steroidal anti-inflammatory drugs (NSAIDs):** Do not affect the outcome, but do help to control symptoms
   a. **Aspirin:** Inexpensive; 3000–6500mg/day in 3–4 doses. Use of enteric coated Aspirin helps to decrease GI side effects
   b. Other NSAIDs have not been proven to be more effective than Aspirin, but may have less side effects
   c. COX-2 inhibitors (Celebrex, Vioxx) have similar efficacy as traditional NSAIDs. Their advantage is a reduced rate of adverse events, especially upper GI bleeding
   d. GI prophylaxis with chronic NSAID use: First line is **Misoprostol (Cytotec)**. H_2 blockers and Carafate do not reduce the frequency of gastric ulceration, but do reduce dyspepsia and may be used if Misoprostol is contraindicated or not tolerated
   e. **Misoprostol (Cytotec)**
      i. Indications: Should be given to patients at high risk for GI toxicity (see below)
         a. Age older than 75
         b. Concomitant use of steroids, use of NSAIDs greater than 3 months, use of more than 1 NSAID or large doses of NSAIDs
         c. History of peptic ulcer disease or GI bleeding
         d. Significant cardiovascular disease
      ii. Dose: 200mcg PO QID (may decrease to 100mcg QID or 200mcg BID if not well tolerated)
      iii. Side effects: Diarrhea and bloating. Note: Absolutely contraindicated in pregnancy
2. **Glucocorticoids**
   a. Indications
      i. Used as a bridge between NSAIDs and until onset of action of the DMARDs (see below)
      ii. For refractory disease when the NSAIDs and DMARDs have failed
      iii. For severe extra-articular manifestations (pericarditis, perforating eye lesions, etc.)
   b. Dose: Use the lowest dose possible—10mg PO QD or less (preferably 5–7.5mg QD). When discontinued, should be slowly tapered down
3. **Disease-modifying antirheumatic drugs (DMARD)**
   a. Have potential for modifying course of disease
   b. Consider starting within 2 months of diagnosis to reduce the possibility of irreversible joint destruction
   c. Should be prescribed by someone with experience with this category of drugs
   d. Require several months before effect is seen and require close monitoring for side effects
   e. Include **Methotrexate** (most frequently prescribed), **Cyclosporine, Hydroxychloroquine, gold salts, oral gold, Sulfasalazine, Azathioprine, D-penicillamine** (see table)

GEN

DISEASE-MODIFYING ANTIRHEUMATIC DRUGS
USED IN TREATMENT OF RHEUMATOID ARTHRITIS

Drug	Approximate Time to Benefit	Usual Maintenance Dose	Toxic Effects
Hydroxychloroquine	2–4 months	200mg twice daily	Infrequent rash, diarrhea, rare retinal toxicity
Sulfasalazine	1–2 months	1000mg 2 or 3 times daily	Rash, infrequent myelosuppression, GI intolerance
Methotrexate	1–2 months	7.5–15.0mg/week	GI symptoms, stomatitis, rash, alopecia, infrequent myelosuppresion, hepatotoxicity, rare but serious (even life-threatening) pulmonary toxicity
Injectable gold salts	3–6 months	25–50mg IM every 2–4 weeks	Rash, stomatitis, myelosuppression, thrombocytopenia, proteinuria
Oral gold	4–6 months	3mg daily or twice daily	Same as those of injectable gold but less frequent, plus frequent diarrhea
Azathioprine	2–3 months	50–150mg daily	Myelosuppression, infrequent hepatotoxicity, early flu-like illness with fever, GI symptoms, elevated results on LFTs
D-penicillamine	3–6 months	250–750mg daily	Rash, stomatitis, dysgeusia, proteinuria, myelosuppression, infrequent but serious autoimmune disease

From American College of Rheumatology Ad Hoc Committee of Clinical Guidelines: Guidelines for the management of rheumatoid arthritis. Arthritis Rheum 39:723–731, 1996.

New DMARDs

Drug	MOA	Dose	Side-Effects
Etanercept (Enbrel)	TNF - antagonists	25mg SQ 2x/week	Reactions at injection site, flu-like symptoms
Inflixmab (Remicabe)	TNF - antagonists	3mg/kg IV Q 8 weeks	Flu-like symptoms, development of auto antibodies
Leflunomide (Arava)	Pyrimidine Synthesis inhibitor	100mg/day x 3 days then 10-20mg/day	Thrombocytopenia, hepatotoxicity, diarrhea, monitor CBC & AST Q 4-8 weeks

CLINICAL PEARLS
- Asking about length of morning stiffness, e.g., "How long does it take in the morning for you to feel as good as you'll be?" is a useful way of following the severity of the disease as the duration of morning stiffness correlates with the degree of joint inflammation
- Since Methotrexate is teratogenic, male patients should wait 3 months after stopping therapy, and female patients should wait at least 1 ovulatory cycle before attempting to get pregnant
- Synovial fluid does not have a low concentration of glucose, therefore if the glucose is low, need to exclude a septic joint

References
Möttönen T, et al. Comparison of combination therapy with single-drug therapy in early rheumatoid arthritis: a randomised trial. Lancet May 8, 1999;353:1568–73.

Pincus T, et al. Combination therapy with multiple disease-modifying antirheumatic drugs in rheumatoid arthritis: a preventive strategy. Ann Intern Med Nov 16, 1999;131:768–74.

Medical Letter consultants. New drugs for rheumatic arthritis. Med Lett Drugs Ther Nov 20, 1998; 40 (1040):110–2.

Ytterberg SR, et al. Codeine and oxycodone use in patients with chronic rheumatic disease pain. Arthritis Rheum Sep 1998;41:1603–12.

Schiff M. Emerging treatment for rheumatoid arthritis. Am J Med 1997;102(Suppl 1A):11–5.

American College of Rheumatology Ad Hoc Committee of Clinical Guidelines. Guidelines for the

GEN

management of rheumatoid arthritis. Arthritis Rheum 1996; 39:723–31.

Rheumatoid Arthritis. Primer on the rheumatic diseases, 10th ed. Atlanta, GA:Arthritis Foundation, 1993:86–99.

Smith CA, Arnett FC. Diagnosing rheumatoid arthritis: current criteria. Am Fam Phys 1991; 44:863.

Steve Brook, MD
Thomas D. Armsey, Jr., MD

67. GOUTY ARTHRITIS

I. DEFINITION

A. Gout: A common inflammatory disease characterized by the deposition of monosodium urate crystals within the kidneys, subcutaneous tissues, or joints. Most commonly seen in ages 30–50, with men affected more commonly than women. May be classified as either primary (resulting from inborn errors of metabolism) or secondary (resulting from medications or other medical conditions). Four stages of gout:

1. Asymptomatic hyperuricemia
2. Acute gouty arthritis
3. Interval gout
4. Chronic tophaceous gout

B. Hyperuricemia: Defined as a level greater than 7.0mg/dL and resulting from either overproduction or underexcretion of uric acid. Although hyperuricemia and gout are frequently associated, the two conditions are not mutually exclusive—some patients with gout have normal uric acid levels, and some patients with hyperuricemia never develop gout

II. ETIOLOGY

A. Primary Gout

1. Underexcretion of uric acid (90% of patients): Primary idiopathic
2. Overproduction of uric acid (10% of patients)
   a. Primary idiopathic
   b. Hypoxanthine-guanine phosphoribosyltransferase deficiency
   c. Phosphoribosylpyrophosphate synthetase overactivity

B. Secondary Gout

1. Underexcretion of uric acid
   a. Renal disease (chronic renal failure, renal insufficiency, lead nephropathy)
   b. Medications (ASA, diuretics, Niacin, Levodopa, Ethambutol)
   c. Alcohol
   d. Dehydration
   e. Starvation
   f. Hypertension
   g. Obesity
   h. Hypothyroidism
2. Overproduction of uric acid
   a. Purine-rich diet (organ meats, sardines, anchovies, bacon, turkey, venison, veal, scallops)
   b. Alcohol
   c. Obesity
   d. Exercise
   e. Myeloproliferative disorders
   f. Lymphoproliferative disorders
   g. Hemolytic disorders
   h. Psoriasis

III. DIFFERENTIAL DIAGNOSIS

A. Infectious arthritis
B. Cellulitis
C. Bursitis
D. Tendonitis

GEN

   E. Osteoarthritis, rheumatoid arthritis
   F. Pseudogout
   G. Amyloidosis
   H. Type IIa hyperlipidemia

IV. SIGNS AND SYMPTOMS: Differ depending on the stage
   A. Asymptomatic hyperuricemia
      1. No symptoms present
      2. Serum uric acid level elevated (greater than 7.0mg/dL)
   B. Acute gouty arthritis
      1. Classic presentation: Acute, nocturnal onset of pain, swelling, warmth, and erythema in the first MTP joint (podagra)
      2. Monoarticular involvement is most common, with the first MTP joint affected in 50% of cases. Other joints affected include the forefoot, heel, ankle, wrist, fingers, and elbow
      3. Fever and chills may be present in severe attacks
      4. Peak intensity occurs within 24–36hrs
      5. Resolution of symptoms without treatment occurs in days to weeks
      6. Absence of symptoms between acute attacks (termed interval gout)
   C. Interval gout
      1. The asymptomatic period between acute attacks. May last weeks to years (50% patients experience another acute attack within 1 year)
      2. Tophi (subcutaneous or interosseous collections of urate crystals) may be present if the disease has progressed to the chronic stage
   D. Chronic tophaceous gout
      1. Increasingly rare due to modern therapy
      2. Tophi are present in 90% of patients. Locations include: ear helix, proximal ulnar olecranon, achilles tendon, and prepatellar bursa
      3. Acute exacerbations are frequent and often polyarticular
      4. Morning stiffness and joint deformity are common

V. EVALUATION
   A. Joint aspiration
      1. Joint aspiration should take place after the acute attack has subsided to avoid patient discomfort. Include a gram stain and culture of the fluid to rule out infection
      2. The presence of monosodium urate crystals confirms the diagnosis of gout
      3. Crystals are needle-shaped and negatively birefringent under polarized light
      4. The white blood cell count may also be elevated within the synovial fluid (10,000–60,000) with neutrophils predominating
   B. 24hr urine for uric acid
      1. Important test to direct treatment and determine if the patient is an overproducer or underexcretor of uric acid. Perform after an acute attack resolves
      2. Patients on a normal diet with a 24hr uric acid excretion >800mg are classified as overproducers. A value of <600mg classifies a patient as an underexcretor
   C. Other labs
      1. Serum uric acid: Often not helpful in the diagnosis of acute gout (normal in 10% of patients). Useful in monitoring the response to urate-lowering therapy
      2. Creatinine, CBC, LFTs, lipid profile, and UA
   D. Imaging
      1. Plain radiographs are not useful in diagnosing acute gout. Usually only soft tissue swelling is seen
      2. Classic radiographic findings in chronic gout: "punched-out" bony lesions, cortical erosions with overhanging margins, and joint space preservation

VI. MANAGEMENT
   A. Asymptomatic hyperuricemia
      1. No medical treatment is indicated
      2. Secondary causes of hyperuricemia should be sought and adjusted accordingly:
         a. Weight loss
         b. Reduction in dietary purines

      c. Reduction in alcohol consumption

      d. Avoidance of diuretics

B. Acute gouty arthritis

  1. Treatment should be initiated as early as possible (preferably within 24hrs). Immobilization and ice are important adjuncts to medical therapy

  2. NSAIDs: drugs of choice, with the exception of ASA. Use with caution in the elderly and patients with PUD, renal, hepatic, and cardiac disease. Examples:

      a. Indomethacin: 50mg PO QID for 2 days then 25mg PO QID until complete resolution (usually within a week)

      b. Naproxen: 500mg PO BID for 2 days then 250mg PO BID until complete resolution

      c. Ibuprofen: 800mg PO QID for 2 days then 400mg PO QID until complete resolution

  3. Alternative therapies: use if NSAIDs contraindicated

      a. Colchicine: 1.2mg PO initially, then 0.6mg PO every hour until improvement (do not exceed 10 doses). Usually terminates acute attacks within 10hrs. Therapy should be stopped when the maximum dosage is reached, the acute attack subsides, or side effects occur (nausea, vomiting, diarrhea). IV **Colchicine** is available but is associated with bone marrow suppression and renal or hepatic cell damage

      b. Corticosteroids: Oral Prednisone 40–60mg PO QD for 5 days then tapered over 10 days. Alternatives to oral therapy are **Triamcinolone Acetonide** 60mg intramuscularly, or **Triamcinolone Acetonide** 10mg intra-articularly

C. Interval gout/Chronic tophaceous gout

  1. Once the acute attack has subsided, the physician and patient should decide if chronic treatment is required. Some patients choose to treat acute attacks as they arise

  2. Indications for chronic therapy:

      a. Two or more acute attacks

      b. Visible tophi

      c. Radiographic evidence of urate deposits

      d. Renal stones

      e. Renal damage

  3. Overproducers of uric acid (>800mg uric acid in 24hr urine) should be treated with xanthine-oxidase inhibitors—

      Allopurinol: 100mg PO QD increased by 100mg every week until a serum uric acid level of 6mg/dL or lower is achieved. The maximum dose is 600mg/day, but response is typically seen at 300mg/day. Dosages above 300mg should be given BID. Adjust dose for creatinine clearance

  4. Underexcretors of uric acid (<600mg uric acid in a 24hr urine) should be treated with a uricosuric agent—

      Probenecid: 250mg PO BID increased by 500mg every 2 weeks until a serum uric acid level of 6mg/dL or lower is achieved. The maximum dose is 3g/day, but response is typically seen at 2 g/day. (**Allopurinol** should be used in underexcretors with a creatinine clearance of <50 mL/min or history of renal calculi)

  5. Low dose **Colchicine** (0.6mg PO BID) or low dose NSAIDs should be initiated a week before therapy as prophylaxis against acute attacks and continued for 3–6 months

D. Indications for rheumatologic referral

  1. Early onset

  2. For documentation of gout in difficult to aspirate joints

  3. Treatment of polyarticular gout

  4. Treatment of refractory gout

  5. Therapeutic guidance in patients with organ failure

GEN

CLINICAL PEARLS

- Any therapy for gout should include lifestyle modifications such as weight loss, low purine diet, and reduction in alcohol consumption
- Never begin therapy with Allopurinol or Probenecid during an acute attack as they can worsen symptoms
- If patients currently treated with Allopurinol or Probenecid experience an acute attack do not adjust the doses. Treat with NSAIDs or Colchicine
- If gout is present in patients younger than 30 years old, consider a genetic disorder

References
Harris MD, et al. Gout and hyperuricemia. Am Fam Phys 1999;59:925–34.
Pittman JR, et al. Diagnosis and management of gout. Am Fam Phys 1999;59:1799–1806.
Gall EP. Hyperuricemia and gout. Decision making in medicine—an algorithmic approach. 2nd ed. St. Louis, Mo:Mosby Inc, 1998:442–443.
Wortmann RL. Gout and other disorders of purine metabolism. Harrison's principles of internal medicine. 14th ed. New York, NY:McGraw-Hill, 1998:2158–66.
Canoso JJ. Crystal-induced arthritides. Rheumatology in primary care. 1st ed. Philadelphia, PA: W.B. Saunders, 1997:150–161.
Buckley TJ. Radiographic features of gout. Am Fam Phys 1996;54:1232–8.

Laurie Dangler, MD
Miriam Chan, PharmD

68. OSTEOPOROSIS

I. DEFINITION: Decrease in density (mass/unit volume) of normal bone and microarchitectural deterioration of bone tissue. Osteoporosis is a progressive disease

  A. WHO definition of osteoporosis: Bone mineral density 2.5 standard deviations below the mean for normal healthy young adults aged 30–40 years

  B. WHO definition of osteopenia: Bone mineral density between 1.0 and 2.5 standard deviations below the mean for normal healthy young adults ages 30–40

  C. Primary osteoporosis: Age-related bone loss in men or women, esp. estrogen-deficient postmenopausal women

  D. Secondary osteoporosis: Osteomalacia, multiple myeloma, hyperparathyroidism, nutritional deficits, endocrine disease (e.g., hyperthyroidism), metabolic (e.g., diabetes, pregnancy), immobility, and medications including glucocorticoids, Cyclosporine, excessive thyroid, prolonged heparin, Phenytoin, Methotrexate when combined with steroids, Phenobarbital

  E. Risk factors for osteoporosis
   1. Female, white or oriental race
   2. Smoking or excessive alcohol
   3. Early menopause
   4. Nulliparity
   5. Lack of exercise
   6. Low body weight
   7. Low calcium intake
   8. Family history of osteoporosis

II. SIGNS AND SYMPTOMS: Often asymptomatic
  A. History
   1. Chronicity and location of fractures
   2. Previous treatment of osteoporosis
   3. Menstrual and menopausal history (early age of menopause, etc.)
   4. Endocrine abnormalities
   5. Alcohol or drug use
   6. Steroid use
   7. Level of physical activity
   8. Diet
   9. Peak adult height
   10. Family history of osteoporosis

  B. Physical examination
   1. Patient's current height and weight
   2. Physical findings of systemic disease (see secondary causes listed above)
   3. Kyphosis, scoliosis, loss of lordotic curve: Dorsal kyphosis (dowager's hump)—result of multiple anterior compression fractures of thoracic spine
   4. Gait, balance, strength, vision

GEN

5. Vertebral Compression Fracture: Often patient can pinpoint exact area of fracture and onset of pain; intense pain for 2–3 weeks followed by gradual regression over 3–4 months

C. May have "early" symptom of upper or mid-thoracic back pain associated with activity, aggravated by long periods of sitting or standing, and easily relieved by rest in the recumbent position

D. **Hip fractures:** Serious complication; mortality rate as high as 20% in first 6 months following hip fracture; large contributor to the $7–10 billion annual cost of osteoporosis in the US

III. DIAGNOSIS

A. Dual energy x-ray absorptiometry

1. Measurement of bone mineral density at both spine and hip. The most accurate diagnosis (has supplanted radiogrametry, quantitative CT and single energy x-ray absorptiometry). Less radiation exposure than a chest x-ray
2. Indications
   a. Estrogen deficient women or women with premature menopause considering therapy
   b. Patients with osteopenia or vertebral fractures revealed on radiographs
   c. Patients with loss of height considering therapy
   d. Patients on long term glucocorticoid therapy (greater than 1 month of therapy and ≥ 7.5mg Prednisone QD)
   e. Symptomatic primary hyperparathyroidism with consideration of surgery
   f. Monitoring therapeutic response in patients undergoing treatment for osteoporosis if result of the test would change management
3. Results: The T-score measures the distance of the measured bone density from the peak value of a young normal population in terms of units of standard deviation for the same young population. Fracture risk approximately doubles for each decrease in T-score unit
   a. T score above –1: A bone density that is not more than 1 standard deviation below the young adult mean (normal)
   b. T score between –1 and –2.5: A bone density that lies between 1 and 2.5 standard deviations below the young adult mean (osteopenia)
   c. T score less than –2.5: A bone density that is more than 2.5 standard deviations below the young adult mean (osteoporosis)

B. Plain radiography: May be diagnostic if shows vertebral fracture, but generally not sensitive enough as screening since bone loss not apparent until 30% or more of bone is lost

C. Labs: To screen for secondary causes if indicated

1. CBC, chemistry
2. Alkaline phosphatase and serum calcium, TSH
3. Urinalysis
4. If suggested by clinical findings: ESR, serum parathyroid hormone concentration, serum 25-hydroxyvitamin D concentration, 24hr urinary calcium excretion, serum/urine protein electrophoresis, bone marrow examination/biopsy
5. **Biochemical Markers:** Osteocalcin, and telopeptides of type I collagen likely to be powerful tool for diagnosis and treatment in future, but currently limited by large diurnal variation and poor reproducibility (15–20%)

IV. MANAGEMENT

A. Exclude secondary causes of osteoporosis (see above) and halt progression through prevention (i.e., stop smoking, decrease alcohol intake, modify risk factors)

B. Calcium and Vitamin D: Calcium, 1000–1500mg/day with Vitamin D, 400–800 IU daily should be taken in the diet or given as supplements concurrently with any of the above treatments. Both are inadequate alone in majority of patients

C. Exercise: Weight-bearing exercise maintains bone density and recommended for both prevention and treatment of osteoporosis (walk, jog, row, weight training)

D. Estrogen Replacement Therapy (ERT): See Chapter 25, Menopause & HRT

1. Conjugated Estrogens (**Premarin**): 0.625–1.25mg PO QD or transdermal Estrogen 50–100μg QD
2. **Medroxyprogesterone** (**Provera**): 2.5–5.0mg PO QD in conjunction with estrogens if intact uterus to reduce risk of endometrial hyperplasia and cancer
3. Greatest benefit if begun early in menopause because greatest rate of bone loss is in first 5–7 years of menopause; also greatest benefit may be after 10 years or more of therapy
4. Contraindications: History of breast cancer, estrogen-dependent neoplasia, undiagnosed abnormal genital bleeding, history of or active thromboembolic disorder

E. Raloxifene (Evista)

GEN.

1. A selective estrogen receptor modulator (SERM) which acts on the bone, but does not stimulate the endometrium or breast
2. Indicated for the prevention and treatment of postmenopausal osteoporosis
3. Dose: 60mg PO QD
4. Side effects: Hot flashes, leg cramps, risk of thromboembolic events

F. Oral Bisphosphonate: Alendronate (Fosamax), Risedronate (Actonel)
1. Mechanism: Inhibits osteoclast-mediated bone resorption; has been shown to achieve bone stabilization, increase bone density and decrease fracture risk when given continuously for 3 years
2. Indications
   a. Treatment and prevention of postmenopausal osteoporosis (Bone mineral density 2.5 standard deviations below the mean for normal healthy young adults ages 30–40)
   b. Paget's disease
   c. Steroid-induced osteopososis
3. Contraindications
   a. Esophageal abnormalities which may delay esophageal emptying (achalasia, stricture)
   b. Creatinine clearance < 35mL/min
   c. Hypocalcemia
4. Dose:
   a. Treatment: **Fosamax** 10mg PD QD, **Actonel** 5mg PO QD
   b. Prevention: **Fosamax** 5mg PO QD, **Actonel** 5mg PO QD
5. Administration: Fosamax or Actonel should be taken with 6–8 oz of plain water (not mineral water which contains calcium) to be taken 30 minutes before eating any food. May sit down, but should not lie down (to decrease esophageal irritation). Do not give concurrently with anything which may contain calcium. Coffee and tea may decrease absorption by up to 50%. Ensure adequate intake of calcium and vitamin D
6. Side effects: GI discomfort including nausea and vomiting, dyspepsia, diarrhea and constipation

G. Calcitonin-Salmon (Miacalcin)
1. Mechanism: Thought to inhibit osteoclastic resorption of bone, but this is uncertain at dose of 200 U/day. Also produces an analgesic effect for bone pain
2. Indications: Should be second line after alendronate or risedronate for postmenopausal osteoporosis
   a. Postmenopausal osteoporosis (Bone mineral density 2.5 standard deviations below the mean for normal healthy young adults aged 30–40 years)
   b. Management of bone pain following an osteoporotic fracture
3. Dose: Ensure adequate intake of calcium and vitamin D
   a. Intranasal: 200 U QD to alternate nostrils QOD
   b. Intramuscularly or subcutaneously: 50–100 U QD (consider performing skin test prior to parenteral therapy)
4. Side effects
   a. Intranasal: Nasal irritation/ulceration
   b. IM or SC: Transient vasomotor symptoms (flushing of hands and face), dizziness, GI discomfort including nausea and vomiting (rare with dose of 200 U/day)

CLINICAL PEARLS
- The risk of fracture doubles with every standard deviation of bone mineral density below the mean for normal healthy young adults ages 30–40 years
- With estrogen replacement therapy, the risk of hip and wrist fractures is reduced about 50% and the risk of vertebral fractures is reduced about 75%. This effect is lost if not continued beyond 5 years
- The best protection for osteoporosis is development of largest peak bone mass within individual genetic potential by maintaining adequate body weight, providing adequate calcium intake, and mechanical loading with weight-bearing exercise
- 1000–1500mg elemental calcium is equivalent to four 8 oz glasses of milk per day

References
Ettinger B, et al. Reduction of vertebral fracture risk in postmenopausal women with osteoporosis treated with raloxifene. Results from a 3-year randomized clinical trial. JAMA 1999;282:637–45
Greenspan SL, Greenspan FS, The effect of thyroid hormone on skeletal integrity.Ann Intern Med 1999;130:750–8.

GEN

Cummings SR, et al. Effect of alendronate on risk of fracture in women with low bone density but without vertebral fractures. Results from the Fracture Intervention Trial. JAMA Dec 1998;280:2077–82, and Heaney RP. Bone mass, bone fragility, and the decision to treat [Editorial]. JAMA December 1998;280:2119–20.

Eastell R. Treatment of postmenopausal osteoporosis. N Engl J Med 1998;338:736–46.

Koziol-Ehni LR. Osteoporosis: current perspectives and management. Resident Reporter 1997;2:20–6.

Moussa J, et al. Osteoporosis: prevention and treatment in the primary care setting. Primary Care Reports 1997;3:1–8.

Karpf DB, et al. Prevention of nonvertebral fractures by alendronate. A meta-analysis. JAMA 1997;277:1159–64.

Bellantoni ME. Osteoporosis prevention and treatment. Am Fam Phys 1996;54:986–91.

Ivan Wolfson, MD
Michael B. Weinstock, MD

69. URINARY TRACT INFECTIONS

I. ACUTE UNCOMPLICATED UTI (CYSTITIS)

A. Etiology: *E. coli* 80%, *Staphylococcus saprophyticus* 15%, *Proteus, Klebsiella, Pseudomonas*

B. Signs and symptoms

1. Up to 30% of patients diagnosed with cystitis-like syndrome may have *subclinical upper tract disease*, therefore they need to be questioned for risk factors for complicated UTI
2. Dysuria, urinary frequency, urgency, hesitancy
3. Hematuria
4. Back pain, fever, chills,
5. History of recent UTI, kidney stone, catheterization
6. Recent treatment
7. Abdominal pain, bladder distension, back pain (CVA tenderness)
8. History of congenital abnormality, unilateral kidney, vesicourethral reflux, renal scarring
9. Vaginal discharge, lesions, mass, bleeding
10. Last menstrual period

C. Laboratory

1. Urinalysis: Cost effective and safe because causative organisms and susceptibility profiles are very predictable. Leukocyte esterase is 75–90% sensitive, although it is not very specific as normal vaginal leukocytes may produce a positive result. If negative, check spin urine and examine under a microscope for WBCs, RBCs, and bacteria. Nitrate has a 10–30% false negative rate. Patient has UA suggestive of UTI if:
   a. WBC > 5–8 / high power field
   b. Bacteriuria is present (any amount)
2. Urine culture: Only necessary if there is no pyuria on dip/micro, atypical clinical features, suggestion of a complicated UTI, patient is a child, is immunosuppressed, has recurrent UTIs, or is status post ATB treatment of UTI
3. Follow-up: For uncomplicated UTIs, no follow-up culture or visit is necessary unless symptoms persist or recur

D. Management: For pain relief, may use urinary antiseptic concurrently with antibiotics (See below)

1. Duration of therapy
   a. A **3 day course** is as effective as 7 days with half the number of side effects. Single dose therapy is no longer recommended
   b. A **10 day course** is recommended for an uncomplicated UTI if patient:
      i. Is diabetic
      ii. Is age > 65
      iii. Is febrile
      iv. Is pregnant (7 days)
      v. Has had a UTI within 6 weeks
      vi. Has had symptoms > 5 days

vii. Is a diaphragm user

viii. Is a child

2. Antibiotics

  a. **TMP/SMZ (Septra, Bactrim):** *1st line empiric therapy* (5–15% resistance)

    i. Adults: 1 DS tab PO BID

    ii. Children > 2 months: 8mg/kg/day **TMP** and 40mg/kg/day **SMZ** in 2 divided doses ×
7 days (**SMX** 200mg/ **TMP** 40mg/5cc)

  b. **Trimethoprim (TMP) (Proloprim, Trimpex):** Adults 100mg PO BID

  c. **Fluoroquinolones:** Less than 5% resistance, but more expensive. Indicated for patients
with recurrent, chronic, or complicated UTIs. Not for use if patient is age < 18

    i. **Ciprofloxacin** 250–500mg PO BID

    ii. **Levofloxacin (Levaquin)** 250–500mg PO QD

  d. **Nitrofurantoin (Macrodantin, Macrobid):** Use for 5–7 days (15–20% resistance)—
Pregnancy

    i. Adults: **Macrodantin** 50mg PO QID—*or*—**Macrobid** 100mg PO BID

    ii. Children > 1 month old: 5–7mg/kg/day in 4 divided doses × 7 days

  e. **Amoxicillin:** 500mg PO TID (33% resistance): *pregnancy*

3. Relief of dysuria

  a. **Pyridium:** 200mg PO TID, maximum 3 days therapy when used with antibacterials

  b. **Urised:** 2 tabs PO QID (PC and HS)

II. COMPLICATED UTIs

A. Definition:

1. Patients with functionally, metabolically, or anatomically abnormal urinary tract (stones,
obstruction, DM, sickle cell disease, polycystic kidneys)

2. Patients with UTIs caused by pathogens resistant to ATB

3. Clinically, these diagnoses range from mild cystitis to life threatening urosepsis

B. Laboratory: Obtain urine cultures and sensitivities

C. Treatment: Begin while awaiting culture and sensitivities. Treat for 10–14 days

1. **TMP/SMZ (Septra, Bactrim):** DS 1 PO BID

2. **Ciprofloxacin:** 250–500mg PO BID

3. **Levofloxacin (Levaquin):** 250–500mg PO QD

D. Hospitalization: Severely ill patients should be hospitalized and covered for *Pseudomonas* and
Enterococcus

III. RECURRENT UTIs

A. Incidence: Occur in ~20% of young women

B. Pathophysiology: 90% are due to exogenous reinfection, typically months apart. They are rarely
due to anatomic or functional abnormalities of urinary tract, therefore imaging studies (urog-
raphy, cystography, cystoscopy) are of little use. Inquire about hygiene, diaphragm use, relation to sexual intercourse, wiping pattern (back to front). If diaphragm and spermicide are
used, consider another form of contraception

C. Laboratory: Obtain culture and sensitivity

D. Treatment

1. Relapses

  a. Recurrent infection is usually by original pathogen, usually within 2 weeks

  b. Seek occult source or urogenic abnormality

  c. Treat for 2–6 weeks

2. If patient has 1 or 2 UTIs per year, consider patient-initiated treatment for 3 day course of
ATB. (See Acute Uncomplicated UTI, I)

3. If 3 or greater UTIs per year:

  a. Consider QD or 3 ×/week prophylaxis with **TMP/SMZ** ½ tab DS, **Trimethoprim** 100mg,
or **Nitrofurantoin** 50–100mg. Consider discontinuing after 6 months to see if patient
remains symptom free

  b. If UTIs are related to coitus, try early post-coital voiding and/or post-coital prophylaxis
with single dose of: **TMP/SMZ** 1 tab DS —*or*— **Nitrofurantoin** 50–100mg

IV. ACUTE UNCOMPLICATED PYELONEPHRITIS
  A. History and physical examination: ranges from dysuria symptoms with mild flank pain to gram negative septicemia
  B. Etiology: *E. coli* (80%), *Proteus, Klebsiella, Enterobacter*
  C. Laboratory: Pyuria almost always present; gram negative bacteria, WBC casts may be present. Culture urine on all patients. Blood cultures of hospitalized patients are positive 15–20% of the time
  D. Indications for hospitalization
    1. Nausea/vomiting
    2. Ill appearing/dehydrated
    3. Age > 65
    4. Pregnancy
    5. Immunosupression
  E. Outpatient treatment: Treat for 10–14 days
    1. **Ciprofloxacin:** 250–500mg PO BID
    2. **Levofloxacin (Levoquin):** 250–500mg PO QD
    3. **TMP/SMZ (Septra, Bactrim):** DS 1 PO BID
    4. **Amoxicillin** and first generation cephalosporins are *not recommended* as first line treatment as there is a 20–30% incidence of resistance

V. UTIs IN YOUNGER MEN
  A. Risk factors: Homosexuality, uncircumcised, sexual partner with vaginal colonization by uropathogen, immunosupressed
  B. Incidence: Rare if age < 50
  C. History and physical examination: Patients present with symptoms of cystitis, but may mimic urethritis with urethral discharge. Need to differentiate from prostatitis and STD by obtaining a good sexual history and performing a rectal examination
  D. Laboratory: Obtain urine culture and sensitivity on all patients. If there is urethral discharge, obtain culture before obtaining urine specimen. It was thought formerly that UTIs in men were caused by urologic abnormalities, but recent studies suggest that these UTIs are due to the same strains of *E. coli* that affect women
  E. Management
    1. Treat with 7 day course of antibiotics: **TMP/SMZ** is first line therapy
    2. Adult men who respond to antibiotics with their first UTI do not need further urologic evaluation. Subsequent UTIs do need further work-up
    3. If indicated, further work-up includes renal ultrasound, IVP, and cystourethrogram

VI. UTIs IN CHILDREN
  A. Indications for diagnostic evaluation
    1. Boys: Initial infection with all ages
    2. Girls
      a. < 6 years: 1st infection
      b. > 6 years: 2nd infection
  B. Laboratory: Obtain culture and sensitivity on all patients
  C. Treatment: After diagnosing a UTI, begin antibiotic treatment as outlined in section I. Treat for 7–14 days
  D. Diagnostic evaluation: If indicated, obtain diagnostic evaluation after urine culture turns sterile, even if antibiotic therapy is not completed
    1. Renal ultrasound: To detect dilation of the collecting system (suggesting obstruction) or an anatomic abnormality of the kidney—*and*—
    2. Voiding cystourethrogram (VCUG): To detect vesicoureteral reflux and abnormality in urethral anatomy
    3. If vesicoureteral reflux or dilation of the collecting system is found, a 99mTc-DMSA renal scan is indicated to rule out renal scarring or interstitial pyelonephritis
  E. Management of vesicoureteral reflux
    1. Reflux is usually a medical problem and should be treated with antibiotic prophylaxis (**TMP/SMZ** or **Nitrofurantoin**) to prevent renal scarring

GEN

2. Up to 80% of cases will resolve with growth
3. Indications for anti-reflux surgery
   a. Breakthrough infections
   b. Antibiotic intolerance
   c. Significant preexisting reflux-related renal damage
   d. Reflux unlikely to resolve
   F. If diagnostic evaluation is negative, consider these causes of UTIs:
   1. Encopresis
   2. Infrequent voiding syndrome
   3. Improper voiding hygiene
   4. Bathing with bubble bath
   5. Diarrhea
   6. Cystitis cystica (cystitis with multiple submucosal cysts in the bladder wall)

VII. UTIs ASSOCIATED WITH CATHETERS
A. Prevention: Sterile insertion, prompt removal, and use of a closed collecting system
B. Bacteriuria: If catheter is in > 30 days, most such patients will have bacteriuria
1. Intermittent catheterization has resulted in lower rates of bacteriuria than long-term indwelling catheter
2. Antibiotic prophylaxis reduces bacteriuria in patients undergoing intermittent catheterization
   a. Antibiotic prophylaxis is indicated for patients performing intermittent catheterization with recurrent UTIs. Consider **TMP/SMZ** or **Nitrofurantoin** QD (See III, Recurrent UTIs, infra)
   b. Asymptomatic bacteriuria: No prophylaxis
3. Distinguish between bacteriuria and infection (pain, fever, CVA tenderness, etc.)
C. Treatment
1. Indicated for *symptomatic patients* with culture showing >100,000 CFU: Treat with **TMP/SMZ** or a **Quinolone** for 10–14 days
2. Asymptomatic bacteriuria: No treatment (still being studied)

VIII. ASYMPTOMATIC BACTERIURIA
Screening is of little use except:
A. Prior to urologic surgery
B. Pregnancy (major cause of maternal and fetal morbidity)
1. Symptomatic bacteriuria
   a. 7 day course of **Nitrofurantoin** or **Amoxicillin**
   b. Fluoroquinolones are contraindicated in pregnancy
   c. Re-culture after therapy to ensure success
2. Asymptomatic bacteriuria
   a. 3 day course of **Nitrofurantoin** or **Amoxicillin**
   b. Screen with Q month cultures
3. If more than 1 UTI or asymptomatic bacteriuria: Need prophylaxis for duration of pregnancy

CLINICAL PEARLS
- Dysuria may also be secondary to urethritis infections, irritant, contact, vaginitis, prostatitis, renal stone, hematuria, or concentrated urine
- Children/infants may present with fever and/or irritability instead of urinary symptoms
- Leukocytes and/or leukocyte esterase may be from vaginal leukocytes and not from cystitis

References
Delzell JE, LeFevre ML. Urinary tract infections during pregnancy. Am Fam Phys 2000;61:691–700.
McCarty JM, et al. A randomized trial of short-course ciprofloxacin, ofloxacin, or trimethoprim/ sulfamethoxazole for the treatment of acute urinary tract infection in women. Am J Med Mar 1999;106:292–9.
Ross JH, Kay R. Pediatric urinary tract infection and reflux. Am Fam Phys 1999;59:1472.
Altieri MF. Pediatric urinary tract infections. Emergency Med Rep 1998;19:1–7.
Stamm WE, Hooton TM. Management of urinary tract infections in adults. N Engl J Med 1993; 329:1328–39.
Johnson MA. Urinary tract infections in women. Am Fam Phys 1990;41:565–71.
O'Brien WM. Gibbons, MD. Pediatric urinary tract infections. Am Fam Phys 1988;38:101–12.

GEN

70. HEMATURIA

DEFINITION: The presence of red blood cells (RBCs) in the urine

I. INDICATIONS FOR WORKING-UP HEMATURIA
A. > 3 RBCs/HPF on 2 of 3 clean catch specimens
B. 1 episode of gross hematuria
C. 1 episode of large microhematuria (> 100 RBCs/HPF)

II. HISTORY
A. Genitourinary history
1. Dysuria, nocturia, or increased frequency
2. Vaginal or penile discharge (obtain sexual history)
3. Recent trauma or vigorous exercise
4. Previous urologic surgery
5. Flank pain or prior nephrolithiasis
6. Last menstrual period

B. Painful vs. painless hematuria
1. Etiologies of painful hematuria: UTI, endometriosis, nephrolithiasis, papillary necrosis, obstruction, passage of clots, glomerulonephritis
2. Etiologies of painless hematuria: Bladder tumor, staghorn calculus, polycystic kidneys, hydronephrosis, sickle cell anemia, hypercalciuria, anticoagulation

C. Recent Infections
1. Fever, sore throat, or rash
2. Tooth extraction or other invasive procedures
3. Recent travel (schistosomiasis)

D. Relation of gross hematuria to urinary stream
1. Initial: Distal urethra
2. Terminal: Bladder neck or prostatic urethra
3. Total: Upper tract or bladder proper

E. Clots
1. Large and thick: Bladder
2. Small and stringy: Ureter (upper tract)

F. Family history
1. Renal disease
2. Sickle cell anemia
3. Deafness (Alport's syndrome—familial nephritis)
4. Bleeding disorders (hemophilia, von Willebrand's disease, vitamin K deficiency, liver disease)

G. Medications: Many drugs (including Cyclophosphamide, Warfarin (Coumadin), NSAIDs, and PCN) may cause hematuria

H. Risk factors for urologic cancer: Age > 40, tobacco use, exposure to rubber or aniline dyes, schistosomiasis, pelvic radiation, family history of urologic cancer, or analgesic abuse

III. THE ABCs OF HEMATURIA: A mnemonic to remember the differential diagnosis
A = Anatomic (renal cysts, AV malformation, obstruction with hydronephrosis, BPH)
B = Boulders (nephrolithiasis, hypercalciuria, hyperuricosuria)
C = Cancer (renal cell, bladder, prostate in adults; Wilms' tumor or leukemia in children)
D = Drugs (prescribed and illicit drugs)
E = Exercise (contact and noncontact sports)
F = Foreign body or familial (indwelling catheter, trauma, Alport's syndrome)
G = Glomerulonephritis (post-strep, Goodpasture's, SLE, Berger's, Henoch-Schönlein purpura)
H = Hematology (hemoglobinopathies, coagulopathies)
I = Infection (bacterial, viral or fungal)

IV. PHYSICAL EXAMINATION

A. **Vital signs:** Temperature and blood pressure
B. **Oropharynx:** Tonsillar enlargement
C. **CV:** Murmur
D. **Abdomen:** Masses, hepatomegaly, or suprapubic tenderness
E. **Back:** CVA tenderness
F. **Extremities:** Supraclavicular, axillary, or inguinal adenopathy
G. **Skin:** Rash or ecchymoses
H. **Rectal:** Masses and prostate size; Guaiac stool

V. EVALUATING HEMATURIA

Directed by results of the history and physical examination
A. **Asymptomatic microscopic hematuria**
   1. Obtain UA and screening chemistries (See below)
   2. If negative UA and screening chemistries, repeat UA in 3 months
   3. If microscopic hematuria persists, then obtain radiologic study (IVP or U/S, with or without tomograms) and consider urologic consult
B. **Asymptomatic gross hematuria**
   1. Obtain UA and screening chemistries (See below)
   2. Obtain radiologic study (IVP or U/S) and obtain urologic consult for cystoscopy
C. **Laboratory**
   1. Urinalysis (consider gram stain and/or C&S)
      a. Pyuria, WBC casts (infection)
      b. Proteinuria, RBC casts (glomerular disease)
   2. Screening chemistries, as clinically indicated
      a. BUN, creatinine, electrolytes, calcium, uric acid
      b. CBC, platelets, PT/PTT
      c. PSA
   3. If evidence of glomerular disease (i.e., presence of proteinuria or RBC casts):
      a. Serum ANA, Anti-GBM (glomerular basement membrane—Wegener's disease), C3, C4, ASO titers (post-strep), ESR, and serum protein electrophoresis
      b. 24hr urine for protein and CrCl
D. **Radiology**
   1. Intravenous pyelography (IVP)
      a. Useful in defining the anatomy of the urinary tract and evaluation of obstruction
      b. Increase sensitivity by adding renal CT scan (will detect smaller lesions or those not encroaching the collecting system)
      c. Consider ultrasound if contrast nephropathy is a concern
   2. Spiral CT
   3. Renal ultrasound
      a. Studies suggest diagnostic yield is similar to IVP without the risk of contrast nephropathy
      b. Defines masses as either cystic or solid
E. **Endoscopy—Cystoscopy**
   1. Useful in evaluating the lower urinary tract (sensitivity 87% for bladder CA)
   2. Patients who have a negative IVP and/or CT with persistent microscopic hematuria probably will not benefit from cystoscopy
   3. Patients who have a negative IVP and/or CT with persistent gross hematuria should undergo cystoscopy
F. **Pathologic**
   1. Urinary cytology
      a. Useful in detecting transitional cell cancer of the bladder
      b. With in situ bladder lesions, cytology is often positive before visualization via cystoscopy
      c. False positives can occur with nephrolithiasis or UTIs
   2. Renal biopsy
      a. Indications are unclear
      b. May not affect prognosis or treatment unless hematuria is accompanied by HTN, proteinuria, or decreased CrCl

GEN

VI. FOLLOW-UP EXAMINATIONS

Patients with a negative initial work-up will need close follow-up

A. **Urologic cancer** has been found on follow-up exam in 1–3% of patients with microscopic hematuria and 18% of patients with recurrent gross hematuria

B. **The following should be considered** as long as hematuria persists:
1. Every 6 months: Urinalysis and cytology
2. Every year: IVP and cystoscopy

CLINICAL PEARLS

• *Serratia marcescens* may cause a "red diaper" in healthy infants. Performing a UA proves the absence of hemoglobin in the urine

• Consider factitious hematuria (narcotic seekers complaining of kidney stones or Münchausen's disease) in patients with persistent undiagnosed hematuria

• A positive urine dipstick but negative microscopic exam may be caused by hemoglobinuria/ myoglobinuria (porphyria, rhabdomyolysis) or certain foods (beets, rhubarb, fava beans, or food colorings)

• Coumadin and Pyridium may cause a red-orange discoloration of alkaline urine

References

Thaller TR, Wang LP. Evaluation of asymptomatic microscopic hematuria in adults. Am Fam Phys 1999;60:1143–54.

Neiberger RE. The ABCs of evaluating children with hematuria. Am Fam Phys 1994;49:623–8.

Bartlow BG. Microhematuria: picking the fewest tests to make an accurate diagnosis. Postgrad Med 1990;88(4):51–61.

Schroeder PL, Francisco LL. Evaluating hematuria in children: where to start and how to proceed. Postgrad Med 1990; 88(8):1716.

Sutton JM. Evaluation of hematuria in adults. JAMA 1990; 263(18):2475–9.

Beth Weinstock, MD

71. PROTEINURIA

I. DEFINITION

A. **Normal excretion of protein in urine**
1. Less than or equal to 150mg/day
2. Total protein excretion comprised of 5–15mg albumin, >30 different plasma proteins, and glycoproteins from renal cells, i.e., Tamm-Horsfall protein (most prevalent, excreted at 50–75mg/day)

B. **"Pathologic" proteinuria:** Greater than or equal to 150mg/day. Massive proteinuria is defined as >3.5gm/day. This leads to large albumin loss and other manifestations of nephrotic syndrome (edema, hypoalbuminemia, hyperlipidemia)

II. DETECTION

A. **Urine dipstick** (only picks up albumin)
1. Registers a "trace" result with as little as 10mg/deciliter protein
2. 1+ protein = 30mg/deciliter
3. False positive result: May be due to highly concentrated urine, gross hematuria, pH> 8.0, alkaline urine (i.e., UTI, HCO_3 supplementation)
4. False negative: Diluted urine. Early morning specimen is most accurate because of concentration

B. **Sulfasalicylic Acid Test:** Will pick up all proteins, including Bence-Jones protein. May be useful if suspicious of multiple myeloma due to patient's symptoms, and the urine dip is negative

C. **24-hour urine collection:** Should be ordered if urine dip measures 1+ or greater proteinuria (depending on patient's age)
1. Instructions for patient on collection of 24hr urine:
   a. Empty bladder on awakening in AM, discarding initial specimen and noting the time

  b. Put all subsequent voided specimens in collection bottle for next 24hrs, including the last void

2. Results
   a. Total volume/24hrs
   b. Total protein/24hrs: >150mg/24hr meets criteria for "proteinuria"
   c. Urine creatinine
   d. Creatinine clearance (Cr Cl) = $\dfrac{\text{Urine Cr} \times \text{Urine volume}}{\text{Plasma Cr}}$
   e. Reliability of the 24hr collection can be approximated by measurement of the total 24hr creatinine excretion in the specimen. The total daily creatinine excretion should be in the range of 15–20mg/kg lean body weight per day in women, 20–25mg/kg lean body weight per day in men. If the calculated Cr Cl from specimen is way outside of this range (< 700 or > 1400mg/24hrs), then specimen was probably not collected correctly
   f. Cr Cl declines by 1mL/min/year over the age of 40

3. Differential diagnosis of 24hr urine results:
   a. If > 2g/24hrs
      i. Nephrotic syndrome (see below)
      ii. Glomerular (diffuse disease)
         aa. Primary (usually diagnosed definitively by kidney biopsy)
            1. Minimal change disease
            2. Focal segmental glomerulosclerosis
            3. Membranoproliferative GN
         bb. Secondary
            1. Diabetes mellitus
            2. Malignancy
            3. Morbid obesity
            4. HIV
            5. SLE
            6. Amyloidosis
            7. Pre-eclampsia
            8. Drug toxicities
   b. If < 2g/24hrs
      i. Transient
         aa. Fever
         bb. Stress
         cc. Exercise
      ii. Tubular (see Mechanism of protein loss, III, infra)
         aa. Multiple myeloma
         bb. Rhabdomyolysis
      iii. Orthostatic (see below)
      iv. Focal Glomerulonephritis
      v. Long-standing HTN or DM
      vi. Polycystic kidney disease (check family history)

III. MECHANISM OF PROTEIN LOSS

A. Tubular: Low-molecular weight proteins (β_2 microglobulin, lysozyme, light chains, insulin) are usually filtered by glomeruli and reabsorbed by tubules. If tubules are damaged, these proteins are excreted, usually in the range of 1–3g/24hrs. (Edema and lipid disorders usually do not occur in this range.) High serum protein levels can also "overwhelm" tubules and overflow into urine—i.e., Bence-Jones protein associated with multiple myeloma, myoglobin. Urine electrophoresis will show migration in α and β regions, with little or no migration in albumin region

B. Glomerular: Normal glomeruli filter little albumin or globulin (due to albumin's anionic quality which causes it to be repelled by anionic glycoprotein matrix structure of basement membrane). Glomerular disease disrupts this barrier; excretion of mostly albumin on urine electrophoresis signifies a glomerular lesion

IV. APPROACH TO EVALUATION AND MANAGEMENT

A. If Dipstick >1(+) proteinuria, then collect 24hr urine

GEN

B. If proteinuria >2g/24hr urine collection:
1. History: Pre-existing disease, HIV risk factors, systemic complaints (fatigue, polydipsia, polyuria, back pain, joint pain, weight loss, rash), family history (diabetes)
2. Physical exam: Blood pressure, weight, funduscopic exam, edema, breast exam (to screen for malignancy as etiology of membranous glomerulonephropathy), skin and joint exam (vasculitis/rheumatologic disease), ophthalmologic exam for diabetic retinopathy
3. Labs
    a. Microscopic exam of urine sediment (casts, crystals):
        i. Casts: Formed when proteins gel inside renal tubules, trapping WBCs and RBCs
            aa. Hyaline casts: Found with concentrated urine, fever, diuretic use
            bb. RBC casts: Glomerulonephritis
            cc. WBC casts: Pyelonephritis, interstitial nephritis
            dd. Renal tubular casts: ATN, interstitial nephritis
            ee. Coarse granular casts: Degeneration of cast with cellular elements, non-specific
            ff. Broad waxy casts: Chronic renal failure. Stasis in collecting tubule
        ii. Crystals: Should be visualized when urine is freshly voided and still warm. Uric acid, phosphate, and oxalate crystals are seen in normal patients as well as stone formers
    b. BUN and creatinine, CBC
    c. Serum protein immunoelectrophoresis (SPE) to identify any paraproteins in the serum which could be overwhelming the tubules. Obtain urine protein electrophoresis simultaneously to quantify the amount of each protein type in the urine (important to consider in patient age > 40)
    d. ANA, Hepatitis B, Hepatitis C, cryoglobulins, complement levels (C3 and C4) to screen for vasculitis as etiology of glomerular damage (depending on patient's associated symptoms)
    e. HIV test (with suspicion)
    f. Blood glucose, Hemoglobin A1C
    g. Blood cultures: Screen for subacute bacterial endocarditis (can cause only proteinuria and/or hematuria)

C. If < 2g/24hrs
1. History: Recent fever, increase in exercise, other systemic complaints (back pain or other bone pain, fatigue) to screen for multiple myeloma
2. Physical: Same as above
3. Labs: Same as above
4. Transient proteinuria
    a. Associated with fever, stress, exercise (within last 48hrs)
    b. Recheck after confounding factors have resolved
    c. If < 150mg/24hrs, then no work-up
    d. If > 150mg/24hrs, then check yearly BP, UA, and Cr
5. Orthostatic proteinuria: Usually a benign process
    a. < 1g/24 hrs; if greater, should consider other etiologies
    b. More common in children and adolescents
    c. Can obtain urine dipstick on first void in AM, then check again after patient has been upright for 2hrs
    d. Should follow yearly BP, UA, and creatinine, especially in children

D. Nephrotic Syndrome
1. Common end point due to a variety of disease processes: DM, amyloidosis, SLE, idiopathic renal disease such as focal glomerular sclerosis, membranous nephropathy, nil disease, etc. Arises due to an alteration in the permeability of the glomerular capillary wall
2. Definition: Proteinuria >3.5g/24hrs, hypoalbuminemia (serum albumin < 3.0g/dL), edema, and hyperlipidemia (fasting level >200)
3. Common to all diseases causing nephrotic syndrome is the presence of oval fat bodies seen on microscopic exam of urine; caused by degenerating tubular epithelial cells filled with cholesterol esters. Under polarized light will see Maltese Cross
4. Loss of antithrombin III and other proteins can lead to a hypercoaguable state, particularly venous involvement (DVT, PE, renal vein thrombosis)

V. SPECIFIC DISEASES

A. Diabetes Mellitus

1. Most common cause of end-stage renal disease in US. Higher incidence of renal complications in Hispanics, blacks, and Native Americans
2. 20–30% risk of developing diabetic nephropathy
3. Early renal changes of increased GFR, increased renal blood flow, and renal hypertrophy can be reversed with good glycemic control. Sustained hyperglycemia and HgbA1C >9 correlates with hyperfiltration and hypertrophy
4. Recommendation: *Yearly urine microalbuminuria screening.* Allows for detection of small amounts of albumin which are not detected on routine urine dipstick test. Persistent or increasing microalbuminuria indicates early diabetic nephropathy
5. 24hr urine should be obtained if urine microalbumin screen is positive
6. ACE inhibitor should be initiated in both hypertensive and normotensive diabetic patients with urine microalbuminuria. Blood pressure should be aggressively reduced to <135/85. Check creatinine and potassium one week after initiating ACE inhibitor
7. Blood glucose should also be aggressively controlled to delay progression to persistent proteinuria
8. Microalbuminuria is highly predictive for subsequent retinopathy development

B. Hypertension

1. Hypertensive patients constitute 20% of the dialysis population. The 2 groups at highest risk for hypertensive ESRD are blacks of all ages and the elderly
2. A complete urinalysis should be performed yearly on all hypertensive patients. If positive for protein, a 24hr urine should be obtained. Other causes of proteinuria should also be considered. In addition to aggressive blood pressure management, patient should follow a no-added salt restriction
3. Medications: Diuretics and ACE inhibitors are most beneficial for patients with renal damage secondary to hypertension
4. Should consider renal artery stenosis as a possible diagnosis in elderly hypertensives with unexplained deterioration of renal function

CLINICAL PEARLS

- In patients with proteinuria and altered renal function, try to avoid NSAIDs
- Smoking cessation has been shown to decrease albumin excretion
- When to refer to a nephrologist: Proteinuria greater than 1g/24hrs, unless the etiology is known (i.e., diabetes mellitus) and already being aggressively treated

References

Orth SR, Ritz E. The nephrotic syndrome. N Engl J Med 1998;338:1202–11.

Giatris I, et al. ACE inhibitors and nondiabetic renal disease. Ann Intern Med 1997;127:337–45.

Bennett PH, et al. Screening and management of microalbuminuria in patients with diabetes mellitus: Recommendations to the Scientific Advisory Board of the National Kidney Foundation from an Ad Hoc Committee of the Council on Diabetes Mellitus of the National Kidney Foundation. Am J Kidney Dis 1995;25:107–12.

GEN

Daniel M. Neides, MD
Kathy Provanzana, MD

72. BENIGN PROSTATIC HYPERTROPHY

DEFINITION: Nodular enlargement of the prostate occurring in the periurethral region of the gland generally among men over age 50

I. DIAGNOSIS

A. Symptoms of prostatism: Frequency of urination, nocturia, urgency, straining to void, weak stream, hesitancy, and a sensation of incomplete voiding

B. The American Urologic Association Symptom Index: Patient Self-Screening Form, quantifies the severity of symptoms. (See table on following page)

II. INITIAL EVALUATION

A. Medical history: Medical problems, previous surgery, and history of any urinary tract problems

B. Physical examination

　1. Includes a digital rectal examination (DRE) to document size of the prostate as well as any palpable abnormalities

　2. Focused neurologic exam

　3. Exclude other etiologies: UTI, neurogenic bladder, urethral stricture, and prostate cancer

C. Urinalysis: Dipstick urine to rule out hematuria or UTI

D. Laboratory: Consider serum creatinine to assess renal function

E. Prostate specific antigen (PSA): This is *optional* in the initial evaluation

　1. Will increase detection rate of cancer over DRE alone and tends to detect cancer at an earlier stage

　2. Age specific PSA: New guidelines using age in determining a normal range:

Age (years)	Normal PSA range
40–49	0–2.5 ng/ml
50–59	0–3.5 ng/ml
60–69	0–4.5 ng/ml
70–79	0–6.5 ng/ml

　　a. If the PSA is increased by age (See table above) or if the PSA has increased by ≥ 0.8 from the previous year, treat the patient for 4 weeks with **TMP/SMX** (**Bactrim, Septra**) **DS** 1 PO BID *or* **Doxycycline** 100mg PO BID

　　b. Repeat the PSA test 1 week after the course of antibiotics is finished

　　　i. If normal, continue routine checks

　　　ii. If still elevated, consider referring patient to a urologist for transrectal ultrasound (TRUS) and biopsy

III. ADDITIONAL TESTING TO AID IN DIAGNOSIS

A. If the diagnosis is uncertain after the initial work-up, consider further testing: uroflowmetry, postvoid residuals, pressure-flow studies, urethrocystoscopy, ultrasonography, cystometography, or urethrocystoscopy

B. *Results from these tests do not define BPH and their use is not mandatory prior to treatment*

IV. TREATMENT OPTIONS

A. No treatment: Will be an appropriate strategy for many patients. Periodic reassessment of symptoms, physical examination, laboratory work, and optional diagnostic procedures should be performed

B. Behavioral modification

　1. No fluids after 7 PM

　2. Decrease caffeine and alcohol intake. No caffeine after noon

PATIENT SELF-SCREENING FORM

Name: _____ Date of Birth: _____ Today's Date: _____

A. For each of the seven questions below, please check the one box that best describes your symptoms. (Note: Numbers within boxes are for health care provider's use only.)

Over the past month...	Not at All	Less Than 1 Time in 5	Less Than Half the Time	About Half the Time	More Than Half the Time	Almost Always
1. How often have you had a sensation of not emptying your bladder completely after you finished urinating?	0	1	2	3	4	5
2. How often have you had to urinate again less than 2 hours after you finished urinating?	0	1	2	3	4	5
3. How often have you found you stopped and started again several times when you urinated?	0	1	2	3	4	5
4. How often have you found it difficult to postpone urination?	0	1	2	3	4	5
5. How often have you had a weak urinary stream?	0	1	2	3	4	5
6. How often have you had to push or strain to begin urination?	0	1	2	3	4	5
7. How many times did you most typically get up to urinate from the time you went to bed at night until the time you got up in the morning?	0 (None)	1 (1 time)	2 (2 times)	3 (3 times)	4 (4 times)	5 (5 or more times)

Instructions to Health Care Provider: To calculate the patient's total AUA Symptom Score, add up the numbers for all boxes checked in questions 1 through 7.
AUA Symptom Score: _____ Degree of Severity: ❏ Mild ❏ Moderate ❏ Severe
(0-7)   (8-19)   (20-35)

Original source for information: Barry MJ, Fowler FJ Jr, O'Leary MP, et al. The American Urological Association symptom index for benign prostatic hyperplasia. J Urol. 1992;148:1549-1557. Used with permission.

B. Please answer the following question by checking the appropriate box.

Quality of Life due to Urinary Symptoms	Delighted	Pleased	Mostly Satisfied	Equally Satisfied and Dissatisfied	Mostly Dissatisfied	Unhappy	Terrible
If you had to spend the rest of your life with your urinary condition just the way it is now, how would you feel about that?	0	1	2	3	4	5	6

C. Medications

1. α-adrenergic antagonists: **Doxazosin (Cardura), Terazosin (Hytrin)** or **Prazosin (Minipress)**
   a. Start with 1mg QHS for 7 days. If well tolerated, increase to 2mg QHS
   b. Have patient follow-up in 1 month. If 2mg was well tolerated, then increase to 4mg QHS for Doxazosin and 5mg for Terazosin
   c. **Doxazosin** can be increased up to 8mg QHS; Terazosin up to 10mg QHS
   d. Start with Doxazosin because it is less expensive than Terazosin
   e. Should increase peak urinary flow while decreasing obstructive and irritative symptoms
   f. Will lower BP in hypertensive patients but should *not* alter BP in normotensive patients
   g. Check orthostatic pressures before starting for elderly patients
   h. Side effects: Orthostatic hypotension, dizziness, fatigue, and headache
2. **Finasteride (Proscar):** *Second line therapy.* Acts as a 5-α-reductase inhibitor (blocks conversion of testosterone to dihydrotestosterone)
   a. Dose is 5mg PO QD
   b. This should increase flow rate while decreasing prostate size
   c. Patients usually do *not* receive immediate benefit; it needs to be continued for at least 6 months
   d. PSA should be reduced by 50% if taking Proscar for 1 year. If at 1 year the PSA is not reduced, further work-up (i.e., for cancer) is indicated
   e. Finasteride may only be effective in men with very large prostates
   f. Side effects: Impotence (3.7%), decreased libido (3.3%), decreased volume of ejaculate (2.8%)

D. Surgery: Offers the best opportunity for symptom improvement, but has the highest rate of complications, including erectile dysfunction and incontinence. Does not need to be a "last resort"—some patients may prefer surgery to other treatment options

1. Transurethral resection of the prostate (TURP): The most commonly used surgical treatment for BPH
2. Transurethral incision of the prostate (TUIP): Limited to patients whose estimated resected prostate tissue weighs < 30g; has the lowest morbidity and ejaculatory disturbance rate; can be performed in ambulatory settings or during a 1-day hospitalization
3. Open prostatectomy: Performed on patients with very large prostates

E. Balloon dilation: Less effective than surgery but is associated with fewer complications. Improvement seems to be temporary; recurrence of symptoms may be seen within 2 years

CLINICAL PEARLS

- Utilize the symptom assessment to quantitate and follow prostatism
- For mild symptoms, reassurance and reassessment are appropriate management
- Educate each patient about treatment options, reviewing risks and benefits of each

References

McConnell JD, et al. The effect of finasteride on the risk of acute urinary retention and the need for surgical treatment among men with benign prostatic hyperplasia. N Engl J Med 1998;338:557–63.

Hicks RJ, Cook JB. Managing patients with benign prostatic hyperplasia. Am Fam Phys 1995;52:135–42.

BPH guideline panel. Benign prostatic hyperplasia: diagnosis and treatment. Am Fam Phys 1994;49:1157–65.

Monda JM, Oesterling JE. Medical treatment of BPH: 5 alpha reductase inhibitors and alpha adrenergic antagonists. Mayo Clin Proc 1993;68:670–9.

Carter HB, et al. Longitudinal evaluation of prostate-specific antigen levels in men with and without prostate disease. JAMA 1992;267:2215–20.

Barry MJ, Fowler FJ Jr, O'Leary MP, et al. The American Urologic Association symptom index for benign prostatic hyperplasia. J Urol 1992;148:1549–57.

Lepor H, et al. A randomized, placebo-controlled multicenter study of the efficacy and safety of terazosin in the treatment of benign prostatic hypertrophy. J Urol 1992;148:1467–74.

Gormley GJ, et al. The effect of finasteride in men with benign prostatic hyperplasia. N Engl J Med 1992;327:1185–91.

Linda Stone, MD
Michael B. Weinstock, MD
Daniel M. Neides, MD

73. CONSTIPATION IN ADULTS

I. HISTORY AND PHYSICAL EXAMINATION
A. History
1. Decreased number of stools, which are hard and infrequent
2. Ask about rectal bleeding, weight loss, and abdominal bloating or cramping
3. Past medical history
   a. Previous patterns of bowel activity
   b. Current medications
   c. History of malignancy
   d. History of radiation therapy
   e. Previous surgeries
B. Physical examination
1. **Abdomen:** Note any surgical scars. Palpate for masses (stool) and hepatosplenomegaly. Check for hernia. Examination results are often normal
2. **Rectal:** Determine presence of stool (and guaiac) and palpate for rectal mass

II. ETIOLOGY
A. **Pain on defecation:** External hemorrhoids; anal fissure or stricture
B. **Medications:** Narcotic analgesics, antihypertensives (Ca^{+2} channel blockers), tricyclic antidepressants, phenothiazines, aluminum hydroxide (antacids), iron supplements
C. **Neurologic dysfunction:** Diabetes mellitus, Hirschsprung's disease, multiple sclerosis
D. **Metabolic and endocrine:** Hypothyroidism, hypercalcemia, hypokalemia
E. **Mechanical difficulties:** Colorectal cancer, hernia, diverticulitis, irritable bowel syndrome (IBS), adhesions, stricture, torsion, volvulus

III. EVALUATION
Direct evaluation based on findings in history and physical examination
A. **Fecal occult blood test:** Perform during examination and send 3–4 home for patient to check and return
B. **Blood chemistry:** Electrolytes, Ca^{+2}, or thyroid function tests
C. **Radiologic/endoscopic:** If colon cancer is suspected
   1. Flexible sigmoidoscopy *and* air contrast barium enema—*or*—
   2. Colonoscopy

IV. MANAGEMENT
If history, physical, and evaluation are all negative:
A. Lifestyle
1. Exercise (walking, jogging, swimming, etc.) for 30 minutes 3–4 ×/week
2. Increase fluids intake: 6–8 glasses (8 oz) of water or fruit juice per day
3. Increase bulk (fiber) in diet: fruits, vegetables, cereals, etc.
B. Medications
1. **Metamucil (Psyllium):** 1 Tbl in 8oz water or 1 wafer QD–TID
2. **Colace (Docusate Sodium):** 100mg PO QD–BID (stool softener)
3. **Pericolace (Docusate Sodium** and **Casanthrol):** 1–2 caps PO QHS (stool softener and laxative). Also available in liquid: 15–30mL PO QHS
4. **Dulcolax (Bisacodyl):** 1 tab QD–TID or 1 rectal suppository QD–BID
   Note: rectal suppository is safer to use if bowel obstruction is suspected
5. **Perdiem (Senna-fiber):** 1 tsp PO QD (may increase to 2 tsp PO QID)
6. Enema: Fleets or mineral oil

GEN

CLINICAL PEARLS

- New onset of constipation is a warning sign for cancer. Screen for colon cancer with selected patients
- Consider irritable bowel syndrome (IBS) as the cause of constipation
- Educate patient on diet and exercise

Reference

Rogers AI. Constipation in gastrointestinal symptoms: clinical interpretation. In: Berk JE, Haubrich WS, eds. Bockus gastroenterology. Philadelphia: BC Decker, 1991.

Michael B. Weinstock, MD
Linda Stone, MD

74. HEMORRHOIDS

I. DEFINITION

A. Hemorrhoids (piles) are varicosities of the rectal venous plexus. They can occur internally (above the pectinate line) or externally (below the pectinate line)

B. Internal hemorrhoids are covered by viscerally innervated mucosa. Uncomplicated internal hemorrhoids are not painful. Internal hemorrhoids are referred to as complicated when the patient presents with painless bleeding, prolapse or thrombosis. Internal hemorrhoids may occasionally become strangulated (massive prolapse and thrombosis, necrosis and ulceration) and the patient presents with severe pain and inability to sit down or defecate

C. External hemorrhoids are covered by somatic innervated mucosa. They may be painful or painless. Complications include acute thrombosis or rupture with hematoma formation

II. CLASSIFICATION OF INTERNAL HEMORRHOIDS

A. First degree: Do not protrude, cannot be palpated by digital rectal exam (DRE), require anoscopy for diagnosis

B. Second degree: Protrude, reduce spontaneously

C. Third degree: Protrude, require manual reduction

D. Fourth degree: Prolapsed, irreducible

III. HISTORY AND PHYSICAL EXAMINATION

A. History

1. Common complaints: Rectal itching, straining with stool, a lump at the rectum, history of constipation
2. Rectal bleeding: Consider evaluation with flexible sigmoidoscopy and air contrast barium enema or colonoscopy to exclude colon cancer, neoplastic polyps and inflammatory bowel disease (IBD)
3. Pain: Signals an evaluation for fissure, thrombosis, ulceration or infection. Consider performing anoscopy

B. Physical examination

1. Inspect the rectum for external hemorrhoids or prolapsed internal hemorrhoids with the patient at rest and while straining. Hemorrhoids are usually painless, red or purplish, and protruding from the anus. Examine for fissures, dermatitis, fungal infection and herpes
2. Digital rectal examination (DRE): Detects only thrombosed internal hemorrhoids
3. Anoscopy
   a. Gently insert a lubricated anoscope
   b. Ask the patient to "bear down" (not too forcefully)
   c. Slowly withdraw the anoscope
   d. Watch for internal hemorrhoids to bulge into the anorectal lumen

IV. MANAGEMENT

A. Initial management: For first to third degree hemorrhoids. If these conservative measures are unsuccessful, then consider definitive management

1. Lifestyle changes to avoid constipation (See Chapter 73, Constipation in Adults)
   a. Defecation: Patients should not suppress the urge to defecate or strain while defecating

b. Modify diet to increase intake of fiber, fluids, and fruit juices. Decrease fats and meats

c. Increase exercise

2. Sitz bath: Sitting in a warm or cool tub for 20 minutes BID–TID in the acute phase

3. **Anusol-HC** cream or suppositories (**Hydrocortisone Acetate**) 1 PR BID × 2 weeks. For severe cases, may increase to TID

B. **Definitive management:** Patients with acute thrombosis and prolapse of internal hemorrhoids may require hospitalization and treatment with bed rest, analgesics, stool softeners and often hemorrhoidectomy. Definitive therapy is indicated for fourth degree hemorrhoids and first to third degree hemorrhoids which are not amenable to the above measures

1. **Sclerotherapy:** For first degree and small second degree bleeding *internal* hemorrhoids. A sclerosing agent (e.g., quinine urea hydrochloride or phenol) is injected into the superior aspect of the hemorrhoid *above the pectinate line*. Injection may need to be repeated in several months

2. **Ligation:** Best suited for third and fourth degrees *internal* hemorrhoids. Should *not* be used for external hemorrhoids or internal hemorrhoids complicated by abscess, thrombosis, cryptitis or anal fissure. Cure rates about 80–90%. The hemorrhoid is strangulated by placing a rubber band at the base. Complications include pain (6%), bleeding (3%), and perianal hematoma (3%). May require 2–3 separate ligations. Fatal septicemia has been reported after ligation and may present with the triad of perianal pain, fever and urinary hesitancy

3. **Incision and evacuation:** Indicated for large painful thrombosed *external* hemorrhoids. (Small thrombosed external hemorrhoids may respond to conservative management.) Patient is placed in the fetal position, anesthetized (local), and the hemorrhoid is removed with an elliptical incision and removal of the hemorrhoidal mass en bloc or with a single radial incision over the hemorrhoid and with expression of the clot. Neither technique requires sutures

CLINICAL PEARLS

• About ½ of Americans over 50 will seek medical advice for hemorrhoids

• The most common cause of painless rectal bleeding is internal hemorrhoids. It is important to exclude rectal cancer, colon cancer, neoplastic polyps and inflammatory bowel disease (IBD) with flexible sigmoidoscopy and air contrast barium enema or colonoscopy. Cancer and hemorrhoids may exist concurrently

• Hemorrhoids are unusual in children and should be viewed with an eye toward other disease

• Rectal pruritus may be the initial complaint with hemorrhoids, but consider other causes such as fissures, dermatitis (contact or seborrheic), psoriasis, pinworm, *Candida*, herpes, neurodermatitis, and squamous cell cancer. Examine the rectum!

References

Pfenninger JL, Surrell J. Nonsurgical treatment options for internal hemorrhoids. Am Fam Phys 1995;52:821.

Leibach JR, Cerda JJ. Hemorrhoids: modern treatment and methods. Hosp Med 1991;27(8):53–8.

Ann Aring, MD
Beth Weinstock, MD

75. CALCIUM DISORDERS

— PART ONE: HYPERCALCEMIA —

I. DEFINITION: Total calcium > 10.5mg/dL or ionized calcium > 5.3mg/dL. False positives may be caused by hemoconcentration during blood collection or elevation in serum proteins, particularly albumin

II. ETIOLOGY: Most common etiologies are malignancy and hyperparathyroidism (~90%)

    A. Malignancy: Breast, lung, renal, pancreas, ovarian, myeloma, lymphosarcoma, Burkitt's lymphoma, adult T-cell lymphoma. Caused mostly by secretion of PTH-like substances and increased bone resorption

    B. Hyperparathyroidism: (Most common etiology in ambulatory care centers; 25% of all hypercalcemia)—parathyroid adenoma (80%), parathyroid hyperplasia

    C. Sarcoidosis: (occurs secondary to increased absorption of calcium) and other granulomatous diseases

    D. Paget's disease

    E. Immobilization (due to suppression of the parathyroid-vitamin axis)

    F. Vitamin D intoxication (due to increased absorption of calcium) and milk-alkali syndrome

    G. Medications: Thiazide diuretics (increased renal reabsorption of calcium) and Lithium

    H. Other causes: Addison's disease, renal failure, familial hypocalciuric hypercalcemia, hyperthyroidism, vitamin A intoxication, disseminated SLE, pheochromocytoma, prolonged immobilization

    I. Multiple endocrine neoplasias (MEN) syndromes

        1. MEN I: Parathyroid, pituitary and pancreatic islet cell adenoma

        2. MEN IIA: Hyperparathyroid, pheochromocytoma, medullary cell CA of the thyroid

III. HISTORY AND PHYSICAL EXAM: Most patients are asymptomatic at the time of the diagnosis. Symptoms vary with degree of hypercalcemia and rapidity of development, but are usually evident when serum calcium > 12mg/dL

    A. General: Weakness, fatigue, pruritis, hypertension, myopathy, weight loss, night sweats (malignancy)

    B. Duration of symptoms (primary hyperparathyroidism is usually etiology of symptoms present greater than 6 months without obvious cause)

    C. Diet: Intake of milk and antacids (milk-alkali syndrome), Thiazides, vitamin A or D, Lithium

    D. Evidence of neoplasm: (breast, ovarian) or ectopic soft tissue calcification

    E. CNS: Confusion, depression, psychosis, stupor, coma, headache, hyporeflexia, hypotonia, apathy, mental retardation (infants)

    F. GI: Constipation, nausea, vomiting, anorexia, abdominal pain (pancreatitis, PUD)

    G. GU: Nephrolithiasis, nocturia, polyuria, urinary frequency

    H. Musculoskeletal: Bone pain (metastatic disease, multiple myeloma), deformities, fractures, myopathy, pseudogout, muscle atrophy, bone pain with palpation, proximal muscle weakness

    I. Eye: Band keratopathy (found in the medial and lateral margin of the cornea)

    J. Family history: MEN syndromes, familial hypocalciuric hypercalcemia

IV. LABORATORY DATA AND OTHER TESTS

    A. Lab

        1. Initial lab tests

            a. CBC, electrolytes, BUN, creatinine (renal insufficiency)

            b. Serum calcium, albumin, phosphate, magnesium, alkaline phosphatase

            c. 24hr urine calcium

            d. PTH level: Distinguishes primary hyperparathyroidism from hypercalcemia caused by malignancy when serum calcium is > 12mg/dL. Below this value there is considerable overlap and differentiation may be difficult. If PTH is low or undetectable, screen carefully for malignancy

GEN

2. With history of excessive ingestion of fat soluble vitamins (vitamin D), obtain 1, 25-dihydroxyvitamin D

B. ECG: Shortening of QT interval, wide T waves, Digoxin sensitivity

C. Bone survey: May show subperiosteal bone resorption (PTH excess)

D. Bone scan: May show lytic lesions

V. MANAGEMENT: Differs between acute symptomatic hypercalcemia and chronic hypercalcemia

A. **Acute hypercalcemia:** Symptomatic patient or serum calcium > 13mg/dL. Patients need to be admitted for close observation

1. Hydration with normal saline

2. **Bisphosphonates**: Inhibit osteoclast activity. In-hospital management:

   a. **Pamidronate**: Inhibits bone resorption. Drug of choice for acute management of hypercalcemia

   b. **Etidronate Disodium (Didronel):** Inhibits bone resorption by osteoclasts

   c. **Calcitonin:** Inhibits bone resorption and increases calcium excretion. Only indicated after saline and Furosemide are not effective. Very useful in hypercalcemia associated with hyperphosphatemia. Safe to use in renal failure

   d. **Plicamycin (Mithracin):** Inhibits bone resorption. Restricted to emergency treatment of malignant hypercalcemia. Avoid using in patients with myelocytic chemotherapy, renal or hepatic failure, or bleeding disorders

   e. Hemodialysis: Temporarily lowers serum calcium if a calcium free dialysate is used. Use in patients with oliguric renal failure that cannot be treated with normal saline

B. **Chronic hypercalcemia**

1. High fluid intake: Unless contraindicated, patients should consume 3–5 L/day of fluids to increase renal calcium excretion and sodium chloride > 400mEq/day

2. Glucocorticoids: Inhibit intestinal absorption of calcium and increases urinary calcium excretion. Effect usually evident after 48–72hrs. Effective in hypercalcemia due to myeloma, hematologic malignancies, breast cancer, vitamin D intoxication and sarcoidosis

   a. Dose: Initial dose **Hydrocortisone** 3–5mg/kg/day IV then **Prednisone** 30mg PO BID

   b. Side effects: Water retention, weight gain, psychosis, avascular necrosis. Toxicity limits usefulness in chronic management

3. Oral phosphates: Promotes calcium deposition in bone and soft tissue as well as inhibiting GI calcium absorption. Use only in patients with normal renal function and serum phosphorus less then 3mg/dL. Follow phosphate levels along with calcium levels; patient should be kept normophosphatemic. Calcium lowering will not be apparent for 2–3 days. PTH levels will increase with this therapy

   a. Dose: 1–3g/day in divided doses

   b. E.g., **Neutra-Phos, Phos-tabs, Fleets phospho-soda**

   c. Side effects: Diarrhea, nausea, soft tissue calcification

4. Dietary Calcium restriction

C. **Hypercalcemia due to specific conditions**

1. Vitamin D toxicity: Treat with a low calcium diet (<400mg/day). May take up to 2 months for effects of vitamin D to subside

2. Sarcoidosis: **Prednisone** 10–20mg/day. Avoid excessive sunlight exposure and limit vitamin D/calcium intake

3. Primary hyperparathyroidism: Parathyroidectomy. This is the only effective treatment for primary hyperparathyroidism. Indications for surgery include symptoms of hypercalcemia, nephrolithiasis, bone mass reduction greater than 2 standard deviations, age < 50, serum calcium more than 12mg/dL

4. Malignancy: Interval between detection of hypercalcemia and death is often less than 6 months

— PART TWO: HYPOCALCEMIA —

I. DEFINITION: Serum calcium < 9mg/dL or ionized calcium < 4.6mg/dL

II. ETIOLOGY

A. **Hypoalbuminemia:** Most common cause of low total serum calcium. Each decrease of 1g in serum albumin will decrease serum calcium by 0.8mg/dL, but will not change free (ionized)

GEN

calcium
   B. **Renal insufficiency:** Decreased production of 1,25-dihydroxyvitamin D, increased serum phosphate levels cause calcium deposits in bone and soft tissue
   C. **Vitamin D deficiency:** Malabsorption, decreased production of 1,25-dihydroxyvitamin D, inadequate intake
   D. **Hypomagnesemia:** Decreased PTH secretion
   E. **Hyperphosphatemia**
   F. **Drugs:** Pentamidine, Ketoconazole, Foscarnet, Cisplatin, Cytosine Arabinoside
   G. **Other:** Acute pancreatitis, rhabdomyolysis, tumor lysis syndrome, pseudohypoparathyroidism (PTH resistance), multiple citrated blood transfusions, sepsis

III. **HISTORY AND PHYSICAL EXAM:** Symptoms vary with the degree and rate of onset. Alkalosis facilitates calcium binding to albumin and increases the severity of the symptoms
   A. **General:** Weakness, depression, lethargy
   B. **Neuro:** Paresthesias, impaired cognitive function, seizures
   C. **Psychiatric:** Depression
   D. **Musculoskeletal**
      1. Symptoms consistent with pseudohypoparathyroidism: Short metacarpals and short stature
      2. Symptoms consistent with idiopathic hypoparathyroidism: Hypothyroidism, candidiasis, vitiligo, adrenal failure
      3. Soft tissue calcifications
   E. **Neurological:** Tetany, seizures, psychosis
      1. Chvostek's sign: Facial twitching after tapping the facial nerve
      2. Trousseau's sign: Carpopedal spasm after inflation of blood pressure cuff (over the patient's systolic blood pressure) for 2–3 minutes
   F. **Cardiovascular:** Dysrhythmias, CHF, hypotension
   G. **Ophthalmologic:** Cataracts
   H. **Past history:** Previous neck surgery
   I. **Family history** of hypocalcemia

IV. **LABORATORY:** Alkalosis facilitates calcium binding to albumin and increases the severity of the symptoms—serum albumin, serum free (ionized) calcium, magnesium, phosphorus, BUN, creatinine, alkaline phosphatase, serum PTH level

V. **ECG:** Prolonged QT interval

VI. **MANAGEMENT**
   A. **Severe acute hypocalcemia**
      1. Tetany, seizures, arrhythmias
      2. **Calcium Gluconate** 10%: Dose 93–186mg (10–20mL) over 10–15 minutes, then 10–15mg/kg over 4–6hrs. Onset immediate
   B. **Hypomagnesemia**
      1. Severe hypomagnesemia (with serum calcium < 0.8mg/dL): Treat as a medical emergency in hospital setting
      2. Moderate hypomagnesemia (with serum calcium 0.8–1.3mg/dL): Give one 2mL ampule of 50% magnesium solution IM. May repeat dose in 4–6hrs
      3. Chronic hypomagnesemia: **Magnesium Oxide** 400mg PO BID–QID
   C. **Chronic hypocalcemia:** The objective is to maintain serum calcium levels between 8–9mg/dL. If hypercalciuria develops at serum calcium levels < 8.5mg/dL, **Hydrochlorothiazide** 50mg PO QD can be used to reduce urinary calcium excretion
      1. PO: **Calcium Carbonate (Tums, OsCal, Biocal, Caltrate)**
         a. Dose: 500–1000mg PO TID
         b. Onset < 1hr
      2. Renal failure
         a. Use phosphate binding antacids to reduce hyperphosphatemia (e.g., **Amphojel**)
         b. Oral calcium supplementation 0.5–1.0g PO TID with meals. Tums provides 500mg elemental calcium and is the least expensive
         c. For long term therapy, vitamin D supplementation with **Calcitriol (Rocaltrol)** is the

GEN

best choice for most patients due to its lower risk of toxicity. Initial dose is 0.25µg PO QD. Most patients are maintained with 0.5–2.0ug PO QD

3. Hypoparathyroidism or vitamin D deficiency: Vitamin D and oral calcium supplementation as noted above

CLINICAL PEARLS

- 20% of patients with gram negative sepsis have hypocalcemia
- Calcium is 2% of the normal body weight

References

Guise TA, et al. Evaluation of hypocalcemia in children and adults. Journal of Clinical Endocrinology and Metabolism 1995;80(5):1473–8.

Kaye TB. Hypercalcemia: How to pinpoint the cause and customize treatment. Postgrad Med 1995;97:153.

Bourke E, et al. Assessment of hypocalcemia and hypercalcemia. Clinics in Laboratory Medicine 1993; 13(1):157–81.

Michael B. Weinstock, MD

76. DISORDERS OF POTASSIUM METABOLISM

GEN

— PART ONE: HYPERKALEMIA —

I. SIGNS AND SYMPTOMS

Patient may have weakness and flaccid paralysis, abdominal distension and diarrhea. Primarily diagnosed by laboratory and ECG changes (See below)

II. DIFFERENTIAL DIAGNOSIS/ETIOLOGY

A. Excessive potassium intake: Salt substitutes, potassium replacement, foods rich in potassium (e.g., soybeans, garbanzo beans, papaya)

B. Decreased potassium excretion: Acute or chronic renal failure, potassium sparing diuretics (spironolactone, triamterene), ACE inhibitors, NSAIDs, aldosterone deficiency (Addison's disease), adrenal insufficiency, dehydration

C. Intra/Extracellular shift (total body potassium is normal): Metabolic acidosis (e.g., DKA), insulin depletion, ß-blockers, Digoxin intoxication

D. Pseudohyperkalemia: Thrombocytosis and leukocytosis, hemolysis (tourniquets, finger stick, delay between blood draw and analysis in lab)

E. Tissue damage: Crush injuries, rhabdomyolysis

F. Other causes (mechanism not clear): Lupus nephritis, chronic pyelonephritis, renal transplantation, acute glomerulonephritis

III. DIAGNOSIS

A. Review history looking for iatrogenic or physiologic reasons for hyperkalemia

B. Obtain stat ECG: Almost half of patients with serum potassium > 6.5 will show no ECG changes

1. Tall, narrow, peaked T waves: First change seen
2. Widening of QRS $\geq$ 0.10 seconds
3. Wide, flat P waves
4. Bradyarrhythmias, tachyarrhythmias, AV block, ventricular fibrillation, sinusoidal wave pattern, cardiac arrest

C. Repeat test if laboratory does not correlate with clinical picture (rule out hemolysis or laboratory error). Make sure patient does not clench fist during venipuncture and that repeated specimen is taken immediately to the lab

D. Do not delay ECG and/or treatment while waiting for repeat labs to come back!

IV. MANAGEMENT

A. Emergency management: Indicated for hyperkalemia associated with cardiac toxicity, muscular paralysis or with severe hyperkalemia (>6.5–7.0) without ECG changes. Items 1–4 are to be used first and in the order listed here. They must be used in conjunction with definitive treatment (**Kayexalate** or dialysis). Look for reversible causes!

Drug	Dose	Onset	Duration	Action
1. Calcium chloride 10%	1 ampule IV (10mL=1g)	0–5 minutes	1 hour	Stabilizes cardiac membranes
2. Bicarbonate	1–2 ampules (44–88mEq) IV	15–30 minutes	1–2 hours	Shifts K⁺ into cells
3. Regular Insulin	5–10 units IV	15–60 minutes	4–6 hours	Shifts K⁺ into cells
4. D50 (dextrose)	1 ampule (25g) IV	15–60 minutes	4–6 hours	Works with insulin
5. **Kayexalate***	15–60g in 20% sorbitol PR or PO	1–4 hours	This is the **definitive** treatment May repeat Q6 hours	
6. **Hemodialysis*** — Indicated for refractory cases or in patients with renal failure.				

* These are the **definitive** treatments that will remove potassium from the body. Insulin and D50 should be used together

B. Non-emergency management

Drug	Dose	Action
Kayexalate	PO: 15–30g in 20% sorbitol Rectal: 15–60g in 20% sorbitol	Binds potassium in bowel
Loop diuretic	**Furosemide (Lasix)** 40–160mg IV or PO	Increased renal potassium excretion
Hemo or peritoneal dialysis — Patients in acute or chronic renal failure		

Source: Adapted from Cogan MG, Papadakis MA. Fluid and electrolyte disorders. In: Tierney LM, et al. Current medical diagnosis and treatment, 34th ed. Norwalk, CT: Appleton & Lange, 1995:751.

CLINICAL PEARLS
- If the history and clinical picture could correlate with hyperkalemia (i.e., a renal patient with a widened QRS), don't wait for the lab value to treat! No harm will be done, and a cardiac arrest could be prevented
- Treat underlying cause, i.e., metabolic acidosis. Discontinue any offending agents

— PART TWO: HYPOKALEMIA —

I. SIGNS AND SYMPTOMS
Muscle weakness, ileus, absent or decreased deep tendon reflexes

II. DIFFERENTIAL DIAGNOSIS/ETIOLOGY
A. **GI loss:** Vomiting, diarrhea (profound loss in watery stools), villous adenoma, laxative abuse
B. **Renal:** Metabolic alkalosis, increased mineralocorticoid effects: primary or secondary aldosteronism (Conn's, Bartter's, malignant HTN, licorice), renal tubular disease (RTA) (leukemias, antibiotics), magnesium depletion, Cushing's syndrome
C. **Cellular shift:** Metabolic alkalosis, periodic paralysis, insulin effect
D. **Iatrogenic/drugs:** Potassium wasting diuretics, Amphotericin B, aminoglycosides, high dose Penicillin, corticosteroids, Digibind

III. DIAGNOSIS
A. Review history looking for iatrogenic or physiologic reasons for hypokalemia
B. If *unexplained* hypokalemia (e.g., young patient taking no meds, no history of vomiting), obtain a urinary potassium before repleting (hyperaldosteronism). If patient is hypertensive, obtain a renin and aldosterone level (mineralocorticoid excess)
C. Consider checking ABG (pH and bicarbonate) in the *unexplained* hypokalemic patient
D. **ECG changes** associated with hypokalemia
   1. Flattening and inversion of T wave
   2. Prominent U wave
   3. ST depression
   4. Ventricular ectopy and AV block

    E. **Hypokalemia** greatly increases the incidence of Digitalis toxicity including junctional rhythms or heart block

IV. **THERAPY**

    A. Mild hypokalemia which is *not* symptomatic can be treated with PO replacement; KCl being the most effective in alkalosis. Potassium Gluconate and carbonate salts also available

      1. **K-Dur** 20–40mEq PO QD—Sustained release: Not to be used in critical situations

      2. **Slow-K** 8mEq—Sustained release: Not to be used in critical situations

      3. **K-Lyte** (powder) 25–50mEq PO/NG: May be used for treating hypokalemia acutely

    B. If the patient is severely hypokalemic (under 3.0), or with evidence of cardiac symptoms, replacement should be IV (on telemetry) with frequent lab checks. Maximum replacement is 20mEq/hr peripherally and 40mEq/hr centrally. The order may be written for 40mEq KCl in 100mL D5W IV over 1hr *per central line—or—*20mEq KCl in 100–250mL D5W IV over 1–2hrs *per peripheral line*

    C. Potassium deficit by level of serum potassium:

      1. $K^+ = 3.0–3.5$ Replace with 50–75mEq KCl

      2. $K^+ = 2.5–3.0$ Replace with 100–150mEq KCl

      3. $K^+ = 2.0–2.5$ Replace with 150–250mEq KCl

    D. If magnesium level is low, then replace with

      1. PO: **Magnesium Oxide** 400mg PO TID × 3–5 days—*or*—

      2. IV: **Magnesium** 1g in 100mL NS IV over 1hr. May be repeated 1–2 times

CLINICAL PEARL

    • Consider replacing magnesium or calcium in patients with refractory hypokalemia because potassium replacement will be ineffective if the patient is also hypomagnasemic or hypocalcemic

Miriam M. Chan, PharmD

77. DRUG INTERACTIONS AND TOXICITIES

I. **DRUG INTERACTION MECHANISMS**

    A. Absorption of 1 drug can be reduced by another drug, e.g., Cholestyramine

    B. Protein/tissue binding displacement can be important especially if the displacing drug also reduces the elimination of the object drug

    C. Metabolism of 1 drug can be enhanced by an "enzyme-inducing" agent, e.g., Phenobarbital

    D. Many commonly prescribed medications interfere with or are metabolized by the hepatic cytochrome P-450 enzyme system. The Cyt P-450 system refers to a collection of isoenzymes that are responsible for the oxidative metabolism of many endogenous and exogenous compounds

    E. Altered renal excretion can be caused by reduced excretion or change in urinary pH

    F. Pharmacodynamic interaction occurs when drugs with either additive or antagonistic properties are given concomitantly

II. **SELECTED CLINICALLY RELEVANT DRUG INTERACTIONS**

The following table is not comprehensive. Drugs in parentheses are important examples of that class of drug

OBJECT DRUG	PRECIPITANT DRUG	EFFECT/ACTION
ACE inhibitors	K+ sparing diuretics (amiloride spironolactone), K+ supplements	↑ serum K+, especially in the presence of significant renal impairment. Monitor serum K+
Antiarrhythmics, Type 1C: Encainide, Mexiletine, Propafenone	*Enzyme inhibitors:* Cimetidine, Quinidine, SSRIs (Fluoxetine, Paroxetine)	↑ antiarrhythmics plasma levels. Monitor patient carefully if used concurrently
Antidiabetics agents: Insulin, Sulfonylureas	β-blockers, e.g. Nadolol, Propranolol, Timolol	Alternation of glycemic control and/or masking of some signs of hypoglycemia (e.g. tachycardia, tremor)
Antifungal agents: Itraconazole, Ketoconazole	*Gastric alkalinizers:* H2-blockers, antacids, Omeprazole	↓ absorption of Itraconazole and Ketoconazole
Benzodiazepines: Alprazolam (Xanax), Triazolam (Halcion)	*Enzyme inhibitors:* Ketoconazole, Itraconazole, Nefazodone	↑ benzodiazepine levels, may lead to unexpected CNS impairment or other toxic effect. Contraindication
β-blockers	Diltiazem, Verapamil	↑ risk of bradycardia and AV block. Avoid combination
β-blockers, non-selective: Nadolol, Propranolol, Timolol	Epinephrine	Severe hypertension and bradycardia secondary to unopposed α-stimulation. Avoid use in patients prone to anaphylaxis because they might not respond to Epinephrine
Carbamazepine (CBZ)	*Enzyme inhibitors:* Cimetidine, Erythromycin, Diltiazem, Fluoxetine, INH, Propoxyphene, Verapamil	↑ serum CBZ levels significantly within 2–3 days. Monitor serum CBZ levels and signs of CBZ toxicity (e.g. drowsiness, ataxia, nystagmus, blurred vision, nausea)
Digoxin	*↓ renal and non-renal clearance:* Antiarrhythmics (Amiodarone, Propafenone, Quinidine), Ca-channel blockers (Verapamil)	↑ Digoxin serum levels. Amiodarone and Quinidine can cause a ≥ 2-fold increase in Digoxin levels. Effects of Propafenone and Verapamil may be less. Patients starting on these drugs should have Digoxin dosage reduced by 50%. Additional dosage adjustment may be necessary. Monitor serum Digoxin concentrations and signs of toxicity (e.g. GI upset, CNS disturbances, arrhythmias)
Digoxin	K+ wasting diuretics (Furosemide, HCTZ)	Digoxin toxicity can occur secondary to hypokalemia. Monitor serum K+ level and replace K+ as needed
HMG CoA reductase inhibitors	Erythromycin, Gemfibrozil (Lopid), Niacin Cyclosporin	Myopathy, ↑ risk of rhabdomyolysis. Close monitoring is required
Lithium	*↓ renal clearance:* NSAIDs except Sulindac, Thiazide diuretics	↑ serum Li+ levels within days. Monitor serum Li+ levels and signs of toxicity (e.g. muscle twitching, confusion)
MAO inhibitors	Cold/cough medicines (Dextromethorphan, sympathomimetics), Meperidine, SSRIs (e.g. Fluoxetine, Paroxetine, Sertraline). Food rich in tyramine (e.g. cheese, red wine, smoked fish)	Severe reactions (shivering, seizures, agitation, delirium, and death). Avoid combination
Oral contraceptives	*Enzyme inducers:* Carbamazepine, Phenobarbital, Phenytoin, Primidone, Rifampin, *↓ enterohepatic recycling:* Ampicillins, Tetracyclines, Griseofulvin	↓ efficacy of oral contraceptives, resulting in break-through bleeding or pregnancy. Use another method of contraception
Phenytoin	*Enzyme inhibitors:* Amiodarone, Cimetidine, Fluconazole, Fluoxetine, Isoniazid, Omeprazole)	↑ serum phenytoin levels. Monitor serum phenytoin levels and signs of toxicity (e.g. ataxia, nystagmus, mental impairment)
Protease inhibitors: Ritonavir (Norvir), Indinavir (Crixivan), Saquinavir (Invirase), Nelfinavir (Viracept)		See chapter 110, Ambulatory HIV/AIDS Management, for further information
Quinidine	*Enzyme inducers:* Phenobarbital, Phenytoin, Rifampin	↓ serum quinidine levels. Adjust Quinidine dose as needed when initiating or discontinuing enzyme inducers
Quinolones (e.g. Cipro, Floxin)	*Chelating effect:* Antacids, Sucralfate	↓ bioavailability of Quinolones. The antibiotic should be given 2 hrs before or 4 hrs after a dose of antacid

GEN

Table continued on following page

OBJECT DRUG	PRECIPITANT DRUG	EFFECT/ACTION
Theophylline	*Enzyme inhibitors:* Cimetidine, Ciprofloxacin, Erythromycin, Fluvoxamine, Tacrine, Ticlopidine, Verapamil, Zileuton (Zyflo)	↑ serum Theophylline concentrations, leading to toxicity within 2–3 days. Theophylline dose may need to be adjusted by 30–50%. Monitor serum Theophylline levels and signs of toxicity (e.g. tachycardia, nausea, tremor)
Theophylline	*Enzyme inducers:* Carbamazepine, Phenobarbital, Phenytoin, Primidone, Rifampin	↓ serum Theophylline concentrations gradually over 1–2 weeks. Monitor serum Theophylline levels and adjust dose as needed
Tramadol (Ultram)	*Enzyme inhibitors:* Phenothiazines, SSRIs, TCAs	↑ serum Tramadol levels and ↑ risk of seizures. Avoid combination
Tricyclic antidepressants: Amitriptyline, Imipramine, Nortriptyline	*Enzyme inhibitors:* Cimetidine, Fluconazole, Propoxyphene, Quinidine, SSRIs (Fluoxetine, Paroxetine)	↑ tricyclic antidepressant serum concentrations possibly leading to toxicity. Monitor closely
Warfarin (Coumadin)	*Enzyme inhibitors:* Amiodarone, antimicrobials (Quinolones, Erythromycin, Fluconazole, Itraconazole, Ketoconazole, Metronidazole, Rifampin, sulfa antibiotics), Cimetidine, Cisapride, Disulfiram, Omeprazole, Propafenone, Zafirlukast (Accolate), Zileuton (Zyflo). *Inhibit platelet function:* NSAIDs, salicylates *Unknown mechanism:* Androgens, Clofibrate, Gemfibrozil (Lopid)	↑ hypoprothrombinemic response of Warfarin and ↑ risk of bleeding. Concurrent use of Clofibrate should be avoided if possible due to the difficulty in the management of these interactions. Amiodarone may produce a large increase in INR over a period of weeks. When Amiodarone is added to therapy, a 50% reduction in Warfarin dose may be needed. NSAIDs also increase the risk of GI bleeding in anticoagulated patients. Use conservative Warfarin dosing, monitor INR more frequently, and monitor for clinical sign of bleeding. It may take 7–10 days to reach a new steady state anticoagulant response
Warfarin (Coumadin)	↓ *GI absorption:* Bile acid sequestrants (Cholestyramine, Colestipol) *Enzyme inducers:* Carbamazepine, Phenobarbital, Phenytoin, Primidone, Rifampin ↑ *Vitamin K:* Vitamin K-rich foods (green vegetables, enteral feeding, green tea)	↓ hypoprothrombinemic response of Warfarin. Monitor INR more frequently and watch for excessive anticoagulant effect when the inducer is discontinued. Avoid use of Rifampin with Warfarin if possible due to the difficulty in the management of these interactions.

III. EXAMPLES OF DRUGS THAT MAY CAUSE RENAL TOXICITY

A. NSAIDs: decrease renal perfusion, may cause interstitial nephritis and nephrotic syndrome

B. ACE inhibitors: cause renal failure in patients with bilateral renal artery stenosis

C. Aminoglycosides: direct tubular injury occurring 7–10 days after initiation of treatment

D. Amphotericin B: direct tubular injury

E. Cyclosporine

F. Radiographic contrast dye

G. Foscarnet, Gangciclovir, Pentamidine

IV. EXAMPLES OF DRUGS THAT MAY CAUSE HEPATIC TOXICITY

A. Acetaminophen: Direct toxic reactions

B. Alcohol

C. Amiodarone: Fatty liver and alcoholic hepatitis

D. Estradiol: Cholestatic reactions

E. Isoniazid: Idiosyncratic reactions

F. HMG CoA reductase inhibitors

G. Phenytoin: Allergic hepatitis

H. Sustained-release nicotinic acid

I. Vitamin A: Indolent cirrhosis

CLINICAL PEARLS

• Always be alert for potential drug interactions with drugs that have narrow therapeutic indexes. E.g., antiarrhythmics, anticonvulsants, Cisapride, Lithium, MAOIs, nonsedating antihistamines, Theophylline, and Warfarin

• If the patient is stabilized on the object drug, it may be necessary to adjust the dose when starting, stopping or altering the dose of the precipitant drug

• Monitoring of serum drug concentrations may be useful in adjusting drug dosage

• Educate patient regarding early signs of a possible drug interaction and monitor carefully the clinical response of the patient

• The onset of drug interactions may vary, depending on the time required to reach the steady-state concentration of the precipitant drug

• Alcohol may potentiate the CNS effects of antidepressants, antihistamines, antipsychotics, benzodiazepines, narcotics, and sedatives. Alcohol can cause a disulfiram-like reaction (flushing, palpitations, tachycardia, nausea etc.) when it is taken concurrently with Metronidazole or Chlorpropamide

References

Ament PW, et al. Clinically significant drug interactions. Am Fam Phys 2000; 61:1745-54.

Hansten PD, Hom JR. Drug interactions analysis and management. Applied Therapeutics, Inc., 1997.

Goldberg RJ. The P-450 system. Arch Fam Med 1996;5:406–12.

McEvoy GK, ed. The American hospital formulary service. Bethesda, MD: American Society of Health-System Pharmacists, 1996.

Lee WM. Drug-induced hepatotoxicity. N Engl J Med 1995;333:1118–27.

Michael B. Weinstock, MD

78. MEDICATION COMPLIANCE

I. STATISTICS

A. Approximately 33% of patients do not take their prescribed medications

B. Up to 5–10% of hospital admissions of the elderly may be associated with medication non-compliance

C. In women who begin hormone replacement therapy (HRT), 33% will have stopped taking their medications by 6 months and 75% will have stopped by 3 years

II. HINTS TO IMPROVE MEDICATION COMPLIANCE

A. Minimize the number of medications patients are taking

B. Explain to patients what their medications do and why they need to take them

C. Prescribe medications with minimal side effects

D. Inform patients about potential side effects and how to best manage them

E. Review patients' medications at each visit to ensure the medications they are taking (or not taking) are the same medications you think they are taking (or not taking)

F. Locate patients at high risk for medication non-compliance (illiterate, decreased mobility, ignorant, rebellious (teenagers), and patients on multiple meds). Spend extra time with these patients or enlist the help of ancillary medical personnel (nurses, pharmacists, social workers, home health workers) to help with compliance

G. Minimize the number of times per day that a patient needs to take medications. If a patient is on a TID medication and another medication needs to be added, when possible, prescribe another TID medication instead of a Q6hr medication

H. Instruct, then observe patient taking metered dose inhalers. Use a spacer to increase delivery of the medication

I. Be aware of cost of medications. Often prescriptions will not even be filled when the pharmacist tells the patient the cost. A brilliant diagnosis dims when a patient doesn't take the prescribed medications

J. Refill only enough medications to get the patient to the next appointment

CLINICAL PEARLS

• Be alert for medication toxicity in patients recently admitted to a hospital or extra-care facility. A clinician may have increased the dose of a patient's medication because it was thought ineffective at a lower dose, when, in fact, the patient was not being compliant. When the patient is admitted and receives prescribed dose, toxic levels are achieved. Admission equals compliance!

• Ensure that the benefit of the medication helps the patient more than the side effects harm the patient. Classic examples are antihypertensives (ß-blockers, Reserpine), antilipidemics (niacin, bile acid sequestrants) where the quality of life is decreased to a high degree

• It is easier to swallow a pill when you are prescribing it. Do not judge your patients for lack of compliance

GEN

References

Heyduk LJ. Medication education: increasing patient compliance. J Psychosocial Nursing 1991; 29(12):32–5.

Col N, et al. The role of medication noncompliance and adverse drug reactions in hospitalizations of the elderly. Arch Intern Med 150 Apr 1990:841–5.

Chatham M. Patient education handbook. Englewood Cliffs, NJ: Prentice Hall, 1981.

GEN

VII. Musculoskeletal/ Sports Medicine

MUSC

Steve Markovich, MD

79. DESCRIBING FRACTURES AND DISLOCATIONS

I. NOMENCLATURE: Each fracture can be described using an organized system based on what the examiner sees radiographically. Less frequently fractures can also be described based on the mechanism of injury

    A. Anatomic Location: Name the bone involved and the general location of the fracture. Long bones are generally divided into thirds. Anatomic locations can also be used when appropriate. Examples:

        1. Fracture at the junction of the middle and distal thirds of the humerus

        2. Fracture of the distal radius

        3. Intertrochanteric fracture of the humerus

    B. Describe the direction of the fracture lines

        1. Transverse: Fracture runs 90° to the long axis of the bone

        2. Oblique: Fracture runs less than 90° to the long axis of the bone

        3. Spiral: Torsion results in curved fracture around the bone

        4. Greenstick: Incomplete fracture in children disrupts the periosteum opposite the fracture

        5. Comminuted: More than 2 fracture fragments

        6. Impacted: One fragment is driven into another

        7. Compression: Crush injury usually seen in vertebral bodies and calcaneous

        8. Avulsion: Small fragment of bone pulled off at the site of muscle attachment

        9. Pathologic: Fracture due to diseased or abnormal bone

    C. Describe the relationship of the fragments to each other

        1. Alignment: Alignment of the distal fragment relative to the proximal fragment. E.g., the distal femur fragment is angulated 15° laterally

        2. Displacement: The surface to surface contact of the fracture surfaces. An estimate is generally made of the percentage of the fracture surfaces in contact. A fracture with 100% displacement and shortening is referred to as a *bayonette fracture*

    D. Describe the relationship to the surrounding soft tissue

        1. Closed: Skin is intact

        2. Open: Skin is broken. May be broken from within (by sharp bone fragments) or from the outside (from trauma or puncture)

II. DISLOCATION, SUBLUXATION AND DIASTASIS

    A. Dislocation: The complete disruption of the joint so that articular surfaces are no longer in contact. Description based on placement of the distal bone relative to the proximal bone. E.g., posterior elbow dislocation—displacement of the ulnar olecranon posterior relative to the humerus

    B. Subluxation: Partial disruption of articulating surfaces, loss of contact is incomplete

    C. Diastasis: Disruption of the interosseous membrane between 2 bones

III. TERMINOLOGY: Orthopedics has a unique language to describe bony structures and relationships

    A. Ankylosis: Restricted motion in a joint

    B. Apophysis: Ossification center at the insertion of a tendon

    C. Arthrodesis: Surgical stiffening/fusion of a joint

    D. Diaphysis: Shaft of a long bone

    E. Epiphysis: Ossification center at the end of long bones, separated from the metaphysis by the physis

    F. Genu: Knee

    G. Hallux: Toe

    H. Kyphosis: Curvature of the spine with posterior convexity

    I. Lordosis: Curvature of the spine with anterior convexity

    J. Metaphysis: Widened portion of bone adjacent to the epiphysis

    K. Pes: Foot

    L. Physis: Cartilaginous growth plate

    M. Pollux: Thumb

N. **Salter Classification:** Refers to physeal fractures in children
1. I—Fracture through the physis
2. II—Fracture through the physis which continues towards the metaphysis
3. III—Through the physis, continues towards the epiphysis
4. IV—Through the physis and continues toward both the metaphysis and epiphysis
5. V—Crush injury to the physis

O. **Spondylolisthesis:** Slippage of one vertebra on another
P. **Talipes:** Ankle
Q. **Valgus:** Distal part away from the midline
R. **Varus:** Distal part toward the midline
S. **Volar:** Towards the palmar surface of the hand, opposite the dorsal surface

IV. SPECIAL TERMINOLOGY

A. **Boxer's Fracture:** Fracture of the fifth metacarpal neck with volar displacement of the metacarpal head
B. **Colles' Fracture:** Distal radius fracture with dorsal displacement
C. **Smith's Fracture:** Distal radius with volar displacement
D. **Jones' Fracture:** Diaphyseal fracture of the base of the fifth metatarsal
E. **Lisfranc Dislocation:** Tarsometatarsal dislocation
F. **Maisonneuve's Fracture:** Proximal fibula fracture with syndesmosis rupture and associated medial malleolar fracture or deltoid ligament rupture
G. **Monteggia's Fracture:** Fracture of the proximal third of the ulnar shaft with radial head dislocation
H. **Nightstick Fracture:** Isolated fracture of the ulna due to direct trauma
I. **Rolando's Fracture:** Y shaped intra-articular fracture of the base of the first metacarpal

Brent Cale, MD

80. ANKLE INJURIES

I. **INTRODUCTION:** Although most ankle injuries are simple sprains of the lateral ligaments, a variety of other structures near the ankle may also be injured. Included in the differential diagnosis should be medial ankle sprains, trauma to the Achilles and peroneal tendons, tarsal tunnel syndrome, fractures, syndesmotic sprains and synovial impingement

II. ANATOMY

A. **Ligaments of the lateral ankle**
1. Anterior talofibular ligament
   a. Prevents forward subluxation of the talus/prevents inversion in plantar flexion
   b. Most frequently injured ligament with inversion injury
2. Posterior talofibular ligament
3. Calcaneofibular ligament

B. **Ligament of the medial ankle:** Deltoid ligament (broad ligament with superficial and deep fibers)

C. **Tibiofibular joint/syndesmosis:** The following ligaments connect the tibia and fibula. They form a fibrous joint between the distal tibia and fibula which is called the syndesmosis (see syndesmosis squeeze test below)
1. Anterior tibiofibular ligament
2. Posterior tibiofibular ligament
3. Interosseous membrane

D. **Superficial posterior compartment of the leg:** All of the following muscles insert at the calcaneus through the Achilles tendon
1. Gastrocnemius muscle
2. Soleus muscle
3. Plantaris muscle

III. HISTORY

A. **Mechanism of injury**

1. Was a "pop" felt or heard at the time of the injury
2. Ability to bear weight immediately following the injury
3. Inversion or eversion
4. Force of injury
5. Swelling or ecchymosis, abrasions or lacerations

B. Previous injury in the same location
C. Treatment provided for a previous injury and the current injury
D. Type of employment
E. Level of athlete

IV. PHYSICAL: Patients with acute ankle injuries will most likely have loss of range of motion (ROM) and decreased strength secondary to swelling and pain which may compromise the exam (drawer tests, etc). It may be helpful to reexamine after the swelling has decreased

A. Inspection for swelling and ecchymosis to help localize the site of the injury. *Inspect the unaffected side for comparison.* Ecchymosis extending proximately from the ankle to the leg may indicate a syndesmotic injury

B. Palpation: Gently palpate to find areas of greatest tenderness—start with examining the areas of least suspected tenderness. Particularly observe for tenderness of the malleoli, anterior talofibular ligament, anterior process of the calcaneous, calcaneofibular ligament, deltoid ligament, Achilles tendon, peroneal tendons, tibialis anterior tendon, and navicular and proximal fifth metatarsal

C. Range of motion: Normal is 13–16° of dorsiflexion and 31–44° plantar flexion

D. Pulses: Dorsal pedis and posterior tibial (vascular compromise is usually caused by posterior dislocation)

E. Neurologic: Check sensation (L4:medial leg, L5:lateral leg and great toe, S1:heel)

F. Ankle stress testing: To assess ankle instability. Exam after acute injury may be limited by pain and swelling

     1. Anterior drawer test: To test for laxity or disruption of the anterior talofibular ligament
         a. Method: Have patient sit or lie flat with the legs unweighted. Grasp lower leg with one hand and the heel with the other hand and then, with the ankle in slight plantar flexion, apply anterior force to the calcaneus to displace the talus forward
         b. Results: 4–5mm displacement of the talus with respect to the tibia is probably normal. Remember to compare other side. Displacement of 8–10mm is noted with division of the anterior talofibular ligament, and 10–15mm displacement is noted with tearing of the anterior and posterior talofibular ligament and calcaneofibular ligament
     2. Talar tilt (Inversion test): To test for laxity or disruption of the lateral ligaments
         a. Method: Have patient sit or lie flat with the legs unweighted. Place inversion stress on the ankle
         b. Results: Indicative of anterior talofibular ligament disruption if 10–20° of inversion is noted. Again, compare unaffected side. If talar tilt greater than 20° then calcaneofibular ligament may also be torn
     3. Syndesmosis squeeze
         a. Method: 10cm above the lateral malleolus, compress the proximal fibula against the tibia
         b. Results: If the patient reports localized pain at the distal tibia and fibula during the syndesmosis squeeze, this may be indicative of a fibular fracture, interosseus membrane disruption or distal tibiofibular syndesmosis damage
     4. The Thompson test
         a. Method: Have the patient lie prone with feet off the edge of the table. Compress the mid-calf and observe for plantar flexion
         b. A positive test (no plantar flexion) helps to confirm the diagnosis of an Achilles tendon rupture

V. IMAGING STUDIES

A. Plain x-ray: Not all ankle injuries necessitate obtaining radiographic films. The Ottawa ankle rules apply to patients 18 years or older and suggest that films be obtained:
     1. If the patient is unable to bear weight initially and when examined
     2. Bone tenderness at the posterior edge or tip of the (distal 6cm) medial or lateral malleolus or proximal 5th metatarsal

B. CT: To localize osteochondritis dissecans, loose bodies and subchondral cysts

C. MRI: Osteochondral lesions such as osteochondritis dissecans and talar dome fractures, visualization of achilles, peroneal and posterior tibial tendons

D. Technetium bone scan: To evaluate for stress fractures, infections or degenerative arthritis

E. Arthrography (rarely needed): To diagnose acute disruption to the calcaneofibular ligament, anterior talofibular ligament, deltoid ligament or syndesmosis. Test should be performed 24–48hrs after the injury

VI. MANAGEMENT OF ANKLE SPRAINS

A. Incidence: 85% are lateral sprains, typically involving the anterior talofibular ligament, 10% are syndesmotic sprains, and 5% are medial sprains involving the deltoid ligament

B. Grade the severity of the ankle sprain

Severity	Pathophysiology	Symptoms	Signs	Weight-bearing
Grade I	Minimal tearing of fibers	Minimal pain or instability	Slight edema Anterior drawer and talar tilt test negative	Unimpaired
Grade II	Incomplete rupture of ligament	Moderate pain and disability	Moderate edema and ecchymosis Anterior drawer and talar tilt tests positive	Difficult
Grade III	Complete rupture of ligament	Severe pain with loss of function	Severe edema and ecchymosis Anterior drawer and talar tilt tests positive Possible avulsion fracture	Impossible

*Adapted from table 2—Ankle sprain grading system from Reisdorff, EJ. The injured ankle: New twists to a familiar problem. Emergency Medicine Reports 1995;16(5)

C. Management of Grade I and II sprains
1. Consider non-weight bearing initially (increase gradually over 2–4 days)
2. Support to prevent eversion and inversion and provide early mobilization
    a. Airsplint
    b. Gelsplint
    c. Swedo boot
    d. ROM boot cast
3. RICE : See VI. E. below
4. Medications: See VI. F. below

D. Management of Grade III sprains
1. Non weight bearing
2. Immobilization
    a. Plaster posterior splint
    b. Sugar-tong splint
3 Orthopedic evaluation
4. RICE: See VI. E. below
5. Medications: See VI. F. below

E. RICE (rest, ice, compression and elevation) protocol

1. Rest: Patient should use crutches until he or she is able to bear weight pain-free

2. Ice: 20 minutes 3 × per day. Do not apply ice directly to skin

3. Compression wrap is the most important measure: Use a focal compression device for the first 24–36hrs or until the swelling has stabilized

4. Elevation: Need to elevate the ankle above the level of the heart

F. Medications
1. NSAIDs: E.g., **Ibuprofen** 600–800mg PO TID, **Naprosyn** 375mg PO TID
2. **Acetaminophen**
3. Narcotic pain medications if necessary
    a. **Tylenol #3:** 1–2 tabs PO Q4–6hrs PRN
    b. **Vicodin:** 1–2 tabs PO Q4–6hrs PRN
    c. **Percocet:** 1–2 tabs PO Q4–6hrs PRN

G. Return to function: The goal of any management plan for treating ankle sprains is to preserve as much strength and ROM as possible. A key component to rehabilitation is physical therapy

MUSC

H. Differential diagnosis of non-healing ankle injuries
1. Incomplete rehabilitation
2. Talar dome fracture
3. Reflex sympathetic dystrophy (RSD)
4. Chronic tendonitis
5. Peroneal tendon subluxation
6. Occult fracture (i.e., base of 5th metatarsal)
7. Impingement
8. Neuroma

VII. MANAGEMENT OF ACHILLES TENDON INJURIES
A. Exclude Achilles tendon rupture—Thompson squeeze test
B. Rest
C. NSAIDs
D. Heel lift
E. Iontophoresis
F. Gentle stretching exercises
G. Consider short leg walking cast
H. Avoid steroid injection

CLINICAL PEARLS
- The typical mechanism of injury of a lateral ankle sprain is by inversion, which frequently occurs with some degree of plantar flexion
- Ecchymosis extending proximally from the ankle to the lower leg may indicate a tibiofibular syndesmotic injury. Syndesmotic sprains tend to require a more prolonged recovery time
- The tibiofibular syndesmosis is a commonly associated injury with injury to the deltoid ligament
- Osteochondral fractures of the talar dome are typically diagnosed 4–6 weeks after an ankle "sprain" that does not heal
- In studies of patients with ankle sprains, no difference was found in the number of patient complaints or residual ankle stability between those who were casted and those who were not
- If patients develop chronic ankle instability and pain following a sprain, it is generally because of inadequate rehabilitation

References
Garrick JG. Managing ankle sprains: keys to preserving motion and strength. The Phys & Sportsmed 1997;25(3):56–8.
Rubin A, Sallis R. Evaluation and diagnosis of ankle injuries. Am Fam Phys 1996;54(5):1609–18.
Mercier LR, et al. Practical orthopedics. 4th ed. St. Louis: Mosby-Year book, 1995.
Bates B. A guide to physical examination and history taking. Philadelphia:J.B. Lippincott, 1991;509–10.

Michael B. Weinstock, MD
Ed Boudreau, DO

81. KNEE INJURIES

I. ANATOMY
  A. **Bursae:** Provide lubrication between dynamic components
  B. **Cruciate ligaments**
   1. Anterior cruciate ligament (ACL): Stabilizes knee to prevent anterior motion of the tibia
   2. Posterior cruciate ligament (PCL): Stabilizes knee to prevent posterior motion of the tibia
  C. **External tendons and ligaments**
   1. Patellar tendon
   2. Collateral ligaments
      a. Medial collateral ligament (MCL)
      b. Lateral collateral ligament (LCL)
  D. **Muscles**
   1. Knee flexors
      a. Hamstrings
      b. Gastrocnemius
   2. Knee extensors: Quadriceps (Continues on as the patellar tendon)
  E. **Articulations**
   1. Lateral and medial tibiofemoral articulations
   2. Patellofemoral articulation

II. HISTORY
  A. **Acute trauma:** Pain which began suddenly during a certain activity. Position of the knee when injured (flexed, extended etc), or as a result of a direct blow to a certain area of the knee
  B. **Chronic trauma:** Certain activities (which the patient chronically engages in) which exacerbate the knee pain
  C. **Swelling** immediately after injury: Suggests meniscal or ligamentous injury
  D. **Locking/Buckling of the knee:** Catching or "give way" episodes (meniscal injury)
  E. **History of patellar dislocation**
  F. **Problems elsewhere in the lower extremity:** One joint above and one joint below
   1. Hip problems
   2. Foot problems
   3. New shoes, etc
  G. **Systemic illness**
   1. Polyarthralgias
   2. Fever
   3. Morning stiffness
   4. History of gout, hyperuricemia, rheumatoid arthritis, or pseudogout
  H. **Past history of knee injury**
  I. **Past surgeries on the knee**

III. PHYSICAL: Compare to uninjured side
  A. **Visually inspect knee** for swelling, evidence of past surgeries/injuries, abrasions, contusions, ecchymosis, erythema, patellar location. Visually inspect leg muscles for atrophy, leg length discrepancies, etc.
  B. **Patella**
   1. Palpate for effusion
      a. Inspection: With the patient seated and both knees flexed 90°, observe for a bulge on either side of the patellar ligament in the symptomatic knee
      b. Ballottement: The patient lies supine with knee extended and the examiner's first hand compresses from above and also on both sides of the patella then the examiner's other hand compresses the patella to see if it is ballotable
      c. Carlin maneuver: With patient supine, milk or squeeze the suprapatellar area and with the other hand place fingers on either side of the patellar tendon palpate for fluid

redistribution or bulging of accumulated fluid
2. Evaluate for hypermobility of the patella by attempting to sublux the patella laterally
3. Apprehension sign: Pain and involuntary contraction of the quadriceps with deviation of the patella laterally

C. Lachman test: Test for ACL injury
1. Method: Have the patient supine and the leg in slight external rotation and the knee in 15° of flexion (often the foot is slightly off the edge of the table). Example for left knee: With the examiner on the patient's right, grasp the lateral aspect of the distal thigh with the left hand and the medial aspect of the proximal lower leg with the right hand and pull anteriorly on the lower leg (with the right hand)
2. Results: The test is positive if there is anterior laxity. This is the most sensitive test for ACL injury

D. Drawer tests: Test for ACL or PCL injury
1. Method: Anterior and posterior drawer tests—patient is supine with the hip flexed 45° and the knee flexed 90° and the plantar aspect of the foot resting on the table. The examiner sits on the patient's foot and then grasps the proximal aspect of the lower leg with both hands and attempts to anteriorly or posteriorly displace the tibia on the femur
2. Results: Anterior subluxation of the tibia on the femur suggests injury to the ACL and posterior subluxation suggests injury to the PCL

E. Varus-valgus stress test: MCL or LCL injury
1. Method: Patient is supine with knee flexed about 20° and a varus or valgus stress is placed on the knee with the examiner's hand
2. Results: Laxity with valgus stress suggests injury to the MCL, and laxity with varus stress suggests injury to the LCL

F. McMurray test: Test for meniscus injury
1. Method: With the patient supine and the knee flexed at 90°, externally rotate the foot and then extend the knee. Repeat with the foot internally rotated, and then extend the knee
2. Results: A test is positive with pain and/or a palpable click at the medial or lateral joint lines occurring from the above maneuver

G. Apley grind test: Test for meniscus injury
1. Method: With the patient prone and the knee flexed at 90°, push straight down on the foot and then rotate the foot (compresses the meniscus). Repeat by pulling up on the foot and then rotating the foot
2. Results: If there is pain when the foot is pushed down, but no pain when the foot is pulled up, then consider a meniscus injury

H. Range of motion
I. Crepitus
J. Gait
K. Patellar grind
L. Strength
M. Flexibility
N. Reflexes

IV. RADIOGRAPHY/SPECIAL TESTS

A. Radiography: AP, lateral, patellar sunrise view are standard, both obliques if concerned about tibial plateau fracture. Cross table lateral can be helpful if looking for penetration of joint capsule or occult fracture
B. MRI: Good to evaluate meniscus injury/internal derangement, occult fracture or bone bruise
C. Arthroscopy
D. Arthrogram: Injection of contrast material and air into joint (rarely performed since MRI)
E. Aspiration of knee effusion: Aspirate to evaluate for hemarthrosis, infection (septic joint), fat globules (fracture), and for relief of symptoms

V. DIFFERENTIAL DIAGNOSIS AND MANAGEMENT OF COMMON KNEE PROBLEMS

A. Fracture: Obtain x-ray with appropriate suspicion (mechanism, swelling, deformity, joint tenderness etc.) and orthopedic referral if positive
B. Meniscus injury
1. History
   a. Twisting, flexion injury

  b. Inability to flex knee
  c. Difficulty in bearing weight
  d. Clicking or locking of the knee
  e. If chronic, may see intermittent effusions, locking, and possible quadriceps wasting
2. Physical
  a. Knee effusion
  b. Tenderness over joint line (Medial with medial meniscus injury, lateral with lateral meniscus injury)
  c. McMurray test and Apley test: See above for method
3. Acute management
  a. Rigid knee immobilizer (short term)
  b. Crutches
  c. Ice
  d. Rest
4. Refer to orthopedist if the patient is still symptomatic after 14 days of conservative management for consideration of MRI (sensitivity ~ 90%). Surgical management may include meniscus repair or excision

C. Ligament injuries
1. History
  a. Pain immediately at time of injury (mechanism of injury)
  b. Knee stiffness and tenderness
  c. Knee swelling (occasionally)
2. Physical
  a. Tenderness to palpation of ligament (MCL,LCL)
  b. Lachman test: Positive with ACL injury (see above)
  c. Drawer tests (Test for ACL, PCL injury)
  d. Tests for lateral instability (MCL, LCL)
3. Classification
  a. Grade I—Stretching of fibers without significant damage
  b. Grade II—Partial tear of fibers
  c. Grade III—Complete tear of fibers
4. Management
  a. Ice, elevation, rest
  b. Rigid knee immobilizer or posterior splint
  c. Crutches for grade II and III injuries
  d. Orthopedic/sports medicine referral/surgery
  e. Physical therapy

D. Patellofemoral syndrome
1. Etiology
  a. Lateral subluxation (Hypermobility of the patella)
    i. May be caused by increased angle between the quadriceps and patellar tendon (Q angle). This is called patella alta
    ii. Normal Q angle is up to 20° (women)
    iii. Patella alta can be identified on a lateral knee x-ray where the length of the patellar tendon exceeds the length of the patella by more than 1cm
    iv. Other causes include variation in hip anatomy that results in compensatory tibial torsion
  b. Chondromalacia: Damage to soft cartilage on posterior patella causing crepitus and pain
2. History
  a. Pain worsened by walking or running up or down hills, climbing stairs or kneeling
  b. Pain often disappears during activity and returns just after activity is completed
3. Physical
  a. Patella alta
  b. Hypermobility of the patella
  c. Pain or crepitus with patellofemoral movement
  d. Apprehension sign: Pain and involuntary contraction of the quadriceps with deviation of the patella laterally (associated with predisposition for patellofemoral syndrome, but is not diagnostic)

MUSC

      e. Patellar grind test
      f. Possibly knee effusion
    4. Evaluation in addition to history and physical includes lateral x-ray (to evaluate for patella alta or DJD) and sunrise view of the patella (to evaluate for lateral subluxation)
    5. Management
      a. Rest with possible use of crutches
      b. Ice
      c. NSAIDs
      d. Avoid sports until symptoms have subsided
      e. Physical therapy to strengthen quadriceps: Patellar realignment
      f. Consider orthotic to correct pronation of the foot
      g. Surgical consideration of conservative therapy fails

E. Osgood-Schlatter's Disease (Apophysitis of the tibial tubercle)
    1. General
      a. Common cause of knee pain in adolescents
      b. Secondary to repetitive avulsions of the patellar tendon where it inserts into the growth plate of the tibial tubercle
      c. Pain is at the insertion of the patellar tendon on the tibial tubercle
    2. History
      a. Pain with onset of activity
      b. Often bilateral
    3. Physical
      a. Enlargement and tenderness at the tibial tubercle
      b. Possible quadriceps atrophy
      c. Tightness of the quadriceps and hamstring muscles
    4. Management
      a. Avoid activities that involve knee extension (running, climbing, jumping, kicking) until symptoms have subsided ~6–8 weeks
      b. Range of motion and stretching: Physical therapy
      c. Oral analgesics
      d. Ice after activity
      e. Surgical management if pain persists after ossification is complete

F. Osteochondritis dissecans: Occurs secondary to ischemia
    1. General
      a. Loss of blood supply (avascular necrosis) to an area next to a joint surface
      b. The ischemic/dead bone and overlying cartilage gradually loosen and cause pain
      c. This osteochondral fragment may break loose into the joint and cause locking, sharp pain and effusion
    2. History: Gradual onset of swelling and vague pain. Worse with activity. Insidious onset may be over several months
    3. Physical: Often pain with palpation of the medial femoral condyle (most common site is the lateral portion of the medial condyle). Quadriceps wasting
    4. Management: Orthopedic referral

G. Other
    1. Prepatellar bursitis
    2. Retropatellar bursitis
    3. Patellar tendonitis
    4. Fat pad syndrome
    5. Pes anserinus bursitis
    6. Neoplasm
    7. Loose bodies

H. Arthritis: See Chapter 64, Differential Diagnosis of Arthritis; Chapter 65, Osteoarthritis; Chapter 66, Rheumatoid Arthritis

CLINICAL PEARLS
    • Tears of the medial meniscus are 10 times as common as tears of the lateral meniscus
    • Following meniscectomy, patients may have joint space narrowing and arthritic changes

MUSC

- Osgood-Schlatter's disease occurs most commonly from age 11–15 and affects males more than females
- Osteochondritis dissecans predisposes to degenerative arthritis

References

Juhn MS. Patellofemoral pain syndrome: a review and guidelines for treatment. Am Fam Phys 1999;60:2012-22.

Cutbill JW, Ladly KO, Bray RC, Thorne P, Verhoef M. Anterior knee pain: a review. Clin J Sport Med 1997;7:40-5.

Smith BW, et al. Knee injuries: part I. History and physical examination. Am Fam Phys 1995;51:615.

Smith BW, et al. Acute knee injuries: part II. Diagnosis and management. Am Fam Phys 1995;51:799.

Ruffin MT, et al. Anterior knee pain: the challenge of patellofemural syndrome. Am Fam Phys 1993;47:185.

Doug DiOrio, MD

82. SHOULDER INJURIES

I. SHOULDER ANATOMY AND BIOMECHANICS

A. Introduction: Normal shoulder function is a combination of the anatomic arrangement and the complex action of many muscles. The shoulder is the joint with the largest range of motion, but this allows for more instability. Shoulder injuries are common in the general population but the extra stresses placed on the joint in athletic activities give it high potential for injury and dysfunction. Because of the high degree of functional interplay a single small injury to the shoulder may lead to functional deficit which potentiates damage to other structures

B. Anatomy
1. Sternoclavicular joint (synovial joint)
2. Acromioclavicular joint
3. Glenohumeral joint (golf ball on a tee)
4. Humeral head
5. Glenoid fossa
6. Joint capsule (lax)
7. Glenohumeral ligaments
8. Rotator cuff
9. Scapula rotators (trapezius, rhomboids, levator scapulae, serratus anterior)

C. Biomechanics
1. Elevation
2. Internal and external rotation
3. Horizontal flexion and extension
4. Scapulohumeral rhythm
5. Glenohumeral motion
6. Scapular motion

D. Outline of chapter
1. Shoulder instability/dislocation
2. Rotator cuff disease
3. Acromioclavicular dislocation
4. Adhesive capsulitis (frozen shoulder)
5. Impingement
6. Biceps tendon injuries

II. SHOULDER INSTABILITY

A. Introduction: Shoulder instability (symptomatic abnormal glenohumeral translation) is a common problem, especially in the overhead athlete. Both acute and chronic instability of the shoulder should be considered in athletes with shoulder pain. Anterior instability is the most common and can range from subluxation to complete dislocation. Instability can also result from repetitive microtrauma as the ligaments are stretched

MUSC

B. History
1. Anterior: The shoulder is usually abducted and externally rotated. A force is applied to the arm causing more external rotation and extension. This event is very painful and the athlete may feel the shoulder slide out of place. The athlete may have associated symptoms of a "dead arm" for seconds to minutes following the event. If the shoulder does not relocate spontaneously the athlete will hold the arm abducted and externally rotated
2. Posterior: The shoulder is usually in a flexed, adducted, and internally rotated position and a force applied to the hand causes the posterior dislocation. This happens with falls and in offensive linemen in football. Also with electrical shock and seizures. The arm will be held adducted and internally rotated and the coracoid will be prominent
3. Multidirectional or recurrent: Pain is the usual complaint that brings the patients to see the doctor. These injuries can masquerade as many other injuries because of disrupted biomechanics of the shoulder

C. Physical exam
1. True apprehension sign is the most sensitive exam finding
2. Fowler sign: Relief of apprehension with posterior directed pressure
3. Sulcus sign: Distance between the lateral border of the acromion and the humeral head
4. Load testing
5. For recurrent injuries check for signs of nerve palsies. Also there may be a loss of internal rotation (10°) and crepitus with ROM. Think of impingement as a sign of instability (Injection test)

D. Complications
1. Hill-Sachs fracture of posterior humeral head
2. Bankart fracture of the glenoid
3. Axillary nerve and artery injury
4. Rotator cuff and biceps tendon injury
5. Chondromalacia and AC degeneration

E. Radiography
1. Plain films: AP (look for Hill-Sachs fracture), Transscapular Y view, Axillary (West Point view)
2. MRI: Now becoming the follow-up test of choice over the CT and arthrogram. There is little use for MRI in pre-surgical decision making in open or arthroscopic repair. It is more useful with recurrent instability and determining associated complications (labral tears, chondral defects)

F. Management
1. Dislocation
   a. To reduce "recreate the mechanism" Rowe maneuver (touch opposite ear), Stimson (Prone with traction weights), double sheet, lift. For posterior you need lateral traction followed by extension and adduction. May need open reduction
   b. Post reduction repeat plain films and immobilize 2–6 weeks. Rehabilitation will include early isometrics. Work on regaining external rotation but keep the shoulder below 90° of abduction. Strengthen rotator cuff and internal and external rotators. For posterior dislocation emphasize external rotators and deltoid. Work on coordination and endurance (swimming)
2. Chronic instability
   a. Rehabilitation goals include protecting shoulder from provocative movements, and regaining ROM and normal shoulder function. At first all exercises should remain in the scapular plane. Restoring normal scapulothoracic motion and strength (rowing etc.) will provide a stable base for the glenoid to allow proper humeral movement. Next working with theraband to improve dynamic stabilizers (rotator cuff, biceps, lats). Gradual return to sport specific exercise and play. Plan 3 to 6 months of therapy
   b. Surgical indications: Irreducible acutely, displaced tuberosity fracture, unstable glenoid rim fracture, absolute stabilization needed prior to return to sport, and loss of time not an option. Surgery is much better for anterior instability than posterior or multidirectional

G. Clinical Pearls
1. Need good on-field exam before reduction

MUSC

2. Static and dynamic shoulder stabilizers must function in sync to retain shoulder stability. The inferior glenohumeral ligament is the most important static stabilizer. The scapula is the base for shoulder stability
3. Shoulder pain is the most common symptom of shoulder instability
4. When you think of impingement, think of chronic instability
5. Asymptomatic laxity can be a normal variant, but may lead to chronic instability
6. Do not overlook scapulathoracic function in the rehab of the shoulder

III. ROTATOR CUFF DISEASE

A. History: The patient may present with a wide variety of signs and symptoms. These can range from minimal pain to marked pain, limited function, and decreased range of motion. Special attention should be given to throwing athletes because they are prone to overuse injuries. Chronic tendonitis may present with night pain. The pain is usually difficult for the patient to locate. Rotator cuff tear in patients younger than age 40 requires significant trauma

B. Physical
1. Tenderness over the greater tuberosity of the humerus
2. Painful abduction of the arm and positive drop arm test
3. Positive supraspinator test
4. Positive impingement sign
5. Weakness or pain with internal or external rotation

C. Radiography
1. Plain films: AP and lateral films
2. MRI may be used in either the acute or chronic tear if rehabilitation has failed

D. Management
1. Acute tears: Begin with conservative treatment with rest and ice and NSAIDs. Rehabilitation program to be started in 1 to 2 weeks. Pain and function in the program will be your guide to further treatment. If pain resolves, continue therapy. If no resolution, and function not improved, consider MRI and surgical referral. Part of the management may include arthroscopic surgery
2. Chronic tears: These are the majority of the cases. The rehabilitation program for these patients is most important. Even though the patient feels that this is a new problem you will be trying to correct a long period of compensation and improper biomechanics. Begin with a stretching and strengthening program, avoiding overhead activities. Ice, heat, message and ionophoresis may also have a role. NSAIDs may be used initially and corticosteroid injection may be indicated. If the patient improves, then slowly work in overhead activities and then sport specific activities. Biomechanics and training techniques may need to be examined and changed. If patient continues to have pain and loss of function consider MRI and surgical referral

E. Clinical Pearls
1. Rehabilitation (physical therapy) is the most important part of treatment
2. A partial thickness tear may easily progress to full thickness tear
3. Age is one of the great dividers in this injury

IV. ADHESIVE CAPSULITIS (Frozen shoulder)

A. Introduction: This is a process of capsular thickening and contraction of the shoulder joint that results in pain and limited mobility. It is caused by fibrosis of the subsynovial layer. It is more common in middle aged, women and diabetics. The number one predisposing factor is a prolonged period of inactivity

B. History: The patient almost always has some history of prolonged immobilization of the shoulder in the past. This may have been in the remote past but the patient has a new job or demand on the shoulder that she is unable to do. Other symptoms include nocturnal pain and pain with movement

C. Physical exam: Limited active and passive ROM in all directions especially abduction. In abduction the patient will rely on scapulothoracic movement to abduct the arm. The patient may have tenderness around the capsule and a thickened capsule to palpation

D. Radiology: AP and lateral views of the shoulder should be obtained. A decrease volume of the glenohumeral joint will be present in most cases. Arthrography is also used in evaluation in some cases

E. Management: Treatment begins with NSAIDs and range of motion exercises. Patient should rest the arm in between exercises and sometimes a sling is used. Physical therapy is a must for distinct regimen of increasing ROM. Sometimes the frozen shoulder will resolve spontaneously but in most cases prolonged treatment is needed. Progression should be followed and ROM should be documented. Steroid injections are used commonly but don't always help. In difficult cases manipulation under anesthesia is used. Rarely surgical intervention is needed but it does not have a great success rate

V. IMPINGEMENT

A. Introduction: The theory behind impingement syndrome is based on the fact that there is a fixed space and structures that must fit in that space. There are two reasons for impingement: increase in volume of the structures in the space (muscle hypertrophy, inflammation, trauma) and decreased available space (fibrositis, osteophyte, convex acromion)

B. History: Patients present with a "toothache-like" pain in the shoulder. Worse with overhead movements. Inquire about past history of any injuries to the shoulder (subluxations or rotator cuff) and any medical problems (inflammatory diseases)

C. Physical exam: Findings are consistent with early rotator cuff disease. The patient should not have any weakness of the cuff muscles. There will be a positive impingement sign

D. Radiology: AP and lateral views

E. Management: Relative rest with avoidance of overhead (greater than 90°) movements. Physical therapy for stretching and rehab of muscles. NSAIDs followed by injection of steroids in 2–4 weeks. Surgery may be needed in cases that do not improve or those that have osteophytes as the primary problem

F. Clinical Pearls

1. Think of shoulder instability as possible cause of the problem
2. Impingement is stage 1 of rotator cuff disease and may progress if not treated

VI. BICEPS TENDON INJURIES

A. Introduction: The biceps' primary function is supination of the arm but also acts as an elbow flexor and helps depress the humeral head. There are 3 types of biceps tendon injuries: tendonitis, dislocation and rupture

B. History: Tendonitis can be an overuse syndrome which is found in overhead throwing athletes and carpenters. Also a sudden violent extension of the arm may cause a strain of the tendon. Dislocation of the tendon occurs with a force that interrupts forward movement of the arm while in abduction and external rotation. A classic example is the quarterback getting hit while releasing the ball. This can also occur as an overuse injury. The patient presents with pain in the anterior arm and a clicking sensation. Tendon rupture is usually caused by a force that extends the arm. A snap or pop is felt with immediate pain. The other mechanism for rupture is degenerative rotator cuff tear which progresses and tears the biceps tendon

C. Physical exam: Pain with resisted flexion of the elbow and supination must be present. A positive Yeargason's test. Look for the Popeye deformity with tendon rupture. Palpate for the click and movement of the tendon with flexion and external rotation

D. Radiology: X-rays are not necessary unless other pathology is being ruled out or if surgical intervention is needed

E. Management

1. Tendonitis is managed conservatively with NSAIDs and relative rest. This is followed by physical therapy. Injection of steroids is controversial and not recommended at present
2. Tendon dislocation is treated with relative rest and rehabilitation. If the patient has a shallow bicipital groove and recurrently dislocates, surgery may be needed to repair the transverse humeral ligament
3. Tendon rupture: A surgical consult should be obtained. Acute tears are repairable but conservative treatment is used much of the time. In degenerative tears surgical repair is much more difficult. Usually there is a 10% strength loss of the biceps after conservative treatment

References
Ebenbichler GR, et al. Ultrasound therapy for calcific tendinitis of the shoulder. N Engl J Med May 20, 1999; 340:1533-8.

Winters JC, et al. Treatment of shoulder complaints in general practice: long-term results of a randomised, single blind study comparing physiotherapy, manipulation, and corticosteroid injection. BMJ May 22, 1999;318:1395-6.

van der Windt DA, et al. Effectiveness of corticosteroid injections versus physiotherapy for treatment of painful stiff shoulder in primary care: randomised trial. BMJ November 7, 1998;317:1292-6.

Larson HM, et al. Shoulder pain: The role of diagnostic injections. Am Fam Phys 1996;53:1637.

Rodgers JA, Crosby LA. Rotator cuff disorders. Am Fam Phys 1996;54:127.

Douglas L. Moore MD
Tim Scanlon, PA-C

83. ELBOW INJURIES

I. ANATOMY
A. The olecranon humeral joint is a hinge joint
B. Articulations
    1. Radius articulates with the capitulum and ulna with the trochlea
    2. Proximal articulations between ulna and the head of the radius
C. Lateral joint space is supported by the radial and ulnar collateral ligament complexes
D. The upper extremity is innervated by the 5 nerve branches that originate at the brachial plexus (axillary, radial, musculocutaneous, ulnar and median nerves). The ulnar nerve is found easily by palpation in the groove behind the medial epicondyle
E. Just proximal to the elbow joint, the brachial artery bifurcates into the radial and ulnar arteries, which supply blood to the distal portion of the upper extremities

II. PATHOPHYSIOLOGY
A. In adults most injuries occur to ligaments, tendons, or bone itself
B. In children, the weakest links are the growth plates, apophysis and epiphysis
C. Tendon damage often occurs secondary to overuse and microrupture
D. Repetitive strains may lead to ligament damage, chondromalacia, osteophytes, tendonosis, neuritis, loose bodies, or osteochondritis dessicans
E. Overhead throwing can lead to medial tension overload, lateral compression, and posterior olecranon impaction

III. ELBOW PAIN BY ANATOMIC LOCATION
A. Lateral elbow pain
    1. Lateral epicondylitis (Tennis elbow): Overload of forearm extensors, mainly extensor carpi radialis brevis causing microscopic ruptures and inflammation at the insertion to the bone
        a. History: Patient complains of pain, especially with combing hair, playing tennis or golf, shaking hands
        b. Physical exam: Pain over the tendon about 1–2cm distal to the lateral epicondyle. Pain is exacerbated by active extension of the wrist or passive flexion
        c. Management: Conservative therapy with ice, NSAIDs, and physical therapy is usually successful. If not better after 1–2 weeks consider steroid injection (See Chapter 86, Corticosteroid Injection of Joints). Enforcing proper technique, decreasing string tension on racquet, applying a cushioned grip and use of counter force bracing are also important therapies. Strengthening of the muscle may be accomplished by extending the fingers with an elastic band stretched over them or by reverse wrist curls. If not better after 12–16 weeks, consider surgery
    2. Radial nerve entrapment
        a. History: Patient complains of local pain, paresthesias, dull ache
        b. Physical exam: Pain in forearm often with radiation proximal and distal. Pain exacerbated by supination and resisted extension of middle finger with wrist in neutral position. Tenderness often 2–3cm distal to lateral epicondyle. May be aggravated by counter bracing
        c. Management: Rest, NSAIDs, and rehabilitation. Surgical release for resistant cases

MUSC

       d. Think of radial nerve entrapment in cases of resistant tennis elbow
  3. Radiocapitellar Overload Syndrome
       a. History: Pain with overhead throwing
       b. Caused by radial head impaction on the capitellum during valgus stress of the elbow accompanied by medial instability. May consist of radiocapitellar chondromalacia, radiocapitellar degeneration, osteochondral fracture, or loose bodies
       c. Physical exam: Patient will have lateral pain and occasionally locking of the elbow

B. Medial elbow pain
  1. Medial epicondylitis (Golfer's elbow)
       a. History: Sharp pain, trouble lifting objects
       b. Physical: Pain at the common flexor origin. Sometimes affects pronator teres and flexor carpi radialis as well. Pain with resisted flexion, pronation, and passive extension
       c. Management: If 1 week of conservative treatment (ice, NSAIDs) not helpful, consider steroid injection. Squeezing a soft ball or wrist curls help strengthen the muscles involved. Surgery only in resistant cases
  2. Medial elbow instability
       a. History: Pain over medial elbow usually during acceleration phase of throwing
       b. Physical exam: Focal tenderness 2cm distal to medial epicondyle, decreased range of motion, pain with valgus stress, and asymmetric valgus laxity between elbows
       c. X-ray: May see small avulsion fracture on x-ray. Stress radiographs may help in diagnosis
       d. Management: In acute tears, conservative measures are treatment of choice for non-athletes. Elite athletes may respond better to surgery. About 50% of chronic tears will respond to conservative measures alone. Steroid injection is contraindicated. Return to competition when pain free, full range of motion, full strength, and coordination returned
  3. Ulnar neuritis
       a. History: Localized pain with paresthesia
       b. Acute pain over medial elbow with radiation down arm caused by repeated traction, compression, or friction on nerve
       c. Physical exam: There may be numbness or tingling in the small and ring fingers. The nerve may feel doughy or thick and there may be a positive Tinnel's sign
       d. Management: Conservative measures preferred. May splint at 30° if chronic subluxation of nerve present. If surgery required must be certain to fix any concomitant ulnar collateral ligament damage

C. Posterior elbow pain
  1. Triceps tendonitis
       a. History and physical: Pain over triceps tendon exacerbated by resisted elbow extension
       b. Management: Initial management with ice, NSAIDs, physical therapy. Rupture is rare and treated by direct surgical repair
  2. Valgus extension overload syndrome
       a. Insidious onset of pain with full extension exacerbated by valgus stress. Caused by impingement of the olecranon allowed by ulnar collateral instability and repetitive valgus stress
       b. Physical exam: May find tenderness at the tip of the olecranon with the elbow in 45° of flexion
       c. X-ray: May reveal osteophytes of the olecranon
       d. Management: Conservative measures preferred, but if osteophytes present surgery is required
  3. Stress fracture of the olecranon
       a. Pain over olecranon with throwing. Due to the repetitive sudden snap at full extension. May need bone scan, CT, or tomogram to diagnose if not seen on standard x-ray
       b. Management: Rest if the fracture is stable. Surgery if conservative measures fail
  4. Triceps apophysitis
       a. Seen in children and is similar to Osgood-Schlatter's disease of the knee. The patient has pain with resisted extension and is tender over the olecranon
       b. Management: Internal fixation with bone grafting
  5. Olecranon bursitis
       a. Present with a distended soft posterior elbow
       b. Management: Ice and compression. May aspirate the bursa if the elbow has decreased range of motion. Send for fluid analysis to ensure not infectious. Can inject with steroids

MUSC

D. Anterior elbow pain

1. Anterior capsule stretch or tear: Can occur secondary to fall on extended elbow, resisted flexion, forceful supination, hyper extension, or direct trauma. Conservative measures are recommended
2. Pronator teres syndrome: Radiating forearm pain with numbness and tingling in distribution of median nerve. Physical exam reveals pain with active pronation and resisted long finger extension
3. Distal biceps tendon rupture
    a. Most often occurs when the elbow is flexed to 90° and the contraction is overcome by a sudden extension force
    b. Physical exam will reveal a palpable deformity, balling of the biceps muscle, decreased strength in elbow flexion and supination, and ecchymosis in the antecubital fossa
    c. Acute surgical anatomic repair is treatment of choice
4. Brachialis tendonitis (Climber's elbow)
    a. Secondary to overuse with the elbow in a pronated and semi-flexed position
    b. Management: Conservative

E. Subluxation of the radial head (nursemaid's elbow)

1. Definition and mechanism of injury
    a. Subluxation of the radial head is common among preschool children. Before age 7 the radial head is the same size as the radial neck. After age 7 the radial head is larger than the radial neck and subluxation is not common
    b. Mechanism of injury is sudden traction on the hand with the elbow extended and the forearm pronated. Forceful traction fibers, which encircle the radial neck, slip and become trapped between the radial head and capitellum
2. History
    a. Important to elicit a history of traction on the child's hand; the act may have been unrecognized by the parent or the history withheld because of a feeling of guilt
    b. About 50% of the radial head subluxations present with an atypical history
3. Physical exam
    a. Clinically the child may present irritable, playful or comfortably in the parents' lap. The common symptom is the unwillingness to use the extremity
    b. Any child not using an arm that is flexed and pronated and without signs of signs of trauma should be considered to have a radial head subluxation, unless the history strongly suggests another diagnosis
4. Evaluation: Radiographs are not necessary, unless another diagnosis is being considered or if reduction is not accomplished
5. Management
    a. Reduction is carried out by firmly placing the thumb over the radial head while the other hand is placed on the wrist. The forearm is fully supinated. If a "click" is not felt, the elbow is flexed. This maneuver may be repeated if the initial attempt does not reduce the subluxation
    b. If a second attempt is not successful then x-rays should be taken of the elbow
    c. Reduction as evidenced by a "click" is highly predictive and will result in relief from pain and, shortly thereafter, use of the affected arm
    d. After the first subluxation, no immobilization is required. For recurrent subluxations, the patient's arm should be immobilized in a sling. Should be referred for orthopedic consultation

CLINICAL PEARLS

- Conservative treatment equals PRICEMM; Protection, Rest, Ice, Compression, Elevation, Medicines, Modalities (ultrasound, ionophoresis, electro stimulation)
- "Little League Elbow" is actually a constellation of diseases seen in skeletally immature athletes including medial epicondylar apophysitis, osteochondrosis of the radial head, osteochondrosis of the capitellum, and non union of a stress fracture of the olecranon epiphysis. Due to overuse of overhead throwing
- If triceps tendonitis doesn't heal, consider an olecranon stress fracture
- Always encourage proper sporting technique, stretching, strengthening, and proper fitting equipment

References

Chumbley EM et al. Evaluation of overuse elbow injuries. Am Fam Phys 2000;61:691-700.

Hay EM, et al. Pragmatic randomised controlled trial of local corticosteroid injection and naproxen for treatment of lateral epicondylitis of elbow in primary care. BMJ Oct 9, 1999;319:964-8.

Mahaffey BL, Smith PA. Shoulder instability in young athletes. Am Fam Phys 1999;59:2773.

Calmbach WL, Gomez J. Injuries about the elbow. In: Sallis RE, Massimino F, eds. Essentials of sports medicine. St. Louis: Mosby, 1997:313-24.

Safran MR: Elbow injuries in athletes. Clinical Orthopaedics and Related Research 1995;310:257–77.

Torg JS, Shephard RJ: Elbow. Current therapy in sports medicine. St Louis, Mosby 104–46, 1995.

Foley AE. Tennis elbow. Am Fam Phys 1993;48:281.

Michael B. Weinstock, MD

84. CARPAL TUNNEL SYNDROME

DEFINITION: Syndrome caused by compression of the median nerve as it passes through the carpal tunnel

I. SIGNS AND SYMPTOMS

A. Paresthesias and burning in the fingers of affected hand (particularly the thumb, index, and middle fingers)

B. Symptoms frequently occur at night, which are relieved by shaking or rubbing hands

C. *Tinel's sign:* Tingling sensation (electric shock) in fingers when the anterior aspect of the wrist is tapped with the examiner's fingers

D. *Phalen's sign:* Symptoms reproduced by full flexion of the wrist for 60 seconds

E. Weakness of affected hand

F. Atrophy of thenar eminence

II. ETIOLOGY

A. Repetitive motion injury

B. Trauma, Colles' fracture, degenerative joint disease, rheumatoid arthritis, ganglion cyst

C. Hyperparathyroidism, hypocalcemia

D. Associated with diabetes, hypothyroidism, pregnancy

III. DIAGNOSIS

A. **Clinical diagnosis:** Exclude reversible causes by obtaining thyroid studies and blood sugar

B. **Electromyography:** Will be abnormal > 85% of the time. Will show prolonged distal latency of the median nerve with reduced sensory nerve action potential. The ulnar nerve should also be stimulated to rule out polyneuropathy

IV. DIFFERENTIAL DIAGNOSIS

A. Cervical spondylosis/radiculopathy

B. Generalized peripheral neuropathy

C. Brachial plexus lesion

D. Vascular insufficiency

E. Thoracic outlet obstruction

V. MANAGEMENT

A. **Non-operative:** Reassess efficacy in 4–6 weeks

   1. Splint wrist in extension, especially at night (cock-up wrist splint)

   2. NSAIDs: **Ibuprofen** 400–600mg PO TID–QID, **Naprosyn** 375–500mg PO BID, etc.

   3. Injection of the carpal tunnel with **Hydrocortisone**. Especially useful in pregnancy (See Chapter 86, Corticosteroid Injection of Joints)

B. **Operative**

   1. Provides relief in > 95% of patients

   2. Usually done on an outpatient basis under local anesthesia

   3. The hand may be fully utilized in 4–6 weeks

C. **Prevention:** A break should be taken once per hour when doing repetitive work

References
Dammers JW HH, et al. Injection with methylprednisolone proximal to the carpal tunnel: randomised double blind trial. BMJ Oct 2, 1999;319:884-6.
Chang MH, et. al. Oral drug of choice in carpal tunnel syndrome. Neurology Aug 1998;51:390-3.
Steyers CM. Practical management of carpal tunnel syndrome. Phys & Sports Med 1995;23:83–8.
Katz JN, et al. The carpal tunnel syndrome: diagnostic utility of the history and physical examination findings. Ann Int Med 1990;112:321.

Chuck Levy, MD
Daniel M. Neides, MD

85. LOW BACK PAIN

I. INTRODUCTION

    A. Low back pain (LBP) is one of the most common ambulatory complaints, with a 60–90% lifetime incidence

    B. LBP is the second most common cause of repeat office visits and the most common cause of disability in patients < age 45

    C. It is important to perform a thorough history and physical examination to exclude a systemic disease as an etiology of the pain

II. HISTORY AND PHYSICAL EXAMINATION

The goals are to exclude systemic disease, characterize neurologic deficits, determine the etiology of LBP, and to differentiate mechanical vs. non-mechanical pain

    A. History

      1. Determine mechanism of injury, onset, and duration

      2. Constancy (intermittent, constant, or waxing and waning)

      3. Distribution (focal, extended, or radiating)

      4. Episodic (determine if similar pain has occurred in the past)

      5. Aggravating factors

      6. Positional pain (which positions make pain better or worse)

      7. Presence (or absence) of sciatica

      8. Bowel or bladder dysfunction

      9. Previous drug and/or therapeutic treatments (and their success or failure)

    B. Physical examination

      1. Begin with observation of posture and gait

      2. Motor examination includes hip flexion (L2), knee extension (L3), ankle dorsiflexion (L4), great toe dorsiflexion (L5), and ankle plantarflexion (S1)

GRADING OF MUSCLE STRENGTH

Grade 0:	No movement
Grade 1:	Trace movement without joint motion
Grade 2:	Partially or fully moves body part with gravity eliminated
Grade 3:	Completely moves body part against gravity
Grade 4:	Moves body part against moderate resistance through full range of motion
Grade 5:	Normal

      3. Reflex examination includes patella or knee jerk (L4), hamstring (L5), and Achilles or ankle (S1)

      4. Because the sensory exam can be quite time consuming, instruct the patient to point out areas of sensory deprivation and compare to a dermatomal map

      5. Limitation of lumbosacral range of motion should be noted in extension, flexion, side-bending, and rotation; palpation of the low back and buttocks can help localize pain and detect tender or "trigger points"

      6. Straight leg raise test: Passive elevation of the lower extremity on the symptomatic side to less than 60° while the patient is supine; the test is positive with resulting radicular pain. Sensitivity is 95%, specificity is 40%

III. DIAGNOSTIC STUDIES

    A. Radiologic studies: Generally overused. *If a careful history and physical examination indicate acute musculoskeletal/radicular LBP in a patient age 20–50, radiologic imaging is unnecessary*

MUSC

    1. Indications for plain x-rays—when you suspect:
      a. Neoplasm
      b. Compression fracture
      c. Spondylolisthesis: Usually L5 slips forward on S1 because of fracture or degeneration
        of the articular process of the neural arch
      d. Spondylosis (defect in the neural arch usually in the pars interarticularis)
      e. Trauma
      f. Patient is involved in a legal case
    2. Indications for MRI or CT
      a. When symptoms progress despite appropriate conservative therapy
      b. Prior to surgery
      c. Should only be ordered when results would significantly affect treatment
    3. Bone scan: Indicated to determine the presence of a pars interarticularis stress reaction or to
      determine the acuity of spondylosis
  B. Electrodiagnostic studies (EMG) assess the neurophysiologic status of the nerve fibers
    1. Indications
      a. To establish (or exclude) the diagnosis of radiculopathy
      b. To localize nerve lesions and characterize their extent, severity, chronicity, and prognosis
      c. To search for the presence of "vulnerable nerves" due to peripheral neuropathy
      d. Particularly important if surgery is being considered
    2. Not recommended
      a. Studies earlier than 3 weeks after injury may not show full extent of pathology
      b. If clinical history and examination are strongly suggestive of radiculopathy, conserva-
        tive therapy may be initiated without EMG

IV. TWO CATEGORIES OF LBP
  A. Mechanical/discogenic
    1. Acute undetermined soft tissue injury (LUMBOSACRAL SPRAIN): May present with lum-
      bosacral pain following a traumatic injury or possibly accompanied by a tearing sensation
      while lifting
      a. History and physical examination reveal no evidence of radiculopathy
      b. Treatment
        i. NSAIDs and Acetaminophen to help with pain relief
        ii. Physical therapy emphasizes stretching hamstrings, gluteals, hip flexors, and tensor
          fascia lata
        iii. Instruction on strengthening of extensor muscles (walking, jogging, swimming)
          and proper lifting techniques
    2. Acute discogenic LBP (HERNIATED DISC): Caused by either *disruption of the annular
      fibers of the disc* or *herniation of the disc* with resulting nerve root impingement
      (radiculopathy)
      a. Radiculopathy almost always involves the L5 or S1 nerve root
      b. The peak age for herniated disc disease is age 30–55
      c. History: Usually includes a previous episode of similar LBP that resolved spontane-
        ously in 3–5 days; patients often complain that pain is worse in a seated position;
        occurs after lifting or trauma
      d. Treatment
        i. Bed rest (no more than 7–10 days) with adequate pain control
        ii. A steroid taper or NSAIDs to decrease inflammation and provide relief
        iii. Physical therapy should include passive lumbar extension exercises unless these
          exacerbate symptoms, in which case isometric flexion exercises may be tried
    3. Chronic LBP: Most episodes of acute LBP respond by 10–12 weeks. Pain beyond this time
      frame should result in the following actions
      a. Review the diagnosis to exclude systemic disease
      b. Determine patient compliance with activity modifications and medications
      c. Review the type of treatment the patient is receiving in physical therapy
      d. Screen for an underlying *depression* (See Chapter 100, Depression and Dysthymia) or
        myofascial pain/fibromyalgia
      e. Look for Waddel Signs on physical examination (at least 3 indicate a psychologic or

MUSC

non-organic component of the pain)
    i. Inappropriate or widespread tenderness
    ii. Pain on simulated physical maneuvers
    iii. Inconsistent exam while the patient is distracted
    iv. Regional non-anatomic distribution of pain or weakness
    v. Overreaction to exam (excess moaning or grimacing)

B. Non-mechanical
  1. Cancer: Multiple myeloma, metastatic disease to bone from lung, prostate, kidney, or breast. Inquire about previous cancer history, recent weight loss, failure to improve with conservative therapy, or pain that awakens patient from sleep
  2. Gynecologic: Determine change in menstrual pattern, possibility of pregnancy, risk of pelvic inflammatory disease (PID), and gynecologic malignancy
  3. Renal: Dysuria, hematuria, history of UTIs, or nephrolithiasis
  4. Rheumatoid arthritis: Morning stiffness > 1hr, improvement with exercise, gradual onset of symptoms, and pain duration > 3 months
  5. Gastrointestinal: History or symptoms consistent with peptic ulcer disease (PUD)
  6. Osteoporosis/compression fractures: Determine history of corticosteroid use or osteoporosis (See Chapter 106, Compression Fractures)
  7. Vascular: Abdominal aortic aneurysm (AAA)

V. TREATMENT
  A. NSAIDs: Will help decrease inflammation and alleviate pain. Recommended for both acute (treat for 14–21 days) and chronic LBP
    1. **Ibuprofen** 400–800mg PO TID   6. **Indocin** 25–50mg PO BID–TID
    2. **Ansaid** 100mg PO BID-TID   7. **Lodine** 300mg PO TID or 400mg PO BID
    3. **Clinoril** 150mg PO BID   8. **Naprosyn** 375mg PO TID or 500mg PO BID
    4. **Daypro** 600mg PO QD   9. **Relafen** 500mg PO BID or 1g PO QD
    5. **Feldene** 20mg PO QD   10. **Voltaren** 50mg PO BID–TID
  B. Narcotic analgesics: May be used in the acute setting but not recommended for long-term therapy secondary to abuse potential: **Percocet, Vicodin**, and **Darvocet**. Avoid using longer than 7–10 days
  Note: Elderly patients should receive lower doses of either narcotics or muscle relaxants ($^1/_2$ to $^1/_3$ recommended dose). See Chapter 104, Medication Use in the Elderly
  C. Muscle relaxants: May be used for acute pain but not recommended for long-term therapy. Avoid using longer than 7–10 days
    1. **Flexeril:** 10mg PO TID
    2. **Soma:** 350mg PO QID
    3. **Robaxin:** 750mg PO QID
    4. **Norflex:** 100mg PO BID
    5. **Parafon Forte:** 500mg PO QID
  D. Physical therapy: Communication between the physician and the physical therapist is essential
  E. Surgery
    1. Indications for surgery
      a. Progressive neurological deficit
      b. Incapacitating leg pain with demonstrated neural compromise
      c. Failure of conservative therapy
    2. For lumbar stenosis, indications for surgery include severe nerve root encroachment on imaging studies and incapacitating leg pain and paresthesias which severely restrict ambulation
    3. Prerequisites for surgery include demonstrated disc herniation (CT, MRI, or myelogram), sensory or motor deficits in the appropriate dermatome or myotome, and failure of at least 6 weeks of conservative treatment
    4. The natural history of herniated disc disease is resolution, but even for those with proven radiculopathy and disc herniation, surgery is elective (unless progressive neurologic deficit occurs)
    5. Up to 60% of patients *without* LBP will have evidence of disc bulge or protrusion on CT or MRI. This is not an indication for surgery

MUSC

CLINICAL PEARLS

- Exclude systemic disease as an etiology for back pain
- Low back pain in a patient taking long-term corticosteroids is a compression fracture until proven otherwise
- 98% of clinically significant lumbar disc herniations occur at either the L4–5 or L5–S1 level
- The single most reliable predictor of return to work is job satisfaction
- Screen for depression when pain becomes a chronic problem
- Avoid using narcotics or muscle relaxants for longer than 7–10 days
- If the patient has a claim with Workers' Compensation, assume that the chart will be requested by attorneys and insurance companies (i.e., document completely)
- Consider referring difficult cases to a physiatrist or a doctor specializing in the diagnosis and treatment of musculoskeletal injuries
- Scoliosis is 80% idiopathic. The presence of concurrent back pain is a red flag to look for other causes (cerebral palsy, muscular dystrophy, spina bifida, neurofibromatosis, tumor)

References

Patel AT, Ogle AA. Diagnosis and management of acute low back pain. Am Fam Phys 2000;61:1779-86,1789-90.

Andersson GB, et al. A comparison of osteopathic spinal manipulation with standard care for patients with low back pain. N Engl J Med Nov 4, 1999;341: 1426-31.

Bratton RL. Assessment and management of acute low back pain. Am Fam Phys 1999;60:2299.

Humphreys SC, Eck, JC. Clinical evaluation and treatment options for herniated lumbar disc. Am Fam Phys 1999;59:575.

Moffett JK, et al. Randomised controlled trial of exercise for low back pain: clinical outcomes, costs, and preferences. BMJ Jul 31, 1999;319:279-83.

Vroomen PC, et al. Lack of effectiveness of bed rest for sciatica. N Engl J Med Feb 11, 1999; 340:418-23.

Alvarez JA, Hardy RH. Lumbar spine stenosis: a common cause of back and leg pain. Am Fam Phys 1998;57:1825–34.

Cherkin DC, et al. A comparison of physical therapy, chiropractic manipulation, and provision of an educational booklet for the treatment of patients with low back pain. N Engl J Med Oct 8, 1998;339:1021-9.

Jensen MC. Magnetic resonance imaging of the lumbar spine in people without back pain. N Engl J Med 1994;331:69–73.

Kuritzky L. Primary care approach to low back pain. Handout from the Department of Family Medicine, University of Florida, 1994.

Deyo RA. Clinical strategies for controlling costs and improving quality in the primary care of low back pain. J Back Musculoskel Rehabil 1993;3(4):1–13.

Deyo RA, et al. What can the history and physical examination tell us about low back pain? JAMA 1992;268:760-5.

Jackson RP. The facet syndrome: myth or reality? Clinical Orthopaed Rel Res 1992;279:110–21.

Saal JA, Saal JS. Nonoperative treatment of herniated lumbar intervertebral disc with radiculopathy: an outcome study. Spine 1989;14(4):431–7.

MUSC

86. CORTICOSTEROID INJECTION OF JOINTS

I. INTRODUCTION: Joint aspiration and injection can be a part of any primary care office. Aspiration can give symptomatic relief and a quick diagnosis with fluid analysis. Joint injection can be part of a diagnostic exam of a painful joint (**Lidocaine**) or part of a treatment plan (steroids)

II. GENERAL LIST OF CONDITIONS IMPROVED WITH STEROID INJECTION

Articular conditions

Rheumatoid arthritis

Seronegative spondyloarthropathies
    Ankylosing spondylitis
    Arthritis associated with inflammatory bowel disease
    Psoriasis
    Reiter's syndrome

Crystal-induced arthritis
    Gout
    Pseudogout

Osteoarthritis

Nonarticular disorders

Fibrositis
    Localized
    Systemic

Bursitis
    Subacromial
    Trochanteric
    Anserine
    Prepatellar

Periarthritis
    Adhesive capsulitis

Tenosynovitis/tendonitis
    De Quervain's disease
    Trigger finger
    Bicipital
    Tennis elbow
    Golfer's elbow
    Plantar fasciitis

Neuritis
    Carpal tunnel syndrome
    Tarsal tunnel syndrome
    Costochondritis
    Tietze's syndrome

Source: Pfenninger JL. Injections of joints and soft tissue: Part I. General guidelines. Am Fam Phys 1991;44:1196–1202. Used with permission.

III. CONTRAINDICATIONS TO JOINT INJECTION/ASPIRATION
    A. Cellulitis or broken skin over the entry site
    B. Coagulopathy or uncontrolled anticoagulation
    C. Prostheses
    D. Septic effusion, unstable joints, lack of response to previous injections (steroids)

IV. SIDE EFFECTS
    A. Steroid arthropathy

    B. Tendon rupture
    C. Skin atrophy, depigmentation
    D. Iatrogenic infectious arthritis
    E. Acceleration of cartilage attrition

V. TECHNIQUE: Follow standard sterile procedure for any procedure where skin barrier is broken. Locate your landmarks and mark entry point with thumbnail or pen. Prep area and aspirate the joint. Use hemostat to hold needle in place if syringes are switched to inject joint. With primary injections make sure to pull back on syringe to ensure that you are not in a blood vessel. Never inject directly into a nerve or tendon

    A. Knee: Place the knee in a slightly flexed position by placing a towel under the popliteal space. A lateral or medial approach may be used. Find the superior lateral (medial) border of the patella. Mark a point perpendicular to the border at a level just posterior to the patella. Insert needle at that point keeping the needle perpendicular to the axis of the knee and guide the needle under the patella. There should be no resistance

    B. Subacromial bursa: Locate the lateral edge of the acromion just posterior to the AC joint. There is usually a soft spot just superior to the humeral head. Insert the needle through the deltoid muscle and under the acromion. Needle should move freely in the space

    C. Plantar facia: Medial approach is done by locating the most tender point of the facia's insertion. From the medial side of the foot insert the needle perpendicular to the bottom of the heel and superior to the heel fat pad

    D. Greater trochanter: Insert needle over the point of maximum tenderness making sure that the needle remains perpendicular to the femur. Patient will usually have pain when the needle enters the bursa

    E. Olecranon bursa: Place the elbow at 90° of flexion and insert the needle into the area of most fluid. Tensing the bursa in your opposite hand may help you to localize the best insertion site

    F. Carpal tunnel: Dorsiflex the wrist to 30° and locate the palmaris longus tendon. Insert the needle at the distal palmar crease radial to the palmeris longus. Advance the needle downward at a 45°angle toward the middle finger. Advance the needle 1–2 cm until there is no resistance. If there is any discomfort in the fingers pull back the needle and redirect

VI. GENERAL GUIDELINES FOR EQUIPMENT AND STEROID DOSING
    A. Technique
        1. Mark the injection site
        2. Clean with povidone iodine and then clean with alcohol prep
        3. Consider anesthetizing site with ethyl chloride spray
    B. Components
        1. Steroid (**Kenalog, Decadron, Depo-Medrol**)
            a. **Kenalog** 40mg/mL (K-40)
            b. **Kenalog** 10mg/mL (K-10)
            c. **Depo-Medrol** 80mg/mL (D-80)
            d. **Depo-Medrol** 40mg/mL (D-40)
        2. Anaesthetic (**Lidocaine, Xylocaine, Sensorcaine**)
            a. **Lidocaine 1%** w/o Epinephrine (L)
            b. **Sensorcaine 0.25%** (S)
    C. Materials: Size of needle, type and amount of steroid and anesthetic
        1. AC joint
            a. 22 gauge, 1½" needle
            b. 1mL (K-40) + 1–2mL (L)
            NOTE: This is the *only* injection where you cannot mix these 2 solutions in the same syringe
        2. Shoulder (subacromial bursa; joint)
            a. 22–27 gauge, ⅝"–1½" needle
            b. 1mL (K-40) + 5mL (L) or 1mL (D-40) + 1mL (K-40) or (K-10)+ 3mL (L)
        3. Elbow (olecranon bursa; joint)
            a. 22 gauge, 1"–1½" needle
            b. ½–1mL (K-40) + 1–2mL (L)
        4. Elbow (lateral epicondyle)

MUSC

      a. 25 gauge, $^5/_8$" needle

      b. ½mL (D-80) + 1mL (L)

  5. Wrist (joint)

      a. 25 gauge, $^5/_8$" needle

      b. ½mL (D-80) + ½mL (L)

  6. Wrist (carpal tunnel)

      a. 25 gauge, $^3/_8$"–$^5/_8$" needle

      b. ½mL (D-40) *only*

  7. Hip (pointer)

      a. 18–22 gauge, 1½" needle

      b. 2mL (K-40) + 10mL (L)

  8. Hip (femoral trochanter bursa)

      a. 22 gauge, 1½" needle

      b. 1mL (D-40) + 1mL (K-40 or K-10) + 3mL (L)

  9. Knee

      a. 22 gauge, 1½" needle

      b. 1mL (K-40) + 2–5mL (L)

  10. Ankle

      a. 20–22 gauge, 1½" needle

      b. 1mL (D-40) + 1mL (L)

  11. Heel (spur)

      a. 18–25 gauge, $^5/_8$"–1½" needle

      b. 1mL (K-40) + 2–3mL (L)

  12. Muscle (general trigger pain)

      a. 25 gauge, $^5/_8$" needle

      b. 1mL (D-40) + 2–3mL (L)

References

Pfenninger JL. Injections of joints and soft tissue: Part I. General guidelines. Am Fam Phys 1991;44:1196.

Pfenninger JL. Injections of joints and soft tissue: Part II. Guidelines for specific joints. Am Fam Phys 1991;44:1690.

Gray RG, Gottleib NL. Intra-articular corticosteroids: an updated assessment. Clin Orthop 1983;177:253–63.

VIII. Dermatology

DERM

87. DESCRIBING DERMATOLOGIC LESIONS

I. TYPE OF LESION
A. Macule: A circumscribed area of skin in which the color is different from the surrounding skin. (Can differentiate from papule by oblique lighting). A macule is flat and may measure up to 1cm

B. Patch: A flat area of color change over 1cm in size

C. Papule: A solid lesion, generally less than 0.5cm in diameter, that is elevated above the plane of the surrounding skin. Confluence of papules leads to plaque formation

D. Nodule: A palpable, solid, round or ellipsoidal lesion that is deeper than a papule and is in the dermis or subcutaneous tissue (basically a large papule). These result from infiltrates, neoplasms or metabolic deposits and are often indicators of systemic disease

E. Vesicle: A circumscribed, elevated fluid-containing lesion (blister) less than 0.5cm, often translucent

F. Bulla: A blister measuring greater than 0.5cm. Both bulla and vesicles are formed from a cleavage at various levels of the skin, i.e., epidermal layers or dermal-epidermal interface

G. Pustule: Blister filled with pus

H. Plaque: An elevation above the skin surface that occupies a relatively large area in comparison with its height above the skin

I. Wheal: An edematous pink papule or plaque that is characteristically evanescent, disappearing within hours

J. Crusts: Dried serum, blood or exudate on the surface of the skin
  1. Honey-colored: Impetigo
  2. Thick and adherent over entire epidermis: Ecthyma

K. Erosion: A break in the surface epithelium

L. Ulcer: A skin defect in which there has been loss of the epidermis and dermis. Describe the location, borders, base, discharge and any topographic features

M. Comedone: A plugged pilosebaceous opening, open-blackhead vs. closed-whitehead

N. Burrow: A linear trail produced by parasites

O. Atrophy: Loss of substance in the epidermis, dermis, and/or subcutaneous tissue

P. Telangiectasia: A superficial dilatation of blood vessels

Q. Purpura: Non-blanching red or violaceous lesions

II. COLOR: Of either the skin if diffuse involvement or the lesion
A. White
  1. Hypopigmented
  2. Depigmented (no pigment)

B. Erythema
  1. Pink
  2. Violaceous

C. Brown
  1. Hypermelanosis
  2. Hemosiderin

D. Black, blue, gray, orange, yellow

III. PALPATION
A. Soft, firm, hard, fluctuant, board-like
B. Temperature difference
C. Mobility of lesion
D. Tenderness
E. Depth

IV. SHAPE
A. Round

DERM

B. Oval

C. Polygonal

D. Polycyclic

E. Annular

F. Iris

G. Serpiginous

H. Umbilicated

I. Grouped

    1. Herpetiform

    2. Zosteriform

    3. Arciform

    4. Annular

    5. Reticular (net-like)

    6. Linear

    7. Disseminated (scattered or diffuse)

V. DISTRIBUTION

A. **Extent**

    1. Isolated

    2. Generalized

    3. Localized

    4. Regional or universal

B. **Pattern**

    1. Symmetrical

    2. Exposed areas

    3. Pressure points

    4. Intertriginous areas

    5. Follicular

    6. Random

    7. Photo distribution

CLINICAL PEARLS

- Persistent and unidentifiable nodules should be biopsied and a portion ground and cultured for fungi and bacteria
- If a wheal remains for longer than 72hrs, biopsy is indicated as this can be caused by urticarial vasculitis

Ryan Hanson, MD

88. CONTACT DERMATITIS

I. DEFINITION: Acute, subacute or chronic inflammation of the epidermis and dermis caused by external agents, toxicity or an allergic reaction and characterized by pruritis or burning

II. TYPES

A. **Allergic contact dermatitis:** Cell-mediated type IV hypersensitivity reaction

B. **Irritant contact:** Due to inflammation from a local toxic effect of a chemical on the skin

C. **Contact photodermatitis:** A type of allergic contact dermatitis triggered by ultraviolet light

D. **Contact urticaria:** Wheal and flare reaction—may be allergic (IgE) or nonallergic

III. HISTORY

A. **Family history of atopy**

B. **Exposure history:** Inquire about some of the common irritants (listed below) or any *new* exposures

    1. Nickel: Found in cheap jewelry, metal clothing fasteners, coins

    2. Potassium Dichromate: Found in cement, paper, leather, metal paint, detergent

    3. Paraphenylenediamine: Found in hair dyes, ink, fur dyes, radiographic fluid

DERM

4. Chrome
5. Rhus plants: Poison ivy, oak and sumac
6. Formaldehydes: permanent press fabrics, shampoos, smoke
C. **Duration of lesions** and previous successful or unsuccessful therapy

IV. PHYSICAL EXAM

A. **Acute contact dermatitis:** Vesicles and/or bullae filled with clear fluid or erythematous, edematous skin
B. **Subacute contact dermatitis:** Erythema, minimal edema, multiple papules
C. **Chronic contact dermatitis:** Lichenified plaques with minimal erythema, minimal edema, possible scales
D. **Rhus dermatitis (poison ivy dermatitis—see below):** Vesicular lesions and crusting. Pathognomic lesions are linear vesicles. A rash that seems to be spreading may present as linear vesicles in one area and multiple small vesicles in another area
E. **Attempt to correlate the location of the eruption with exposure** (E.g., dermatitis due to nickel in cheap earrings is present on the earlobes)
F. **Evaluate for secondary infection**

V. PATCH TESTING

A. Patch testing may be performed in patients who are suspected of having contact allergy but no allergen can be elicited by history. This should be done *after* the episode of dermatitis has resolved
B. Apply patch test to skin on back and occlude for 48hrs
C. Interpret in 72hrs
D. Positive test with the development of erythema, papules, vesicles

VI. MANAGEMENT

A. **Identify and eliminate the offending agent,** i.e., remove exposure
B. **Wet compresses for oozing and vesiculation**
C. **Wash BID with soap and water**
D. **Burrow's solution:** Aluminum Acetate tablets in water for wet compresses, then apply steroid cream to suppress inflammation
E. **Topical steroid cream:** Use a stronger cream for areas of thick skin (back of arms, palms, etc.) (See Chapter 92, Topical Steroids, for a listing of different steroid creams). Do not use fluorinated steroid creams on the face as it may result in depigmentation of the skin
F. **Systemic (oral) corticosteroids** for extensive dermatitis. Begin with **Prednisone** 1–2mg /kg/day (40–60mg max) given QD or as a divided dose and taper over 2–3 weeks. Shorter courses may result in a rebound phenomenon
G. **Symptomatic medications**
   1. Adults
      a. **Hydroxyzine (Atarax):** 25mg PO TID–QID
      b. **Diphenhydramine (Benadryl):** 25–50mg PO TID–QID
   2. Children
      a. Younger than 6 years: **Hydroxyzine** (10mg/5cc), 50mg /day PO in divided doses
      b. Older than 6 years: Same as adults

VII. RHUS DERMATITIS: POISON IVY, POISON SUMAC, ETC.

A. **Hypersensitivity reaction** from exposure to *rhus* plants either directly (by contact with a plant) or indirectly (by contact with something which has been exposed to the plant and carries its oils—clothing, gloves, pets, shoelaces, etc.)
B. **Exanthem** develops over 48–72hrs and consists of linear vesicles (with direct exposure) or grouped vesicles (with indirect exposure) which may be weeping. The fluid inside the vesicles is not contagious as it does not contain the plant oils
C. **Complications:** Infection or overwhelming infection in vital structures (eye, throat, etc.)
D. **Management**
   1. Have the patient cut fingernails short (especially in children)
   2. Wash lesions BID with soap and water
   3. Symptomatic medications: Same as above
   4. Cold washcloth or shower will help decrease itching

DERM

5. Topical steroid cream: See above
6. Oral steroids: Indicated for most rhus rashes unless small area (topical) or asymptomatic or contraindicated. Begin with **Prednisone** 1–2mg/kg/day (40–60mg maximum) and taper over 2–3 weeks (to prevent rebound)
7. Patients (especially children) should be educated in identification of plants

CLINICAL PEARLS
- *A rash that seems to be spreading* may be caused by repeated exposure to the plant, exposure to clothes/pets which bear the oils, or different sensitivities of the skin which has been exposed (arm vs. face)
- Contact dermatitis is one of the most common reasons for worker's compensation claims for skin disease

References
Klaus MV, Wieselthier JS. Contact dermatitis. Am Fam Phys 1993;48:629.

Ryan Hanson, MD
Steve Markovich, MD

89. ACNE AND ROSACEA

I. DEFINITION
A. Acne vulgaris: Chronic inflammation of the pilosebaceous units, caused by increased sebum production, abnormal follicles, propionibacterium, and hormonal and immunological factors
B. Rosacea: Chronic acneform inflammation of the pilosebaceous units of the face coupled with an increased reactivity of the capillaries to heat, leading to flushing and telangiectasias
C. Special forms of acne include:
1. Acne conglobata: A severe cystic acne with coalescing nodules, cysts and abscesses
2. Acne fulminans: An acute, severe suppurative cystic acne with fever and generalized arthritis

— PART ONE: ACNE VULGARIS—

II. ETIOLOGY
A. Caused by *Propionibacterium*
B. Endocrine
1. Premenstrual and androgenic disorders such as polycystic ovary, or Cushing's syndrome
2. Menstrual irregularites
3. Hirsutism
C. Environment
1. Humidity
2. Excessive sweating
3. Working in an environment with aerosolized fats (i.e., fast-foods)
D. Mechanical
1. Pressure
2. Constant rubbing of clothes
3. Picking/squeezing: May lead to scarring and worsening
4. Washing with harsh soaps
5. Excessive scrubbing
E. Cosmetics
F. Medications: Steroids, ACTH, androgens, Dilantin, barbiturates, Lithium, Isoniazid, Cyclosporine, iodides and bromides, oral contraceptives with strong androgens and/or anti-estrogenic

III. HISTORY
A. Duration and previous successful and unsuccessful therapies

DERM

    B. Relation to menses

    C. Presence of hirsuitism

    D. Cleansing habits (vigorous scrubbing, etc.)

    E. Environment

    F. Mechanical factors: Tight clothing, constant rubbing of clothes, picking and squeezing

    G. Cosmetics

    H. Medications: Listed above

    I. Seasonal prevalence: Often worse in fall and winter

    J. Diet: There are no firm studies linking diet to acne, but patients may notice worsening of acne after eating certain foods

IV. PHYSICAL

    A. Comedones: Sebum clogged sebaceous follicles, open (blackheads) or closed (whiteheads)

    B. Pustules: Erupting follicular contents

    C. Papules: Inflammatory raised lesions in dermis

    D. Cysts: Deep, intense inflammatory papule progressing to fluctuant, painful area

    E. Seborrhea may also be seen

    F. Inspect face, back, chest and buttocks for lesions and scarring

    G. Severity: To guide treatment

        1. **Type 1—Mild inflammatory acne:** Comedonal, less than 10 lesions, face only, no scarring

        2. **Type 2—Mild papular acne:** Less than 25 lesions, face and trunk, mild scarring

        3. **Type 3—Pustular acne:** More than 25 lesions with moderate scarring

        4. **Type 4—Severe cystic acne:** Nodulocystic with extensive scarring

V. LABS: Indicated in young women who don't respond to therapy

    A. Hormone testing

        1. Androgens

        2. Plasma testosterone

        3. Dihydroepiandrosterone

        4. Partial 11- or 12-hydroxylase block

    B. Genetics: Severe acne in XYY

VI. MANAGEMENT: Listed by type of acne

    A. General

        1. Wash with mild soap (e.g., Dial, Ivory, Phisoderm, Panoxyl, Neutrogena)

        2. If any of the above factors (listed in etiology) are contributing to a worsening of acne, then modify as needed. Avoid foods noted to cause flare-ups, avoid mechanical pressure, vigorous cleansing, etc.

    B. Mild inflammatory acne (Type 1): Topical medications 1st line

        1. **Benzoyl Peroxide** 5% or 10%. Apply to clean, dry skin QHS or BID (Available in 2.5%, 5%, 10%, gels, creams, lotions and soaps. The liquid and cream are less irritating, gel better for oily skin)

        2. **Retinoic Acid (Retin A):** Apply QD. Start with lowest strength and increase after a few weeks if necessary. Again cream is better for dry skin. (Available in .025%, .05% and .1% creams, .01%, .025%, and .1% gel and .05% liquid). Avoid sun exposure

        3. May try Benzoyl Peroxide in the AM and Retin-A in the PM if single therapy fails

    C. Mild papular acne (Type 2): Topical antibiotics with Benzoyl Peroxide or Retin-A

        1. **Clindamycin** 1% lotion or gel. Applied BID to clean and dry skin

        2. **Erythromycin** 2% gel or pledgettes. Applied BID

    D. Pustular acne (Type 3): Oral antibiotics plus topical agents, taper antibiotics after 7–10 days to lowest effective dose

        1. **Tetracycline**

           a. Dose: 250mg PO QID or 500mg PO BID

           b. Note: Do not use in pregnancy or children under 12 years of age

        2. **Erythromycin**

           a. Dose: 250mg PO QID

           b. Note: Pustular acne is more resistant

DERM

3. **Minocycline**
   a. Dose: 50mg PO BID or 100mg QD
   b. Note: Highly effective due to lipophilicity
   c. Side effects include dizziness and color changes
4. **Trimethoprim/Sulfamethoxazole**
   a. Dose: 1 DS tablet QD
   b. Note: For refractory cases (may have severe eruptive reaction)

E. **Severe cystic acne (Type 4)**
   1. **Isotretinoin (Accutane)**: Decreases sebum production
      a. Many side-effects, including teratogenic, thus birth control required 1 month before starting and 2 months after
      b. Should only be prescribed by physicians with experience with the use of this very potent drug
   2. **Steroid injection:** Intralesional triamcinalone can decrease cyst-size in 2–3 days. Use a minimal amount to avoid steroid-atrophy
   3. Systemic hormones
      a. OCPs for low-dose estrogen effect (e.g., **Ortho-tri-cyclen**)
      b. **Prednisone** 5mg/day to decrease adrenal androgen production—bad long-term!
      c. Spironolactone to decrease sebum production

F. **Treatment failure:** If treatment fails after oral antibiotics, consider dermatology referral due to the serious side-effects of the latter therapies and the scarring

— PART TWO: ROSACEA —

I. HISTORY
   A. Usually ages 30–50
   B. Females > Males
   C. Celtic/Northern Europeans much more than pigmented races
   D. Hot liquids/heat may stimulate or worsen
   E. Alcohol increases flushing
   F. Emotional stress may be a factor
   G. Rosacea has now been associated with H Pylori. Treatment of H. Plylori disease has improved co-existing rosacea

II. PHYSICAL
   A. Flushing
   B. Papular and papulopustular lesions
   C. Telangiectasias
   D. Nodules
   E. Absence of comedones
   F. Usually **face only**: cheeks, chin, forehead, nose and rarely neck
   G. Associated rhinophyma
   H. Blepharitis, episcleritis and conjunctivitis may occur

III. MANAGEMENT
   A. Decrease alcohol and hot beverage intake
   B. **Metrogel (Metronidazole 0.75%)**: Apply BID to clean, dry skin. May take 4–8 weeks
   C. If Metrogel fails, then consider **Tetracycline** or **Erythromycin** gels
   D. If topical fails, then consider **Tetracycline** 500mg PO BID or **Minocycline** 100mg PO BID (for Tetracycline failures)
   E. Avoid sun

CLINICAL PEARLS
   • Blepharitis can often be cleared with simple lid scrubs with baby shampoo and PO Tetracycline

References
Russell J. Topical therapy for acne. Am Fam Phys 2000;61:357–66.
Thiboutot DM. Acne rosacea. Am Fam Phys 1994;50:1691.
Nguyen QH. Management of acne vulgaris. Am Fam Phys 1994;50:89.

DERM

Daniel M. Neides, MD
Steve Markovich, MD

90. RASHES IN CHILDREN

I. DESCRIPTION
  A. Maculopapular: a combination of flat and raised lesions < 0.5–1.0cm in diameter
    1. Infectious:
      a. Viral: Measles, rubeola, rubella, erythema infectiosum (fifth disease), roseola, enterovirus, mononucleosis, pityriasis rosea
      b. Nonviral: Scarlet fever, scalded skin syndrome, toxic shock, Kawasaki's, meningococcemia, mycoplasma, Rocky Mountain Spotted Fever (RMSF)
    2. Ingestion: Ampicillin, Penicillin, barbiturates, anticonvulsants, sulfonamides
    3. Other: Sunburn, juvenile rheumatoid arthritis, serum sickness
  B. Vesicular: Raised lesion < 0.5cm in diameter containing fluid
    1. Infectious:
      a. Viral: Varicella zoster, Herpes simplex, Enterovirus, Molluscum contagiosum
      b. Nonviral: Impetigo, *Erythema multiformæ*, scalded skin syndrome
    2. Other: Insect bites, contact dermatitis (poison ivy, etc.)
  C. Petechial: small, flat, nonblanching lesion
    1. Infectious:
      a. Viral: Enterovirus, rubeola, varicella zoster
      b. Nonviral: Meningococcemia, *H. Influenzæ*, pneumococcemia, RMSF, sepsis, gonococcemia, endocarditis
    2. Other: Henoch-Schönlein purpura, idiopathic thrombocytopenic purpura, aplastic anemia

II. COMMON MACULOPAPULAR EXANTHEMS
  A. Measles (Rubeola)
    1. Incubation: 10–14 days
    2. Prodrome: Cough, coryza, conjunctivitis, 3 days high fever; child appears toxic
    3. Exanthem: Erythematous macules and papules appear on upper neck and face, then begin to progress down to extremities. May get a petechial eruption on the soft palate 1–2 days before rash followed by Koplik's spots (blue-white macules with surrounding erythema found on the buccal mucosa adjacent to the second molars. The rash co-exists with fever and lasts 7–10 days
    4. Complications: Pneumonia, encephalitis, otitis media, thrombocytopenia, hemorrhagic measles, pneumothorax, hepatitis
    5. Management: Supportive
  B. Rubella
    1. Incubation: 14–21 days
    2. Prodrome: Usually none; lymphadenopathy (postauricular, suboccipital)
    3. Exanthem: Pink, begins on face and progresses downward, lasts 2–3 days
    4. Complications: Arthritis common in women after 2–3 days of illness (knee, wrist, finger), encephalitis, thrombocytopenia
    5. Management: Supportive—isolate from pregnant women
  C. Erythema infectiosum (*fifth disease*—Parvovirus B19)
    1. Incubation: 7–14 days
    2. Prodrome: None
    3. Exanthem: 2 stages—
      Stage I. Red-flushed cheeks with circumoral pallor (slapped cheek)
      Stage II. Maculopapular eruption on extremities (lacelike)
    4. Complications: Arthritis
    5. Management: Supportive
  D. Roseola (Human Herpes Virus—Type 6): Occurs in children age 6 months to 2 years
    1. Incubation: 10–14 days

DERM

    2. Prodrome: 3–4 days of high fever which precedes rash; child looks great despite fever

    3. Exanthem: Macules with secondary erythema which appears when fever breaks. Initially seen on the chest, it spreads to involve face and extremities. Lymphadenopathy may be present (suboccipitally)

    4. Complications: Febrile seizures

    5. Management: Supportive

E. Scarlet fever (Group A streptococci)

    1. Incubation: 2–4 days

    2. Prodrome: 1–2 days of fever, vomiting, sore throat; toxic appearing

    3. Exanthem: Erythematous, sandpaper texture; starts neck, axillae, inguinal areas and then spreads to rest of body; lasts 7 days and then desquamates

    4. Complications: Rheumatic fever, acute glomerulonephritis

    5. Management: **Penicillin**—See Chapter 7, Pharyngitis, for dosage information

F. Hand, foot and mouth disease (enteroviruses: Coxsackievirus a16, a5, and a10)

    1. Incubation: 4–6 days (exposure through enteric route; oral-oral or fecal-oral)

    2. Prodrome: Low grade temperature, sore throat, malaise, lymphadenopathy

    3. Exanthem: Aphthae-like lesions anywhere in the mouth followed by 3–7mm red macules on the palms and soles. These develop into cloudy vesicles with red halos. Can also see mild peri-orbital edema

    4. Complications: None

    5. Management: Supportive including **viscous Lidocaine** and **Diphenhydramine elixir** —both swish and spit

G. Kawasaki's disease (Mucocutaneous lymphnode syndrome)

    1. Incubation: Unknown

    2. Prodrome: Abrupt, high spiking fever (101–104°F), unresponsive to antipyretics. Occasionally diarrhea, cough or abdominal pain

    3. Exanthem: Within 3 days of fever

        a. Bilateral bulbar conjunctival congestion

        b. Erythematous mouth and pharynx with strawberry tongue and red, cracked lips

        c. Edema of the hands and feet with erythema of the palms and soles

        d. Generalized rash that can be morbilliform, maculopapular, scarlatiniform or may resemble erythema multiforme

    4. Complications: Arthritis, meningitis, cardiac and other organ involvement

    5. Management: Supportive care, detection of coronary disease and anti-inflammatories (IVIG and Aspirin). Hospital admission

III. VESICULAR EXANTHEM

A. Chickenpox (varicella zoster virus)

    1. Incubation: 10–20 days

    2. Prodrome: Malaise; low grade fever

    3. Exanthem: Develops over 3–6 day period usually starting along hairline of face; each lesion begins as a macule that progresses to a papule and vesicle and finally a crusted vesicle; rash emerges in crops over the trunk and finally the extremities; lesions in different stages are present throughout the first week

    4. Complications: Bacterial infection of vesicular lesions, pneumonia, hepatitis, arthritis, glomerulonephritis, CNS disease

    5. Management:

        a. Cut patient's fingernails short to prevent scratching and secondary infection

        b. Wash lesions BID with soap and water

        c. **Benadryl**, cold washcloth or oatmeal baths (aveeno bath) will help decrease itching

        d. **Acyclovir** (**Zovirax**) can be used for high risk patients (immunocompromised)

        e. **Varicella zoster immune globulin** (**VZIG**) is available for patients at risk for developing progressive chickenpox (immunocompromised patients)

        f. VZV vaccine is recommended routine in childhood immunization for susceptible children, adolescents and adults

B. Poison ivy (See Chapter 88, Contact Dermatitis)

DERM

CLINICAL PEARLS

- VZV vaccine if used within 3–5 days postexposure of household or hospital contact may abort infection and reduce symptoms
- The management of most rashes in children is supportive—rule out the "life threatening" causes of rashes with a thorough history and physical exam
- Most petechial rashes are caused by viruses
- The most common vector-borne illness in North America (Lyme disease) is caused by the spirochete *B. burgdorferi* through the bite of an infected Ixodes tick. Lyme disease is largely a clinical diagnosis, with the classic rash being *erythema migrans*. Animal studies documenting a low incidence of Lyme disease when infected ticks are attached for less than 24hrs and a high incidence after 72hrs of attachment have been consistent with human findings

References

Shinefield HR, et al. Safety, tolerability and immunogenicity of concomitant injections in separate locations of M-M-RII, Varivax and Tetramune in healthy children vs. concomitant injections of M-M-RII and Tetramune followed six weeks later by Varivax. Pediatr Infect Dis J Nov 1998;11;980–5.

Centers for Disease Control and Prevention. Measles, mumps, and rubella—vaccine use and strategies for elimination of measles, rubella, and congenital rubella syndrome and control of mumps. MMWR 1998;47(RR-8):24.

American Academy of Pediatrics. 1997 Red book: Report of the Committee on Infectious Diseases. 24th ed. Elk Grove Village, IL: American Academy of Pediatrics, 1997.

Nelson, D.G., et al. Evaluation of febrile children with petechial rashes: is there consensus among pediatricians? Ped Infect Dis J 1998;17:1135.

Ryan Hanson, MD

91. SKIN BIOPSIES

I. INDICATIONS

    A. All lesions suspected of being neoplasms

    B. All bullous disorders: Send for immunofluorescence

    C. Disorders where a specific diagnosis is not possible by clinical exam alone

    D. Cosmesis

II. INFORMED CONSENT: Make certain the patient understands the risk of scarring, bleeding, the indications and alternatives and the general risks. Also, that further treatment may be necessary

III. SITE

    A. Choose well-developed lesions

    B. If a lesion is ulcerated, then biopsy the border

    C. Lesions to avoid (consider referral)

        1. Cosmetically sensitive areas

            a. Face

            b. Hypertrophic scarring areas like upper chest and deltoid region

        2. Excoriated lesions

        3. Secondarily infected areas

        4. High-infection areas: axilla and groin

        5. Lesions overlying vital structures (nerves, arteries, joints)

IV. ANESTHESIA

    A. 1% Lidocaine (Xylocaine) is usually adequate. Use enough to make a good wheal under the skin

    B. Lidocaine with 1:100,000 **Epinephrine**: Useful if hemostasis is an issue or prolonged effect desired

DERM

    1. Wait several minutes for Lidocaine to take effect
    2. NEVER use Lidocaine with Epinephrine in digital or penile block

C. Adjuncts
    1. Topical anesthetics, i.e., EMLA cream (2.5% **Lidocaine**, 2.5% **Prilocaine**): Applied thickly over area with occlusion for *at least* an hour. Not to be used on mucous membranes or broken skin
    2. Cryotherapy
    3. Distraction
    4. Sterile saline or **Diphenhydramine (Benadryl):** 0.5% or 1% in patients allergic to Lidocaine—works by increased turgor pressure
    5. Add 8.4% **Sodium Bicarbonate** to **Lidocaine** at a 1:10 ratio to decrease burning
    6. Inject at a 30° angle to form a wheal under the skin

V. TYPES: Take care with handling so as not to crush sample, place immediately in formalin. Special studies such as immunofluorescence and electron microscopy require special handling and stains

A. Shave biopsy: If the blade is kept parallel to the skin, scarring should be slight
    1. Indications: Removal of protruding portion of superficial raised papular or pedunculated lesions or superficial lesions on a convex surface (pinnae of the ear or nose). (E.g., Milia, warts, seborrheic keratosis, molluscum contagiosum, benign appearing nevi)
    2. Technique
       a. Infuse local anesthetic intradermal to raise the lesion
       b. Stretch the skin on either side of the biopsy site
       c. Use a No. 15 scalpel or a No. 10 scalpel for larger lesions
       d. Keep blade parallel to the skin with the cutting edge upward to prevent penetration into the dermis
       e. Hemostasis (see below)
    3. Tissue diagnosis is compromised when pathology extends deep into the tissue
    4. Never use with a pigmented lesion suspicious for malignant melanoma

B. Punch biopsy: Full thickness cylindric biopsies, 2–8mm in size
    1. Indications: When dermal pathology requires evaluation (E.g., Sarcoidosis, granuloma annulare, sclerosing basal cell CA, psoriasis, *erythema multiforme*, connective tissue disorders, bullous skin diseases). Easy removal of small tumors or when multiple biopsies are needed. If suspicious of malignant melanoma, perform an excisional biopsy
    2. Technique
       a. Usually performed with a 4mm instrument (trephine)
       b. Stretching the skin perpendicular to the tension lines while performing biopsy will result in an oval shaped skin defect which can more easily be closed with sutures
       c. Push vertically into skin with rotational movements until into subcutaneous tissues
       d. Lift specimen with toothless Adson forcep (or 25 gauge needle) and cut the base
       e. Not always necessary to suture with less than 4mm biopsies, but inform patient that there will be a scar—usually a 1–2mm white depression at the site. Close biopsies 4mm or larger with sutures
       f. Hemostasis (see below)

C. Excisional biopsy: Removal of the entire area of pathology
    1. Indications: Removal of tumors of the skin for diagnosis and cure. Diagnosis of pigmented lesions suspicious for melanoma. Any lesion that requires multiple studies
    2. Technique
       a. Elliptic excision oriented parallel to the skin tension lines (Langer's lines)
       b. Length is 3 times the width
       c. If suspicious of melanoma, the excision needs to be at the level of the subcutaneous tissue (to facilitate Breslow score)
       d. Undermining the wound may allow for easier closure (blunt dissection under wound edges to create a plane under the skin to allow the wound edges to be more easily brought together with minimum tension)

DERM

e. Consider layered closure for large defects (absorbable suture such as vicryl for deep and nylon or polypropylene sutures (4–0 to 5–0) for the skin edges)

f. Hemostasis (see below)

D. Incision biopsy: Elliptic specimen taken from within a lesion

1. Indications: For examination of subcutaneous tissues (fibrous tumors, pannicluitis) and when necessary to view transition from normal to abnormal tissue. In pigmented lesions, use only if there are contraindications to excisional biopsy (cosmesis or functional considerations)

2. Technique: Similar to excisional biopsy

a. Narrow elliptic incision

b. Choose location of most raised or most pigmented area of the lesion

c. Technique as above

d. Hemostasis (see below)

VI. HEMOSTASIS

A. Pressure

B. Pinpoint electrodessication

C. Topical solutions

1. **Aluminum Chloride Hexahydrate (Drysol)**

2. **Absorbable gelatin powder (Gelfoam)**

3. **30% Aluminum Chloride**

4. **Monsel's solution (Ferric Subsulfate)**: May leave raised pigmented lesion

5. **Silver Nitrate**

CLINICAL PEARLS

- Never use a shave biopsy for pigmented lesions
- Allergy to Procaine (Novocain) is not a contraindication to use of Lidocaine
- The incidence of melanoma has nearly tripled in the last 3 decades, faster than any other cancer. The poor prognosis makes speed and accuracy of diagnosis essential. The ABCDE's of malignant melanoma are:

    A—asymmetry

    B—border irregularity

    C—color variegation

    D—diameter > 6mm

    E—enlargement, rapid growth over weeks to months

DERM

References

Achar S. Principles of skin biopsies for the family physician. Am Fam Phys 1996;54(8):2411.

Arca M, et al. Biopsy techniques for skin, soft-tissue, and bone neoplasms. Surg Oncol Clin North Am 1995;1:157–74.

Koh HK. Cutaneous melanoma. N Engl J Med 1991;325:171–82.

92. TOPICAL STEROIDS

Classification of topical steroid preparations by potency

LOW POTENCY		
Alclometason diproplonate 0.05% Aclovate (crm, oint) **Fluocinolone acetonide 0.01%** Synalar (soln) **Hydrocortisone base or acetate 0.5%** Cortisporin* (crm)	**Hydrocortisone base or acetate 1%** Cortisporin* (oint) Hytone (crm, lotion, oint) Proctocort (crm) Vytone* (crm)	**Hydrocortisone base or acetate 2.5%** Anusol-HC (crm) Hytone (crm, lotion, oint) **Triamcinolone acetonide 0.025%** Aristocort A (crm) Kenalog (crm, lotion, oint)

INTERMEDIATE POTENCY		
Betamethasone valerate 0.12% Luxiq (foam) **Desonide 0.05%** DesOwen (crm, lotion, oint) Tridesilon (crm, oint) **Desoximetasone 0.05%** Topicort-LP (emollient crm) **Fluocinolone acetonide 0.01%** Derma-Smothe/FS (oil, shampoo) **Fluocinolone acetonide 0.025%** Synalar (crm, oint) **Flurandrenolide 0.025%** Cordran-SP (crm) Cordran (oint)	**Flurandrenolide 0.05%** Cordran-SP (crm) Cordran (lotion, oint) **Fluticasone propionate 0.005%** Cutivate (oint) **Fluticasone propionate 0.05%** Cutivate (crm) **Hydrocortisone probutate 0.1%** Pandel (crm) **Hydrocortisone butyrate 0.1%** Locoid (crm, oint, soln) **Hydrocortisone valerate 0.2%** Westcort (crm, oint)	**Mometasone furoate 0.1%** Elocon (crm, lotion, oint) **Prednicarbate 0.1%** Dermatop (emollient crm) **Triamcinolone acetonide 0.1%** Aristocort A (crm, oint) Kenalog (crm, lotion) **Triamcinolone acetonide 0.2%** Kenalog (aerosol)

HIGH POTENCY		
Amcinonide 0.1% Cyclocort (crm, lotion, oint) **Betamethasone dipropionate, augmented 0.05%** Diprolene AF (emollient crm) Diprolene (lotion) **Desoximetasone 0.05%** Topicort (gel)	**Desoximetasone 0.25%** Topicort (emollient crm, oint) **Diflorasone diacetate 0.05%** Psorcon e (emollient crm, emollient oint) Psorcon (crm) **Fluocinonide 0.05%** Lidex (crm, gel, oint, soln) Lidex-E (emollient crm)	**Halcinonide 0.1%** Halog (crm, oint, soln) Halog-E (emollient crm) **Triamcinolone acetonide 0.5%** Aristocort A (crm) Kenalog (crm)

SUPER HIGH POTENCY		
Betamethasone dipropionate, augmented 0.05% Diprolene (oint, gel)	**Clobetasol propionate 0.05%** Temovate (crm, gel, oint, scalp application) Temovate-E (emollient crm)	**Diflorasone diacetate 0.05%** Psorcon (oint)
		Flurandrenolide 4mcg/sq cm Cordran (tape)
		Halobetasol propionate 0.05% Ultravate (crm, oint)

*Indicates that the product has more that one active ingredient.

The classification is based on vasoconstrictor assays and clinical studies, Potency varies according to the corticosteroid, its concentration, and the vehicle. In general, corticosteroids in lotions, creams gels, and ointments, are increasingly more potent due to increased absorption from these vehicles.

Absorption is increased by prolonged therapy, large areas of skin damage, and the use of occlusive dressings which may cause an increase in the incidence of side effects.

(revised 1/2000)

Source: Monthly prescribing reference. Prescribing Reference, Inc., New York NY Jan 2000;88. Used with permission.

Michael B. Weinstock, MD
Steve Markovich, MD

93. MISCELLANEOUS DERMATOLOGIC THERAPIES

I. TREATMENT OF WARTS

A. Cryotherapy: Scar formation is minimized

1. Begin by shaving the wart
2. Plantar warts often require Q week applications at weekly or biweekly intervals

B. Medical: Begin by shaving the wart as closely as possible, then soaking in warm water to moisten the wart. Vaseline may be applied to areas surrounding the wart to prevent tissue injury

1. **Duofilm:** Apply to affected area QD × 3 months
2. **Trans-Ver-Sal** (Salicylic Acid in a transdermal delivery system): Apply QD × 6 weeks
3. **Topical Retinoids (Retin-A):** Apply BID × 4–6 weeks. Less scarring than other therapies, therefore, good for use on the face
4. Consider **Benzoyl Peroxide, Di- and Trichloroacetic Acid, Podophyllin,** occlusive therapy (occlusion with waterproof tape for 1 week)

II. TREATMENT OF SCABIES

A. Permethrin 5% (Elimite) cream: Apply from head to soles of feet. Rinse after 8–14hrs. 30g is adequate for adults. Drug of choice for children

B. Lindane (Kwell, Scabene) lotion, cream or shampoo. Apply lotion or cream to skin from neck down to feet and rinse in 8–12hrs. Some dermatologists recommend retreating in 7–14 days. Should not be used in children who are premature, malnourished, with underlying skin disease or seizure disorders

C. Treat all intimate contacts and family members. Bed linens, clothing and towels should be washed

III. TREATMENT OF PEDICULOSIS (LICE)

A. Head lice: 1% Permethrin (NIX) or Lindane

B. Pubic lice: Lindane shampoo: Lather from neck to feet and leave on for 10 minutes. May also use **Permethrin** or **Lindane** creams—leave in place for several hours

C. Body lice: Permethrin or **Lindane** cream applied once and left on for several hours

D. Eyelash infestation: Manual removal of lice and nits or apply **Petroleum jelly (Vaseline)** to eyelids TID–QID for 8–10 days. Do not use pediculicides to treat eyelash infestations

IV. ANTIFUNGALS

A. **Treatment of tinea pedis** (4 weeks), **tinea cruris** (2–3 weeks), and **tinea corporis** (2–3 weeks). May require longer treatment based on clinical response
  1. Topical agents: All should be applied to affected areas BID
    a. **Undecylenic Acid (Cruex, Desenex):** Available OTC
    b. **Tolnaftate 1% (Tinactin, Aftate, NP-27):** Available OTC
    c. **Ciclopirox 1% (Loprox)**
    d. **Imidazoles**
      i. **Clotrimazole 1% (Lotrimin, Mycelex):** Available OTC
      ii. **Miconazole 2% (Monostat-Derm, Micatin):** Available OTC
      iii. **Ketoconazole 2% (Nizoral)**
    e. **Allylamines**
      i. **Naftifine 1% (Naftin)**
      ii. **Terbinafine 1% (Lamisil)**
  2. Oral agents (for extensive infections): **Microsized Griseofulvin (Fulvicin-U/F, Grifulvin V, Grisactin)** 10mg/kg/day PO × 4 weeks, usual adult dose is 500mg QD. Available as suspension 125mg/5mL and 250, 500mg tabs. Monitor renal, hepatic and hematopoietic functions periodically and discontinue if granulo-cytopenia occurs
B. **Treatment of *tinea capitis*: Microsized Griseofulvin (Fulvicin-U/F, Grifulvin V, Grisactin)** 10mg/kg/day PO × 4–6 weeks (2 weeks beyond clinical resolution), usual adult dose is 500mg QD. Available in suspension 125mg/5mL and 250, 500mg tabs. Monitor renal, hepatic and hematopoietic functions periodically and discontinue if granulocytopenia occurs
C. **Treatment of *tinea unguium***
  1. Oral agents (for cure): **Sporanox** or **Lamisil**
    a. Fingernails
      1. **Terbinafine (Lamisil):** 250mg PO QD × 6 weeks
      2. **Itraconazole (Sporanox):** pulse therapy 200mg PO BID × 7days, then off for 3 weeks and repeat × 1
    b. Toenails
      1. **Terbinafine (Lamisil):** 250mg PO QD × 12 weeks; monitor LFT
      2. **Itraconazole (Sporanox):** 200mg PO QD × 12 weeks; monitor LFT
  2. Topical agents (for treatment):
    a. **Ciclopirox Topical solution 8% (Penlac nail lacquer):** Apply the lacquer evenly on the entire nail once daily. Once a week, remove the Penlac with alcohol and then apply Penlac once daily. May take 6 months of therapy before initial improvement of symptoms is noticed
  3. Topical agents (for control): Apply BID indefinitely
    a. **Ciclopirox (cream, lotion)**
    b. **Terbinafine (cream, gel)**
D. **Treatment of oral candidiasis**
  1. **Nystatin (Mycostatin** suspension): 5mL PO QID swish and swallow 5–7 days
  2. **Clotrimazole (Mycelex):** 10mg troches, dissolve in mouth 5 ×/day for 14 days
  3. **Fluconazole (Diflucan):** 200mg on day 1, then 100mg PO QD × 2 weeks. Esophageal candidiasis: Same dose for minimum of 3 weeks, continue for 2 weeks after symptoms resolve. Monitor renal and liver function
E. **Treatment of tinea versicolor**
  1. **Topicals:** Apply BID for 1–3 weeks
    a. **Selenium Sulfide 2.5%**
    b. **Ciclopirox 1%**
    c. **Clotrimazole 1%**
    d. **Miconazole 2%**
    e. **Ketoconazole 2%**
  2. **Orals**
    a. **Ketoconazole:** 200mg QD × 7 days (concentrates in sweat, use before exercise)

   b. **Itraconazole:** 200mg/day × 7–10 days
   c. **Fluconazole:** 150–300mg/day × 7–10 days

V. HAIR CHANGES

A. Definition: Hair is a type of keratin generated by the *hair matrix*, which form the shaft and surrounding structures. The scalp has 100–150,000 hairs

B. Types of hair:
   1. Lanugo: Soft silky hair that covers the fetus in utero. Mostly shed before birth
   2. Vellous: Short fine hairs that cover the entire body except for the palms and soles
   3. Terminal: Long, coarse pigmented hair. Before puberty found only on the scalp and in eyebrows and eyelashes. Additionally, after puberty in the axilla, pubic area and on the chest and face in men

C. Growth Cycle: Hair growth and loss is continuous and random, not cyclical or seasonal and can be defined by 3 discrete stages
   1. Anagen: Active growth phase, 0.3–0.4mm/day or 1 cm/28 days. This rate decreases with age. 90% of hairs are in this phase, which continues for 2 to 6 years. Hair on the extremities, lashes and brows has a shorter growth phase and longer resting phase. Plucked hair in this phase has a 2–3mm white sheath at the end
   2. Catagen: Active follicular regression that signals the end of anagen. Lasts 2–3 weeks. Plucked hair has a small white tip at the end
   3. Telogen: A resting phase, all cellular activity stops. Represents 10% of all hair and lasts for approximately 100 days. 25–100 telogen hairs are normally shed each day. Shampooing may dramatically increase this number

D. Approach to the patient with hair loss
   1. Generalized versus discrete areas of hair loss
   2. Rapid versus gradual hair loss
   3. Partial versus complete balding
   4. Changes in hair texture or breakage
   5. Scarring

E. Diffuse, rapid hair loss
   1. Telogen Effluvium: Telogen (resting) hair loss often seen 3 months after pregnancy, fever or severe illness, major surgery or change in diet. Generally over 1–2 months and usually no more than 50% of hairs are affected. Scarring and inflammation are absent. Resolves spontaneously
   2. Anagen Effluvium: Abrupt insult to active growth. Usually due to chemotherapeutics. Only telogenic hairs remain

F. Diffuse, gradual hair loss, often with thinning, restricted to top of scalp
   1. Male pattern baldness: Frontal recession or loss over the temples or crown
   2. Female pattern baldness: Gradual loss on the central scalp with preservation of the frontal hair line
   3. Treatment: Topical **Minoxidil** is indicated for men and women. **Propecia (Finasteride)** is indicated in men only. Surgical options include hair transplants, scalp reductions and flaps and hair weaves

G. Diffuse, gradual hair loss, often with thinning, all over scalp
   1. Diffuse alopecia areata: Alopecia areata is rapid hair loss in a sharply defined, usually round, areas. It rarely occurs in more diffuse distributions with poorer potential for regrowth
   2. Thyroid/Iron deficiency
   3. Drugs: Warfarin, Heparin, Propranolol, vitamin A
   4. Secondary syphilis or S.L.E.
   5. Gradual hair loss with age

H. Discrete balding areas without scarring or scalp inflammation
   1. Alopecia areata: Most common cause in both children and adults. Etiology is unknown. Check for ! shaped hairs at the edge of balding areas. These are short, broken-off hairs where the broken end is thicker and darker than where the hair emerges from the scalp. May be associated with nail pitting and longitudinal striations. Generally resolves spontaneously but can also be treated with intra-lesional steroids

DERM

2. Trichotillomania: Caused by the irresistible urge to pull out longer hairs leaving very short, fine hairs. Often seen in children

I. Discrete balding areas with scarring or scalp inflammation

1. Infection: Tinea Capitis, kerion, bacterial infection, herpes zoster
2. Traumatic: Burns, radiation
3. Neoplastic: Basal cell carcinoma, metastatic disease
4. Systemic: S.L.E., Psoriasis, eczema, lichen planus, scleroderma

J. Excessive hair growth

1. Hirsutism: Excessive terminal hair in a pattern not normal for females (beard or moustache, chest or lower abdomen). May be associated with other signs of virilization including acne, clitoral hypertrophy, decreased breast size, deepening of the voice, increased muscle mass and changes in menstruation. Evaluation should focus on personal and family history, medications, other endocrine abnormalities and the ovary and adrenal glands as possible sources of androgens
2. Hypertrichosis: Excessive hair all over the body. Often lanugo hair. If confined to the lumbo-sacral area it may be associated with spina bifida
3. Treatment: Serious underlying disease must be treated first and cosmetic appearance second. Oral contraceptives reduce free testosterone. Low dose oral steroids suppress adrenal function and lower adrenal androgen production. Spironolactone competes for androgen receptors at the follicle and reduces hair shaft size and pigmentation

References

Pardasani AG, et al. Treatment of psoriasis: an algorithm-based approach for primary care physicians, Am Fam Phys 2000;61:725–33,736.

Chaula EN, et al. Equivalent therapeutic efficacy and safety of ivermectin and lindane in the treatment of human scabies. Arch Dermatol Jun 1999;135:651–5.

Temple ME, et al. Pharmacotherapy of tinea capitis. J Am Board Fam Pract May-June 1999;12:236–41.

DERM

IX. Surgery

SURG

Daniel M. Neides, MD
Eric Bates, PA

94. EVALUATION OF ABDOMINAL PAIN

I. INTRODUCTION: Evaluation of an acute abdomen continues to remain a diagnostic challenge. Abdominal pain is the most common cause for hospital admission, with approximately 57/1000 adult ED visits in 1996, and up to 42–63% of admissions. It is also the most frequent chief complaint of the patient with an acute abdomen

II. HISTORY: Is the most important component in the evaluation of abdominal pain. This information is commonly grouped into the attributes of pain, associated symptoms, and past history
- **A.** Pain
    1. Onset: Sudden vs. gradual, time of onset
    2. Location: Have patient point to where pain is located
    3. Quality/Character: Visceral pain (steady ache or vague discomfort or excruciating or colicky pain); parietal pain (more localized to specific site); referred pain (e.g., renal colic may refer pain to the testicles or labia, biliary pain may be referred to the right infrascapular region)
    4. Severity: Quantify pain on scale of 1–10
    5. Duration
    6. Palliative and provocative factors
    7. Change of any variables over time
    8. History of previous pain
- **B.** Associated symptoms
    1. Fever: Elderly may not mount an appropriate fever response. The measured temperature may be artificially low due to antipyretics or an oral temperature taken in a tachypnic patient
    2. Vomiting: Relationship of abdominal pain and vomiting (e.g., pain usually precedes vomiting by 3–4hrs in patients with appendicitis but is just the opposite in gastroenteritis). Frequency of vomiting along with character (including color and content, i.e., bilious, bloody, coffee ground, etc.)
    3. Anorexia: Usually associated with acute abdominal pain: may precede the onset of pain in appendicitis
    4. Bowels: Constipation, diarrhea, and recent change in bowel habits. Watery diarrhea with crampy pain suggests gastroenteritis. Failure to pass flatus with crampy pain and vomiting suggests mechanical obstruction. Blood in stool
    5. Urination: Dysuria, frequency, urgency, incontinence, hematuria, back pain
    6. Vaginal: Discharge, bleeding,
    7. Menstruation: Last menstrual period (exact dates), frequency, duration, the type of contraception and duration of use
- **C.** Past medical and surgical history
    1. Prior surgeries/hospitalizations help to rule in or out certain diagnoses
    2. History of similar pain suggests recurrent disease
    3. Detailed review of systems
    4. History of chronic diseases (including diabetes, HIV status and risk factors, CNS disease, i.e., multiple sclerosis)
    5. Recent or current medications (including NSAIDs and antibiotics)
    6. Recent trauma
    7. Social history (including use of tobacco, alcohol and other drug usage)
    8. Occupation (including possible toxic exposure)
    9. Living circumstances (e.g., homeless, residing in an unheated dwelling, no running water, other family members with similar symptoms)
    10. Recent out of country travel or exposure to lake, well, or stream water

III. PHYSICAL EXAMINATION
- **A. General:** Patient's appearance, ability to answer questions, position in bed, and degree of discomfort. Dehydration may be suggested by dry mucous membranes, sunken eyes, and by

SURG

rapid and shallow respirations. A patient writhing on the bed or pacing the room may have kidney stones, while a patient lying still is more likely to have peritoneal irritation. Facial expression may indicate pain of a crampy or constant nature. Pallor suggests anemia

B. Vital Signs: Are vital! As with other disease processes tachycardia and hypotension signify hypovolemia and possible shock. A variant in blood pressure and pulse between arms may indicate an acute aortic dissection. An accurate and careful evaluation of respiration can indicate possible compensatory efforts for an underlying metabolic acidosis, or possible peritoneal pain related to diaphragmatic excursion. Temperature changes, while not always a reliable predictor of absence of disease, are an important diagnostic tool

C. Inspection: Visual study of the chest and abdomen. Inquire about every scar. A rash may indicate herpes zoster. Abdominal distention and masses

D. Auscultation: Frequency and pitch of bowel sounds. High pitched bowel sounds may indicate obstruction. Presence or absence of abdominal bruits

E. Percussion and palpation
1. Have patient point "with one finger" to area of greatest pain
2. Begin in the quadrant free of pain and perform lightly (Note voluntary and involuntary guarding, rigidity and rebound)
3. Organomegaly, and other masses including the bladder, and hernias
4. Pulsatile mass may indicate an aortic dissection
5. Costovertebral angle tenderness

F. Genitourinary
1. Umbilical hernia (and inguinal hernia)
2. Examine the testicles for swelling and/or retraction
3. Penis for discharge

G. Pelvic examination
1. Both speculum and bimanual examination
2. Obtain GC and *Chlamydia* cultures in the sexually active female
3. Note cervical motion and/or adnexal tenderness or masses, discharge or bleeding

H. Rectal examination
1. Probe for perirectal mass, fecal impaction, prostate enlargement or irregularity
2. Guaiac stool

IV. DIAGNOSTIC STUDIES

A. Plain abdominal radiograph: While plain films of the abdomen may be helpful in the evaluation of acute abdominal pain, some feel that their usefulness is limited and markedly overutilized. One study concluded that plain films should be used only for suspected obstruction, perforation, ischemia, peritonitis, or renal colic. Both a supine and upright film of the abdomen should be obtained, as well as a PA (+/- lateral) chest film to exclude intrathoracic causes of acute abdominal pain (e.g., lower lobe pneumonia or aortic dissection)
1. Observe for presence of free intraperitoneal air and presence or absence of air and fluid within the small and large intestine (a lateral decubitus film may be more accurate in diagnosing free air)
2. If the psoas shadow is obscured, consider the possibility of retroperitoneal inflammation
3. On plain x-ray look for colonic haustra in order to distinguish large from small bowel
4. Inspect for the presence of foreign bodies and the presence of stones
5. Calcification of the vessels may suggest the possibility of an aneurysm

B. Ultrasonography: Will help in the diagnosing of cholelithiasis, fluid-containing cavities, intraabdominal masses, intrauterine or extrauterine pregnancy, ovarian cyst, and testicular torsion

C. Intravenous pyelogram (IVP) is helpful in diagnosis of renal and ureteral calculi, but is becoming of less value with the advances in helical CT scan

D. CT Scan: Increasing value in detection of renal and ureteral calculi, and is useful in diagnosis of small bowel obstruction, appendicitis, pancreatic necrosis, mass, abscess and when routine radiographic studies are inconclusive

E. Nuclear medicine: Helpful in diagnosing cholecystitis and testicular torsion

F. Laboratory
1. Complete blood count (CBC). Can indicate an infectious process, but if normal does not exclude one. Can indicate anemia and blood loss

2. Urinalysis (urinary tract infection, renal or ureteral calculi)
3. Serum amylase and lipase, (may indicate pancreatitis), SGOT/AST (hepatitis), b-HCG (pregnancy, ectopic), lactic acid (mesenteric ischemia)
4. Serum electrolytes (for fluid management) if surgical intervention is required
5. PT/PTT, type and screen (prior to surgery)

V. CAUSES OF ABDOMINAL PAIN STRATIFIED BY AGE

Final Diagnosis	≤ 50 years old	≥ 50 years old
Biliary tract disease	6%	21%
Nonspecific abdominal pain	40%	16%
Appendicitis	32%	15%
Bowel obstruction	2%	12%
Pancreatitis	2%	7%
Diverticular disease	<0.1%	6%
Cancer	<0.1%	4%
Hernia	<0.1%	3%
Vascular	<0.1%	2%
Acute gynecologic disease	4%	<0.1%
Other	13%	13%

Source: Gallagher J. Acute abdominal pain. In: Tintinalli J, ed. Emergency Medicine: a comprehensive study guide. 5th ed. New York: McGraw-Hill, 2000: 500.

VI. PRESENTATION OF COMMON CONDITIONS LEADING TO AN ACUTE ABDOMEN

DIAGNOSIS	PRESENTATION	EVALUATION
Peritonitis	Diffuse, severe tenderness; guarding or rigidity; absent bowel sounds; rebound	*Diagnosis is clinical;* upright chest film may show free intraperitoneal air
Appendicitis	Focal, lower right quadrant (McBurney's point) tenderness, with rebound; anorexia	*Diagnosis is clinical;* ultrasound, CT, spiral CT or barium enema may aid in diagnosis
Acute Pancreatitis	Diffuse upper abdominal tenderness radiating to the back; mild rebound; ileus; Grey Turner's sign (flank hematoma)	Serum amylase and Lipase; ultrasound or CT
Acute Cholecystitis	Right upper quadrant tenderness; muscle guarding; worse with inspiration	Ultrasound
Diverticulitis	Left lower quadrant tenderness; rebound; guarding; fever; quiet bowel sounds	CT; barium enema (Gastrografin should be used if a perforation is a possibility)
Small bowel obstruction — Proximal	Nausea, vomiting; alkalosis; normal or quiet bowel sounds; NO distension	Abdominal film; upper GI series; endoscopy
Small bowel obstruction — Distal	Nausea, vomiting; tenderness, distension; hyperactive bowel sounds	Abdominal film; angiogram; serum amylase
Cholangitis	Fever, jaundice; right upper quadrant pain	Ultrasound; ERCP; cholangiogram
Ectopic pregnancy	Peritonitis, hypotension; anemia; shock	B-hCG; vaginal ultrasound; culdocentesis
Ruptured Aortic Aneurysm	Upper abdominal tenderness; back pain; pulsatile mass; hypovolemic shock	Angiogram; ultrasound, CT
Diseases related to AIDS: CMV Opportunisitc infections Lymphoma Kaposi's sarcoma of GI tract	Peritonitis Peritonitis Distension; obstipation; GI bleeding Distension; obstipation; GI bleeding	CT; paracentesis CT; paracentesis CT; upper GI series; endoscopy Endoscopy

SURG

VII. NONSURGICAL CAUSES OF ABDOMINAL PAIN

SYSTEM	DISEASE
Cardiac	Myocardial infarction, acute pericarditis
Pulmonary	Pneumonia, pulmonary infarction or embolus, pleural effusion
Gastrointestinal	Pancreatitis, gastroenteritis, hepatitis, inflammatory bowel disease (IBD), peptic ulcer disease (PUD), irritable bowel syndrome (IBS)
Endocrine	DKA, acute adrenal insufficiency, Addisonian crisis
Metabolic	Acute porphyria, familial Mediterranean fever
Musculoskeletal	Rectus muscle hematoma
Neurologic	Nerve root compression, tabes dorsalis
Genitourinary	Pyelonephritis, acute salpingitis, ovarian cyst, prostatitis, nephrolithiasis, endometriosis, dysmenorrhea
Psychologic	Depression, anxiety, somatization

CLINICAL PEARLS

- Pain that is out of proportion to findings on exam may suggest ischemic bowel
- Most common etiologies of small bowel obstruction are adhesions, hernia, and tumor
- Most common etiologies of colonic obstruction are tumor, volvulus, and diverticular disease
- If an abdominal exam is difficult because of increased pain, peritoneal irritation can be demonstrated by having the patient cough and then asking to point to the area of maximum tenderness
- The white blood cell count can be helpful, but may also be misleading. One study (1,800 patients) showed that a WBC > 10,000–11,000 only doubled the odds of appendicitis
- The history and physical are almost worthless in excluding an ectopic pregnancy in a pregnant patient with abdominal pain and/or vaginal bleeding. An ectopic pregnancy cannot be absolutely excluded based on quantitative hCG. A low (or high) hCG should NOT be reassuring to the clinician. Perform vaginal ultrasound in pregnant patients with abdominal pain and/or vaginal bleeding

References

Ahmed A, et al. Management of gallstones and their complications. Am Fam Phys 2000;61:1673–80,1687–8.

Gallagher J. Acute abdominal pain. In: Tintinalli, J ed. Emergency medicine: a comprehensive study guide. 5th ed. New York: McGraw-Hill, 2000: 497–512.

Dart RG, Kaplan B, Varaklis K. Predictive value of history and physical examination in patients with suspected ectopic pregnancy. Ann Emerg Med 1999;33:283–290.

Carrico CW, et al. Impact of sonography on the diagnosis and treatment of acute lower abdominal pain in children and young adults. Am J Roentgenol Feb 1999;172: 513–6.

Sfairi A, et al. Acute appendicitis in patients over 70 years of age. Presse Med Apr 27, 1999; 25(15):707–101.

Coleman C, et al. White blood cell count is a poor predictor of severity of disease in the diagnosis of appendicitis. Am Surg Oct 1998;64(10):983.

Balthazar EJ, et al. Appendicitis: the impact of computed tomography imaging on negative appendectomy and perforation rates. Am J Gastroent May 1998;93(5):768.

Parker LJ, et al. Emergency department evaluation of geriatric patients with acute cholecystitis. Acad Emerg Med Jan 1997;4(1):51–5.

Gupta H. Advances in imaging of the acute abdomen. Surgical Clinics N Am 1997;77(6)1245–61.

Martin, R. The acute abdomen: an overview and algorithms. Surgical Clinics of N Am 1997;77(6) 1227–43.

Parker JS, et al. Abdominal pain in the elderly: use of temperature and laboratory testing to screen for surgical disease. Fam Med Mar 1996; 28(3):193–7.

Smyth E, et al. Prognosis of elderly patients with non-specific abdominal pain. J Accid Emerg Med Jan 1996;13(1):44–5.

95. DIVERTICULOSIS AND DIVERTICULITIS

I. DEFINITION: Colonic diverticula are mucosal protrusions through the muscularis. Diverticulitis refers to inflammation in or around diverticula. 33% of the US population will have diverticular disease by age 45 and 67% by age 85. Diverticulitis occurs in 10–25% of people with diverticulosis

II. PATHOGENESIS
    A. High fat, low fiber diet "Western diet" results in decreased bulk of stool which leads to decreased colon diameter which leads to increased wall tension
    B. Retention of fecal material in a diverticular sac (obstruction of diverticuli) compromises blood flow to the sac and surrounding tissue which leads to inflammation

III. EPIDEMIOLOGY
    A. Incidence of diverticula increases with age (See Clinical Pearls below)
    B. Incidence in left colon is 3 times that of the right colon. Highest incidence is in the sigmoid colon
    C. Incidence in men greater than women
    D. Incidence in the US and Europe greater that in Asia and Africa (genetic vs. diet)

IV. SIGNS AND SYMPTOMS: Patients present because of bleeding and complications of inflammation
    A. Diverticulosis: Usually asymptomatic, but may present with painless hematochezia
    B. Diverticulitis
        1. Fever
        2. Anorexia, nausea, vomiting
        3. Abdominal pain (usually LLQ)
        4. Rebound tenderness
        5. Hypoactive bowel sounds
        6. Leukocytosis with left shift
        7. Guaiac positive stools (rarely gross hematochezia)
        8. Constipation or diarrhea
        9. Tenesmus
        10. Urinary frequency (from irritation of the bladder or ureter)
    C. Complications
        1. Ruptured diverticula/perforation
        2. Fistula between colon and bladder (pneumaturia, fecaluria)
        3. Paralytic ileus
        4. Small bowel obstruction (if loop of bowel becomes narrowed or kinked in the inflammatory mass)

V. EVALUATION
    A. Diverticulosis
        1. If bleeding, then obtain barium enema, colonoscopy or angiography
        2. Diverticulosis is often an incidental finding on colonoscopy, flexible sigmoidoscopy and barium enema
    B. Diverticulitis
        1. Physical Exam
            a. Abdominal exam: Focal guarding or localized rebound, mass
            b. Rectal: May demonstrate tenderness on the left side. May be heme positive
        2. Laboratory
            a. WBC: Normal with diverticulosis, may be elevated with left shift in diverticulitis
            b. H/H: May be decreased with bleeding (chronic diverticulosis)
            c. Urinalysis: May include WBC or RBC with fistula formation
            d. Blood culture: May be positive with perforated diverticular disease
        3. Other studies
            a. Acute abdominal series: Free air (perforation), mass, obstruction
            b. Barium enema: For diagnosis of diverticulosis
            c. Colonoscopy

SURG

d. Angiography: With bleeding
e. Abdominal CT: Evaluate for abscess or fistula

VI. DIFFERENTIAL DIAGNOSIS
A. Colon cancer
B. Appendicitis
C. Inflammatory bowel disease
D. Ischemic colitis
E. Urinary tract infection
F. Ovarian pathology (torsion, cyst)
G. Incarcerated hernia
H. Prostatitis
I. Irritable bowel syndrome
J. Ectopic pregnancy

VII. MANAGEMENT
A. Asymptomatic diverticula
1. Low fat and high fiber vegetable diet
2. Psyllium (Fibercon, Metamucil, etc.)
3. Avoiding seeds and nuts is controversial
B. Bleeding diverticulosis
1. Bowel rest
2. Colonoscopy with cautery
3. Angiogram with vasoconstrictor injection
4. Surgery (80% cease spontaneously)
C. Diverticulitis
1. Outpatient: No signs of peritonitis or systemic infection
   a. Bowel rest: Liquid diet for 48hrs
   b. Antibiotics: Need aerobic and anaerobic coverage. Use 1 of the following antibiotics with **Metronidazole (Flagyl)** 500mg TID or **Clindamycin (Cleocin)** 300mg QID
      i. **Cephalexin (Keflex)** 500mg QID
      ii. **Ciprofloxacin** 500mg BID
      iii. **TMP-SMX DS** BID
      iv. **Amoxicillin** 500mg TID
2. Hospitalization
   a. Indications
      i. Systemic signs or symptoms of infection
      ii. Localized peritonitis
      iii. Inability to take oral meds
      iv. Questionable diagnosis
   b. Bowel rest
   c. Broad spectrum antibiotics

CLINICAL PEARLS
- Irritable bowel syndrome is often diagnosed as diverticular disease
- Bleeding occurs in 5–15% of patients with diverticulosis. Stops spontaneously in 75–95%

References
Chintapalli KN, et al. Diverticulitis versus colon cancer: differentiation with helical CT findings. Radiology Feb 1999;210:429–35.
Conn HF, ed. Conn's current therapy. Philadelphia: W.B. Saunders, 1997.
Jeffers JD, Boynton, SD, eds. Harrison's principles of internal medicine. New York:McGraw-Hill, 1994.
Sleisenger MH, Frodtran JS, eds. Gastrointestinal disease. Philadelphia:W.B. Saunders, 1993.
Emergency medicine—a comprehensive study guide. Colonic diverticular disease New York:McGraw-Hill, 1996:473–6.

SURG

Karen Hazelton, PA

96. MANAGEMENT OF WOUNDS

I. INTRODUCTION: The general goal of suturing is hemostasis, cosmesis, prevention of infection and restoration of function

II. HISTORY: Crushing injuries and puncture wounds are at increased risk for infection
 A. How, when and where did injury occur
 B. Mechanism of injury
 C. How long ago did injury occur
 D. Clean or soiled environment
 E. What was the position of the extremity during the injury (position of a hand is important for locating tendon injury)
 F. Dominant hand
 G. Profession

III. PHYSICAL EXAM
 A. Location, length, shape, depth and tension lines of the wound
 B. Associated tissue injury, such as joint, tendon or ligament involvement
 C. Contaminants and foreign bodies
 D. Neurovascular integrity and function

IV. LABORATORY AND RADIOLOGICAL STUDIES
 A. If wound appears clinically infected, consider aerobic and anaerobic cultures
 B. Radiograph may be needed for suspected radiopaque foreign objects or fracture

V. INITIAL WOUND PREPARATION
 A. Wounds should generally not be closed after 6–12hrs, but in heavily vascularized areas such as the face, wound closure may be attempted up to 12–24hrs
 B. Unless heavily contaminated, anesthetize wound first so wound can be cleansed in a pain free environment. With some highly contaminated wounds, wound preparation may be performed before anesthesia to prevent introduction of bacteria into healthy tissue
 C. Massively contaminated wounds and wounds with extensive macerated tissue may require debridement in the operating room
 D. Most commonly used skin-preparation solution to cleanse the skin *around the wound* is 1% **Povidone-Iodine (Betadine)** solution
 E. Adequate debridement and copious irrigation with normal saline or Ringer's lactate solution reduces risk of infection. Attach a 18–20 gauge needle to a 30–60cc syringe to irrigate heavily contaminated wounds. Irrigation from an IV bag is not adequate
 F. Hair should be cut and not shaved. Do not clip, cut, or shave the eyebrows
 G. Consider temporary short term placement of a tourniquet to obtain a bloodless field

VI. ANESTHESIA
 A. Anesthetic agents
  1. Topical: Contraindicated on mucous membranes and areas of end circulation such as digits, ears, tip of nose, penis
   a. **TAC: Tetracaine (0.5%), Adrenaline (1:2000), Cocaine (11.4%)**
   b. Topical **Lidocaine** (5%)
   c. **Epinephrine** (1:2000)
  2. Infiltrative
   a. **Lidocaine** (1% or 2%): Maximum dose is 5mg/kg (0.5cc/kg of 1%)
   b. **Lidocaine** with **Epinephrine** 1:2000
    i. Maximum dose is 7mg/kg (0.7cc/kg of 1%)
    ii. Contraindicated in areas of end circulation
   c. **Bupivacaine 0.25% (Marcaine):** Maximum dose is 3mg/kg (1.2cc/kg)
  3. Allergy to Lidocaine
   a. Usually due to an allergy to the PABA preservative

SURG

    b. Consider using a preservative-free Lidocaine
    c. Consider using **Diphenhydramine** 1% or 0.5% for infiltration
  4. Nerve blocks: Most commonly used for face, hands, and feet
  5. Sedation: Most commonly used agents are Ketamine, Midazolam (Versed) and Fentanyl
B. **Techniques to reduce pain with infusion**
  1. Use needle ≥ 25 gauge
  2. Inject slowly
  3. Inject through wound (as opposed to intact skin)
  4. Use a buffering agent: Mix 9cc of 1% **Lidocaine** with 1cc of **Sodium Bicarbonate** with a concentration of 44mEq/50mL
  5. Warm anesthetic to 98.6° F
  6. Use topical agents or sedation in children
  7. Regional nerve blocks in highly contaminated wounds
  8. Digital blocks for fingers and toes

VII. WOUND CLOSURE MATERIAL
A. Sutures

REPAIR OF LACERATIONS WITH SUTURES

SITE OF LACERATION	SUTURE*	SIZE OF SUTURE	SUTURE REMOVAL	COMMENTS
Eyelid	Nonabsorbable suture: Prolene monofilament (Prolene) Nylon monofilament (Ethilon)	6-0, 7-0	3 days	Prolene has the least amount of tissue reactivity
Cheek	same	5-0. 6-0	3–5 days	
Nose, forehead, neck	same	4-0, 5-0	5 days	
Ear	same	4-0, 5-0	4–5 days	
Scalp	same	3-0	5–7 days	
Arm, hand	same	3-0, 4-0	7–10 days	
Leg, foot, chest, back	same	3-0, 4-0	10–14 days	
Tendons	Prolene	3-0, 4-0	----	
Deep closure of wounds, intraoral	Absorbable suture: Vicryl Dexon PDS Chromic gut	3-0, 4-0, 5-0 5-0 (intra-oral)	----	Vicryl and Dexon lose 50% of their tensile strength in 14–20 days PDS loses 50% in 5 weeks Synthetic sutures: preferable to gut in acute wounds

*Despite its ease of tying, silk suture should generally not be used because of increased tissue reactivity and chance of infection

B. Tape
  1. Advantages: Minimizes trauma, tension and infection risk
  2. Disadvantages: Cannot produce eversion of wound edges or closure of deep tissues
  3. Potential indications
    a. Superficial lacerations with little tension
    b. Flaps where vascular supply may be compromised by sutures
    c. Patients with thin frail skin secondary to age or chronic corticosteroid use
C. Staples
  1. Advantage: Faster
  2. Precautions: Never use on face
  3. Potential indications: Consider use on scalp, trunk, upper and lower extremities
D. Topical tissue adhesive
  1. Example: 2-octylcyanoacrylate (Dermabond)
  2. Technique: Approximate wound edges and 3 ever larger concentric circles over wound edges
  3. Use only with superficial wounds under low tensile stress

SURG

VIII. SUTURE TECHNIQUE

A. Always use good lighting and be comfortable (easier to sit than stand or bend)

B. Most common suture technique is simple interrupted

C. Sutures should be placed with equal depth and width for best results. Sutures should be placed to evert wound edges without gapping or pulling. Eversion may be accomplished by placing the needle through the skin at a 90° angle and not tangentially

D. Sutures should be used to approximate the wound edges and not to pull the wound together. For wounds with high tension, place deep sutures or mattress sutures

E. Sutures are placed closer together and with smaller bites on the face and neck to minimize scarring

F. When suturing lips, place first suture through vermilion border (junction of lip and skin)

G. Delayed primary closure is preferred in heavily contaminated wounds if no signs of infection are present after 3–5 days

H. Hints for special circumstances

   1. Tape for superficial lacerations with little tension

   2. Staples for selected sites such as scalp

   3. Continuous sutures for longer lacerations of the face and scalp

   4. Deep sutures for high-tension wounds

   5. Vertical mattress sutures for medium deep lacerations

   6. Half buried mattress sutures for flap lacerations

IX. BITE WOUNDS

A. Initial evaluation

   1. Generally, bite wounds are primarily closed in very vascular areas and if cosmetically necessary

   2. Areas usually primarily sutured are face, scalp, and neck. Avoid deep sutures

   3. Consider closing wounds of trunk, arm and legs

   4. Avoid suturing any bite wounds of the hands and feet

B. Wound preparation: See above. Very important to use copious irrigation and debridement of devitalized tissue

C. High risk bite wounds

   1. Location: Hand, foot, wrists, joints. In infants: Scalp or face

   2. Type of wound: Puncture (cat bite) or crush

   3. Patient: Age > 50, asplenic, alcoholic, immunocompromised, diabetic, peripheral vascular disease, chronic steroid use, prosthetic or diseased cardiac valve or joint

D. Human bites

   1. Most common organisms include α-hemolytic *Streptococcus, Staphylococcus, Eikenella corrodens, Corynebacterium* and *Bacteroides*

   2. Carry the highest risk of infection on the hand. About 47% of human bites to hand become infected

   3. If there is invasion of the MCP joint capsule (usually from injuries sustained during a fight), then refer to a hand surgeon for possible debridement in the operating room

   4. Wound closure

     a. Human bites to the hand should not be closed

     b. Those in other areas may be closed if less than 6hrs old after adequate irrigation and debridement

   5. Antibiotic prophylaxis: **Amoxicillin/Clavulanate (Augmentin)** 875mg PO BID × 5 days

E. Dog bites

   1. Most common organisms include *Strep viridans, Pasteurella multocida, S. aureus, E. corrodens, Bacteroides*

   2. Dog bites tend to be more of an open, tearing type of wound

   3. Wound closure

     a. Dog bites to the hand should not be closed

     b. Those in other areas may be closed if less than 6hrs old after adequate irrigation and debridement

   4. Antibiotic prophylaxis

     a. Risk of infection without antibiotics is 9–16%

     b. Prophylaxis should be administered in high risk bite wounds (see above) and optional in other wounds

     c. Give prophylaxis as soon as possible (preferable before repair is done)

     d. Antibiotic prophylaxis: **Augmentin** 875mg PO BID × 3–5 days

     e. Alternative

SURG

      i. Adults: **Clindamycin** 300mg PO QID plus **Fluoroquinalone** (e.g., **Cipro** 500mg BID)

      ii. Children: **Clindamycin** plus **Bactrim**

F. Cat bites

  1. Most common organisms include staph and strep species and *Pasteurella multocida*

  2. Cat bites are usually deep puncture type wounds

  3. Wound closure: Leave all cat bites open to heal by secondary intention

  4. Antibiotic prophylaxis

    a. Risk of infection is ~ 50% without antibiotics

    b. Recommended: **Augmentin** 875mg PO BID × 3–5 days

    c. Alternative: **Cefuroxime (Ceftin)** 500mg PO BID or **Doxycycline** 100mg PO BID

    d. Caution: Do not use **Cephalexin (Keflex)** or **Dicloxacillin**

X. AFTERCARE INSTRUCTIONS

A. General

  1. Dressings

  2. Topical antibiotics

  3. Non adherent dressing

  4. Sterile gauze dressing

  5. Splint lacerations over joints

B. Wound that should be rechecked in 24–48hrs

  1. Hand wounds

  2. Bite wounds

  3. Heavily contaminated wounds

  4. Other wounds requiring prophylactic antibiotics

C. Tetanus prophylaxis

SUMMARY OF TETANUS PROPHYLAXIS FOR THE INJURED PATIENT

History of Adsorbed Tetanus Toxoid (Doses)	Nontetanus-Prone Wounds		Tetanus-Prone Wounds	
	Td[1]	TIG	Td[1]	TIG
Unknown or ≤ three	Yes	No	Yes	Yes
≥ Three[2]	No[3]	No	No[4]	No

1   For children younger than 7 years old: DTP (DT, if pertussis vaccine is contraindicated) is preferred to tetanus toxoid alone. For persons 7 years old and older, Td is preferred to tetanus toxoid alone

2   If only 3 doses of fluid toxoid have been received, a fourth dose of toxoid, preferably an adsorbed toxoid, should be given

3   Yes, if more than 10 years since last dose

4   Yes, if more than 5 years since last dose (more frequent boosters are not needed and can accentuate side effects)

Td Tetanus and diphtheria toxoids adsorbed—for adult use

TIG Tetanus immune globulin — human

CLINICAL PEARLS

    • Lidocaine with Epinephrine should not be used in areas with poor blood supply (nose, fingers, toes, skin flaps, etc.)

    • Wounds should generally not be closed after 6–8hrs, but may be primarily closed up to 24hrs in very vascular areas such as the face and scalp

    • Subcutaneous suture in the hand and any silk suture is generally not used because of increased tissue reactivity and increased risk of infection

    • Shaving the hair around a wound increases the chance of infection

References

Burns TB, Worthington, JM. Using tissue adhesive for wound repair: a practical guide to Dermabond. Am Fam Phys 2000;61:1383–8.

SURG

Hollander JE, Singer AJ. Laceration management. Ann Emerg Med Sep 1999;34:356–67.

Lewis KT, Management of cat and dog bites. Am Fam Phys 1995;52:479.

Mortiere MD. Principles of primary wound management—a guide to the fundamentals. Gaithersburg, MD:PFP Printing,1996.

Noeller T. Laceration repair techniques. Emergency Med Rep 1996:17(21):207–18.

Presutti RJ. Bite wounds: early treatment and prophylaxis against infectious complications. Postgraduate Med 1997:101(4):243–54.

Sanford JP, et al. Guide to antimicrobial therapy. 30th ed. Antimicrobial Therapy, Inc. 2000.

Eisenbud DE. Modern wound management. Columbus, OH: Anadem Publishing, 1998.

Michael B. Weinstock, MD

97. PAIN MANAGEMENT IN ADULTS AND CHILDREN

PAIN MANAGEMENT IN ADULTS AND CHILDREN

Medication	Equi-analgesic dose PO*	Equi-analgesic dose IM/SC	Duration of analgesia** (hours)	Recommended dose in adults and children*** (start with the lowest dose for pain control and then increase dose as needed)
Morphine sulfate	30mg	10mg	3–7	Adults — IM/IV: 2–10mg Q 2–3hrs Children — IM/IV: 0.1–0.2mg/kg/dose **Roxanol** 20mg/mL, 10mg/2.5mL — Titrate to effective dose Q 4 hours PO — Logical starting dose is 10–30mg Q 4hours PO **MS Contin/Oramorph SR** (Sustained release) — 15, 30, 60, 100mg tabs (MS contin has a 200mg tab)
Hydro-morphone (Dilaudid)	4–6mg	1.5–2mg	2–4	IM/IV/SC: 1–2mg Q 4–6 hours PO: 2–4mg Q 4–6 hours (2, 4, 8mg tabs or 5mg/5mL liquid) Rectal: One supp. PR Q 6–8 hours Available 3mg Not recommended for children
Methadone (Dolophine)	5–6mg	2.5–3mg	4–8	Adults — PO: 2.5–10mg Q 3–4 hours
Meperidine (Demerol)	300mg	75–100mg	2–4	Adults — IV/IM/PO: 50–100mg Q 3–4 hours (20, 100mg tabs) Children — IV/IM/PO: 1–1.5mg/kg/dose Q 3–4 hours (Elixir: 50mg/5mL)
Oxycodone (Oxyir, Percocet, Percodan, OxyContin)	30mg	NA	4–6	**Oxyir** (oxycodone 5mg caps or 20mg/mL liquid) **OxyCotin** (controlled release) — every 12 hours available 10, 20, 40, 80mg **Percocet 2.5/325** (oxycodone 2.5mg/acetaminophen 325mg) **Percocet 5/325** (oxycodone 5mg/acetaminophen 325mg) **Percocet 7.5/500** (oxycodone 7.5mg/acetaminophen 500mg) **Percocet 10/650** (oxycodone 10mg/acetaminophen 650mg) **Percodan** (oxycodone 4.5mg/aspirin 325mg)
Hydrocodone (Lorcet, Lortab, Vicodin, Vicoprofen)	30mg	NA	3–8	**Lorcet 10/650** (hydrocodone 10mg/acetaminophen 650mg) **Lorcet plus** (hydrocodone 7.5mg/acetaminophen 650mg) **Lortab 10/500** (hydrocodone 10mg/acetaminophen 500mg) **Lortab 7.5/500** (hydrocodone 7.5mg/acetaminophen 500mg) **Lortab 5/500** (hydrocodone 5mg/acetaminophen 500mg) **Lortab 2.5/500** (hydrocodone 2.5mg/acetaminophen 500mg) **Lortab elixir** (hydrocodone 7.5mg/acetaminophen 500mg/elixir 15mL) **Vicodin** (hydrocodone 5mg/acetaminophen 500mg) **Vicodin ES** (hydrocodone 7.5mg/ acetaminophen 750mg) **Vicoprofen** (hydrocodone 7.5mg/ibuprofen 200mg)
Codeine (Tylenol #2, #3, #4, Empirin #2, #3, #4)	200mg	120mg	4–6	Note: Cough suppressant at 15–30mg Q4 hours Note: PO doses > 65 not recommended due to decreased incremental analgesia. **T#2** = codeine 15mg/acetaminophen 300mg **T#3** = codeine 30mg/acetaminophen 300mg **T#4** = codeine 60mg/acetaminophen 300mg **Elixir:** codeine 12mg/acetaminophen 120mg/5mL
Propoxyphene (Darvon, Darvon-N Darvocet-N 100)	130–200mg	NA	4–6	**Darvon** (propoxyphene 65mg) **Darvon-N** (propoxyphene 100mg) **Darvocet-N 100** (propoxyphene 100/acetaminophen 650mg)
Fentanyl (Duragesic)	Duragesic transdermal system patch 100mcg/hr = morphine 60mg IV/24 hours		72	Patches in doses of 25, 50, 75, 100mcg/hour Note: Should not be used to treat acute pain Dose – give every 3 days

* Consider reducing calculated parental dose when switching from PO to IV/IM to accommodate for cross sensitivity and absorption variation.

** Duration of action is immediate release preparations (not sustained release)

*** All doses are for adults unless otherwise specified. Maximum 4g acetaminophen per day. Medications are generally dosed every 4–6 hours unless otherwise specified.

I. SIDE EFFECTS OF OPIOIDS
   A. Respiratory depression/arrest
   B. Sedation
   C. Nausea and vomiting: May administer an anti-nausea medication concurrently with opioid
   D. Constipation
   E. Tolerance and dependence

II. OVERDOSE—Naloxone (Narcan) 0.4–2mg IV: 1 ampule equals 0.4mg
   A. May be necessary to give more than once
   B. Consider starting with ½ ampule in a post-op patient to avoid *complete* narcotic reversal. After reversal of narcotic, continue to closely monitor the patient as the half-life of the narcotic may be longer than the half-life of the Naloxone

III. NON-OPIOID PAIN MANAGEMENT

NON-OPIOID PAIN MANAGEMENT

DRUG	ADULT DOSE	PEDIATRIC DOSE
Acetaminophen (Tylenol)	650–1000mg Q4–6 hours PRN (Max. daily dose is 4g)	10–15mg/kg/dose Q4–6 hours PRN Supplied: Drops — One dropper-full (0.8mL)=80mg Elixir — 160mg/5mL (One teaspoon) Chewable tablets — 80mg/tab
Ibuprofen	200–800mg Q8 hours (Max. daily dose is 3200mg)	5–10mg/kg/dose Q8 hours PRN Supplied: 100mg/5mL (One teaspoon)
Aspirin	325-650mg Q4–6 hours PRN (Max. daily dose is 3600mg)	For anti-rheumatic doses or for treatment of Kawasaki's dz., consult other sources
Ketorolac (Toradol)	IM: 30–60mg IM loading dose PO: 10mg Q4–6 hours PRN Do not exceed 5 days (injection plus oral)	Not recommended for children
Tramadol (Ultram)	50–100mg PO Q4–6 hours PRN	Not recommended for children

CLINICAL PEARLS:
   • Pain medicines are frequently underdosed. Pain medicines should generally be *scheduled* and given in doses adequate to relieve pain. This practice will reduce the possibility of addiction
   • To initiate pain management, begin with the most benign medicine which will still control the pain. This often involves starting with a non-opioid analgesic and titrating upward. The "comparison of opioid analgesics" is listed from most to least potent
   • When using an opioid analgesic, anticipate constipation and prescribe a laxative
   • It is questionable whether Acetaminophen with Codeine is any more effective than Acetaminophen without Codeine

References
Ricard-Hibon A, et al. A quality control program for acute pain management in out-of-hospital critical care medicine. Ann Emerg Med 1999;34:738.
Drayer, R.A., et al. Barriers to better pain control in hospitalized patients. J Pain Symp Man 1999;17:434.
Becker N, et al. Pain epidemiology and health related quality of life in chronic non-malignant pain patients referred to a Danish multidisciplinary pain center. Pain 1997;73:393–400.
Foley KM. Advances in cancer pain. Archives of Neurology 1999;56:413.
Lipman AG. Opioid analgesics in the management of cancer pain. Am J Hosp Care Jan/Feb 1989;13–23.

SURG

Michael B. Weinstock, MD

98. PREOPERATIVE EVALUATION

I. INTRODUCTON

A preoperative assessment is mandatory to avoid preventable perioperative complications. This is done by first quantitating a patient's known medical problems and discovering unknown medical problems during a preoperative assessment, and then maximally managing these problems before surgery. The preoperative evaluation should be performed within 1 month of surgery

The recommendations that follow are a compilation of several sources, generally taking the more conservative approach

II. HISTORY

A. History: Should be performed in a similar manner to a complete history and physical examination, with an *emphasis on cardiac and pulmonary disease.* Other systemic diseases should be explored including diabetes, thyroid disorders, renal and hepatic disease, signs of dementia (perform mini-mental status exam), and neurological status. Ask if patient may be pregnant

B. Social history: Patient should be thoroughly questioned on other factors that increase perioperative risk, including smoking history, alcohol and drug use. It is recommended that patients stop smoking at 4–8 weeks prior to surgery

C. Past history, medications, allergies: Inquire about past surgeries, anesthetic complications and drug allergies. Determine if patient is taking any medications that require additional lab work pre-op or any special perioperative consideration. These medications include Digoxin, diuretics, corticosteroids, hypoglycemics, β-blockers, anticoagulants, or anticholinergics

D. Code status: Address code status when appropriate

III. PHYSICAL EXAMINATION

A. Vitals: Heart rate and rhythm, BP

B. HEENT: Dentition/dentures, neck examination (thyroid, carotid bruits, pulses)

C. Cardiac: Heart murmurs (AS), gallop, cardiomegaly, JVD, peripheral edema, orthopnea

D. Pulmonary: Rales (CHF), wheezes (COPD), rhonchi, pleural effusions, clubbing

E. Neurological: Mini-mental status examination if applicable, cranial nerve examination

F. General: Jaundice, cyanosis, anemia, dehydration

IV. INDICATIONS FOR LABORATORY, ECG, AND RADIOLOGICAL TESTING

It is important to order only those tests that might affect patient management. Many commonly ordered tests have not been found to be helpful. Below is a table with recommendations for pre-op testing

SURG

To use the following table, order:

1. All tests recommended for patients by age — *plus* —
2. All tests recommended based on the type of surgery — *plus* —
3. All tests recommended based on patients' associated conditions

INDICATIONS FOR PREOPERATIVE TESTING

	Hb/Hct	PT/PTT	Type/screen	Electro-lytes	Creat/BUN	Glucose	CXR	ECG
1) Age < 40 y/o	X							
Age 40–65	X				X	X		X
Age > 65 y/o	X				X	X	X	X
2) All ages, **major surgery** *	X	X	X	X	X	X	X	X
3) *Associated conditions:*								
Cardiovascular					X		X	X
Pulmonary							X	X
Diabetes				X	X	X		
Renal	X			X	X			
Hypertension					X			X
Smoking (>20 pack years)	X						X	
Use of diuretics				X	X			
Use of digoxin				X	X			X
Use of anticoagulants	X	X						
Use of steroids				X		X		
Antiarrhythmics				X				X

* Major surgery—vascular, orthopedic, intrathoracic/intra-abdominal surgery

V. INDICATIONS FOR TESTING IN PATIENTS WITH CARDIOVASCULAR DISEASE

  A. Elective surgery should be delayed for at least 6 months post-MI. (There is a 37% re-infarction rate if surgery is performed within 3 months post-MI. This stabilizes at 5% at 6 months)

  B. Semi-elective surgery may be performed 4–6 months post-MI with intensive monitoring

  C. Stress testing is suggested for all patients prior to peripheral vascular surgery. This will usually be a Persantine thallium test or a Dobutamine ECHO

  D. Stable angina,CHF, and arrhythmias should be maximally medically managed prior to surgery

  E. Obtain an ECG on first postoperative day and within 3–5 days post-op

  F. Indications for cardiac stress testing or cardiac catheterization prior to elective or semi-elective *noncardiac* surgery

    1. **Low risk patient** (No risk factors for CAD, age < 70, active lifestyle): No further cardiac evaluation necessary

    2. **Intermediate risk patient** (1–2 risk factors for CAD, diabetic, symptoms controlled if LV dysfunction is known)

      a. Low risk surgery: Head and neck, prostatic, ophthalmologic: No further cardiac evaluation necessary

      b. High risk surgery: Vascular, orthopedic, intrathoracic/intraabdominal

        i. Perform stress thallium or Dobutamine ECHO

        ii. Decision to proceed to cardiac catheterization based on results of stress test. If stress test is normal, no further cardiac evaluation is necessary

    3. **High risk patient:** History of CAD, 3–6 risk factors for CAD, LV dysfunction which has been recently diagnosed or is poorly controlled: Proceed directly to cardiac catheterization

SURG

G. GOLDMAN CARDIAC RISK INDEX: To determine perioperative risk of cardiac event

Risk category	Points (Total 53)
Age > 70	5
MI within last 6 months	10
S_3 gallop or JVD	11
Important aortic stenosis	3
Rhythm other than NSR or PACs	7
PVC's > 5/minute	7
Poor medical condition:	3
$\quad$ $pO_2 < 60$ or $pCO_2 > 50$	
$\quad$ BUN > 50, Creat > 3.0	
$\quad$ Abnormal SGOT, chronic liver	
$\quad\quad$ disease, bedridden patient	
Intraperitoneal, intrathoracic or aortic surgery	3
Emergency operation	4

CARDIAC COMPLICATIONS BASED ON GOLDMAN CARDIAC RISK INDEX

Patient class	Cardiac complications *
Class I (0–5 points)	1%
Class II (6–12 points)	7%
Class III (13–25 points)	14%
Class IV (≥ 26 points)	78%

* MI, cardiogenic pulmonary edema, V Tach, cardiac death

Source: Adapted from Goldman L, et al. Multifactorial index of cardiac risk in noncardiac surgical procedures. N Engl J Med 1977;297:848. Reprinted with permission of The New England Journal of Medicine, Copyright 1977, Massachusetts Medical Society.

VI. INDICATIONS FOR PULMONARY FUNCTION TESTING IN PATIENTS WITH PULMONARY DISEASE *

$\quad$ **A.** *Pulmonary function testing is indicated if* the patient has a history of COPD, SOB, or orthopnea
$\quad\quad$ —and—
$\quad\quad$ 1. There is a need to determine reversibility of bronchospasm with bronchodilators (reversibility is defined as a 15% improvement in the FEV_1 by the American Thoracic Society);
$\quad\quad\quad$ —or—
$\quad\quad$ 2. A need to determine baseline condition in anticipation of post-op intubation;
$\quad\quad\quad$ —or—
$\quad\quad$ 3. Patient is scheduled for lung resection
$\quad$ **B.** Test results indicating a significantly increased morbidity and mortality following surgery:
$\quad\quad$ 1. If $FEV_1 < 2$ liters
$\quad\quad$ 2. Vital capacity (VC) or MVV < 50% of predicted
$\quad\quad$ 3. Arterial $pCO_2 > 45$mm HG
$\quad$ **C.** With positive test results, it needs to be decided if the risks of surgery outweigh the benefits, or if these patients can be medically managed to decrease the risks of surgery
* Source: Adapted from Miller RD. Anesthesia. New York: Churchill Livingstone, 1994:859. Used with permission.

VII. PREOPERATIVE MANAGEMENT OF DIABETIC PATIENTS

$\quad$ **A.** Instruct patient not to take hypoglycemic agents (oral or parenteral) until in the hospital and an IV is in place
$\quad$ **B.** IV insulin therapy during major surgery is indicated for all patients with IDDM and patients with NIDDM who have chronic hyperglycemia (FBS > 180 and HgbA1C > 10%)
$\quad$ **C.** Patients should generally have their postoperative insulin administered with regular insulin by a sliding scale if they are NPO. If they can eat dinner post-op, they may have their usual evening dose of insulin. Continue to check blood sugar Q4hrs or QAC and QHS and cover additional insulin requirements with a sliding scale

SURG

VIII. PREOPERATIVE ADMINISTRATION OF MEDICATIONS

A. Cardiovascular: Continue all medications including diuretics and especially ß-blockers

B. Pulmonary: Continue all medications, especially bronchodilators

C. CNS: Continue all medications including antiseizure medications and major tranquilizers

D. Gastrointestinal: Continue all medications except antacid suspensions (risk of permanent pulmonary damage from aspiration)

E. Endocrine: Continue steroids and thyroid medications. Administer hypoglycemic agents, oral and parenteral, in the hospital after an IV is in place

IX. INDICATIONS FOR DVT PROPHYLAXIS*

A. High risk—*DVT prophylaxis indicated*:10–20% risk of proximal DVT with 1–5% risk of PE
1. History of DVT or PE
2. Age > 40
3. Surgery > 30 minutes (orthopedic, pelvic, abdominal surgery)
4. Obesity, immobilization, malignancy, varicose veins, estrogen use, paralysis
5. Coagulopathy: Protein C, S or anti-III, anticardiolipin antibodies

B. Moderate risk—*Individualize decision about DVT prophylaxis:* 2–10% risk of proximal DVT with 0.01–7% risk of PE
1. Age > 40
2. Surgery > 30 minutes
3. Obesity, immobilization, malignancy, varicose veins, estrogen use, paralysis

* Source: Adapted from Merli GJ, Weitz HH. Approaching the surgical patient. Clinics Chest Med 1993;14(2):208. Used with permission.

References

Miller RD. Anesthesia. New York: Churchill Livingstone Inc., 1994.

Maxwell LG. Preoperative evaluation of children. Pediatric Clinics N Am 1994;41(1):93–109.

Paul SD, Eagle KA. Assessing the cardiac risk of non-cardiac surgery. Contemp Int Med 1994;6(1):47–58.

Merli GJ, Weitz HH. Approaching the surgical patient. Clinics Chest Med 1993; 14(2):208.

Arron MJ, et al. Perioperative evaluation of the elderly. Comprehensive Therapy 1992;18(11):4–10.

Zuniga RE, et al. Preoperative screening for perioperative cardiac risk. Am Fam Phys 1991; 44:1285–90.

King MS. Preoperative evaluation of the elderly. J Am Bd Fam Prac 1991; 4(4):251–8.

Williams DO, Cugell DW. Pulmonary function tests: indications and interpretation. Hospital Med 1988;24(5):23–53.

Blery C, Szatan M, Fourgeaux B. Evaluation of a protocol for selective ordering of preoperative tests. Lancet 1986;1:139–141.

Goldman L, et al. Multifactorial index of cardiac risk in noncardiac surgical procedures. New Engl J Med 1977;297:845–50.

SURG

X. Care of Patients with Psychiatric Disorders

PSY

Daniel M. Neides, MD
Christine Costanza, MD
Budd Ferrante, EdD

99. ANXIETY DISORDERS

I. INTRODUCTION

    A. Anxiety disorders, commonly seen in the general population, include:

        1. Generalized anxiety disorder (GAD)

        2. Panic disorder

        3. Obsessive-compulsive disorder (OCD)

        4. Adjustment disorder with mixed anxiety and depression

        5. Phobic disorder

        6. Post traumatic stress disorder (PTSD)

        7. Social phobia

        8. Substance induced anxiety disorder

    B. Panic disorder is the most common of the anxiety disorders in which patients will seek treatment and can be very disabling with severe financial, social, and occupational consequences for the patient

    C. Patients with panic disorder often have many physical complaints. Delineate between symptoms resulting from the panic disorder and those which are non-psychiatric in origin

    D. Rule out organic causes for the patient's symptoms of anxiety

II. MEDICAL CAUSES OF ANXIETY

    Before treating a patient for an anxiety disorder, a complete history and physical and lab work (if indicated) will be necessary to rule out other organic causes. The major causes are hyperthyroidism, excessive caffeine intake, unstable angina and substance abuse

    A. Endocrine: *Hyperthyroid*, hypoglycemia, carcinoid syndrome, parathyroid dysfunction, pheochromocytoma, adrenal dysfunction

    B. Inflammatory: Systemic lupus erythematosus (SLE), rheumatoid arthritis (RA), polyarteritis nodosa, temporal arteritis

    C. Neurologic: CNS tumors, migraine, subarachnoid hemorrhage, syphilis, multiple sclerosis, Wilson's disease, Huntington's chorea, seizure disorders

    D. Cardiopulmonary: *Angina*, pulmonary insufficiency

    E. Nutritional: Pellagra, B_{12} deficiency

    F. Metabolic: Porphyria

    G. Pharmacologic: *Alcohol and drug abuse or withdrawal,* amphetamines, *caffeine*, sympathomimetics, tobacco

    H. Assess for other psychiatric disorders such as depression

PSY

III. GUIDELINES FOR TREATMENT OF ALL ANXIETY DISORDERS

    A. Consideration should be given to non-pharmacologic approaches (cognitive-behavior therapy is indicated regardless of pharmacologic or non-pharmacologic approaches)

    B. Define underlying conflicts and stresses as clearly as possible

    C. Evaluate the coping mechanisms and support systems

    D. Consider if psychosocial factors or the patient's personality place the patient at risk for abuse or addiction

    E. Individualize anxiolytic therapy. Patients whose anxiety lasts all day may benefit from a long acting Benzodiazepine (BDZ), whereas patients whose anxiety occurs in acute, situationally related episodes may need a short acting BDZ taken PRN. Warning: Benzodiazepines are extremely addictive

    F. The goal of therapy should be clearly discussed with the patient. Stress that long-term pharmacologic therapy is *not* the goal of therapy

    G. In the elderly:

        1. Start with half dose regimen

        2. Avoid frequent dosing adjustments

        3. Watch for signs of confusion, sedation, ataxia

H. There is no evidence that BDZs (or any other anxiolytics) are more effective than **no** pharmacologic treatment when prescribed for long periods or indefinitely (for GAD)

— PART I: GENERALIZED ANXIETY DISORDER (GAD) —

I. EPIDEMIOLOGY
A. Prevalence is 2–4% of the general population; female to male ratio is 2:1
B. Age of onset is in the 20s, although there is a clear rise in diagnosis of children and adolescents
C. 15–17% of first degree relatives have GAD

II. DIAGNOSIS OF GAD (ADAPTED FROM DSM-IV)
A. Excessive anxiety and worry occur more days than not for at least 6 months
B. The patient finds it difficult to control the worry
C. The anxiety and worry are associated with 3 or more of the following symptoms: muscle tension, restlessness, fatigue, difficulty concentrating, irritability or sleep disturbance
D. The focus of the anxiety and worry is not confined to features of an Axis I disorder—e.g., the anxiety or worry is not about being embarrassed in public (social phobia)
E. The anxiety, worry, or physical symptoms cause clinically significant distress or impairment in social, occupational, or other important areas of functioning
F. The disturbance is not related to the psychological effects of a substance (alcohol, caffeine, drugs, or other medications) or a general medical condition (hyperthyroidism), and does not occur during a mood or psychotic disorder

III. TREATMENT
A. **Remove exacerbating factors:** Caffeine, tobacco, drugs
B. **Psychotherapy:** Cognitive-behavioral therapy or group psychotherapy are a few of the therapies which may help in treating a generalized anxiety disorder
C. **Anxiolytic: Non-benzodiazepine**
  1. **Buspirone (Buspar)** 5mg PO BID–TID (gradually increase to 30–60mg/day). Does *not* have the sedative, *withdrawal*, or abuse potential seen with the Benzodiazepines. Effects of the drug may take several weeks to become evident
  2. Side effects: Dizziness, drowsiness, headache
D. **Benzodiazepines:** Have the potential for abuse and dependence
  1. **Diazepam (Valium)** 2–10mg PO BID–QID
  2. **Clonazepam (Klonopin)** 0.5mg PO BID (may increase to 2–10mg/day)
  3. Side effects: Drowsiness, fatigue, ataxia, unsteadiness
E. **Venlafaxine (Effexor XL):** Recently approved for the indication of GAD. Starting dosage is 37.5–75mg QD × 4–7 days, then increase by 37.5–75mg/day PRN up to 225mg/day. The most frequent side effects: nausea, anorexia, insomnia, headache, increased BP, especially in dose>300mg/day
F. **Propranolol (Inderal):** Starting dose is 10–20mg TID–QID. Useful for patients who have prominent and *somatic* (as opposed to *psychotic*) complaints (i.e., palpitations, trembling, restlessness, motor tension)
Note: Not approved for use for anxiety or other psychiatric problems

— PART II: PANIC DISORDER —

I. EPIDEMIOLOGY
A. 2–4% prevalence in the general population
B. Age of onset: Usually late 20s
C. Female to male ratio: Without agoraphobia (irrational fear of being in open or public places), 1:1; with agoraphobia, 2:1
D. 20% of first degree relatives of agoraphobic patients have agoraphobia
E. Co-morbidity with depression

II. DIAGNOSIS OF PANIC DISORDER (ADAPTED FROM DSM-IV)
A. Recurrent unexpected panic attacks (defined as a period of intense fear or discomfort in which 4 or more of the following symptoms develop abruptly and peak within 10 minutes: palpitations, tachycardia, sweating, trembling, shortness of breath, choking sensation, chest pain, nausea, dizziness, derealization,

depersonalization, fear of losing control or of dying, paresthesias, chills, hot flushes)
B. At least 1 of the attacks has been followed by 1 month or more of at least 1 of the following: persistent concern about additional attacks, worry about the implications of the attack, or a significant change in behavior related to the attacks
C. Agoraphobia may be present or absent
D. The panic attacks are not due to the direct psychological effects of a substance (alcohol, drugs of abuse, or medications) or a general medical condition
E. The panic attacks are not better accounted for by another mental disorder

III. TREATMENT

- Before initiating treatment, discuss previous therapies (psychotherapy or drugs) the patient may have encountered, and the results of the particular therapies
- This condition may be chronic, so rapid resolution of symptoms may not occur

A. Benzodiazepines: Used most often in the acute setting of panic disorder especially when symptoms are severely disabling. Long-term use of this class of drugs is not recommended due to the risks of abuse and/or dependence. Side effects: Drowsiness, ataxia, dizziness, cognitive impairment, hypotension

B. Selective serotonin reuptake inhibitors (SSRIs)
  1. **Sertraline (Zoloft):** Begin 25mg PO QAM × 1–2 weeks, then increase to 50mg QD
  2. **Paroxetine (Paxil):** Begin 10mg PO QD 1 week, then increase to 20mg QD
  3. **Fluoxetine (Prozac):** Begin 10mg PO QAM and gradually increase to 40mg QD
  4. **Citalopram (Celexa):** Begin 10mg PO QAM and gradually increase to 40mg QD

C. Psychotherapy: Cognitive-behavioral therapy, cognitive therapy, or group therapy are some nonpharmacologic options for treating panic disorder

D. Behavioral: Avoidance of places where attacks might occur or if this cannot be done, then brief exposure initially with increases over time

CLINICAL PEARLS

- Separation anxiety disorder in childhood may predispose to panic disorder later in life
- Patients with panic disorder and other anxiety disorders are at increased risk for drug abuse, especially alcohol and anxiolytics
- Depression screening is helpful to reduce the high risk of co-morbidity with anxiety. Treatment of depression can help to reduce anxiety

References
Saeed SA, Bruce TJ. Panic disorder: effective treatment options. Am Fam Phys 1998; 57:2405–12.
Walley EJ, et al. Management of common anxiety disorders. Am Fam Phys 1994;50:1745–53.
American Psychiatric Association. Diagnostic and statistical manual of mental disorders (DSM-IV). 4th ed. Washington, D.C.: American Psychiatric Association, 1994.
Sharma R, et al. Anxiety states. In: Flaherty JA, et al. Psychiatry diagnosis and therapy. Norwalk, CT: Appleton & Lange, 1993:133–4.
Roy-Byrne, et al. Psychopharmacologic treatment of panic, generalized anxiety disorder, and social phobia. Psych Clin N Am 1993;16(4):719–33.

PSY

Peter P. Zafirides, MD
Daniel M. Neides, MD
Mary S. DiOrio, MD
Christine Costanza, MD
Budd Ferrante, EdD

100. DEPRESSION AND DYSTHYMIA

I. INTRODUCTION
    A. Up to 70% of patients with clinical depression do *not* receive treatment for their condition
    B. Proven therapies (pharmacologic and psychotherapeutic) are available, with the majority of patients (85%) responding to treatment

II. EPIDEMIOLOGY
    A. Depression
        1. 5% of the U.S. population is affected by depression at any 1 time
        2. 17–30% of the U.S. population is affected in a lifetime
        3. Female to male ratio is 2–3:1
        4. Increased risk of developing depression for first degree relatives
    B. Dysthymia
        1. Lifetime prevalence is 6%
        2. In children, occurs equally in both sexes
        3. In adults, women are 2–3 times more likely to develop or to report

III. DIAGNOSIS
    A. DSM-IV Criteria for Major Depression
        1. At least 5 of the following symptoms have been present during the same 2 week period and represent a change from previous functioning; at least 1 of the symptoms is depressed mood or loss of interest or pleasure
          a. Depressed mood most of the day
          b. Diminished interest or pleasure in all, or almost all, activities most of the day
          c. Significant weight loss or weight gain or a decrease or increase in appetite
          d. Insomnia or hypersomnia
          e. Psychomotor agitation or retardation
          f. Fatigue or loss of energy
          g. Feelings of worthlessness or excessive or inappropriate guilt
          h. Diminished ability to think or concentrate
          i. Recurrent thoughts of death, recurrent suicidal ideation without a specific plan, or a suicide attempt or a specific plan for committing suicide
        2. The symptoms cause clinically significant distress or impairment in social, occupational, or other important areas of functioning
        3. The symptoms are not due to the direct physiological effects of a substance (drug of abuse or prescribed medication) or a general medical condition
        4. The symptoms are not better accounted for by bereavement
    B. A mnemonic for symptoms of Major Depression is: **SIG E CAPS:**

S	Sleep (insomnia or hypersomnia)
I	Interest (loss of interest)
G	Guilt
E	Energy (feeling of fatigue)
C	Concentration (inability to concentrate)
A	Appetite (increased or decreased)
P	Psychomotor (agitation or retardation)
S	Suicidality (ideation, plan)

PSY

  C. DSM-IV Criteria for Dysthymia

    1. Depressed mood for most of the day, for more days than not, as indicated either by subjective account or observation by others, for at least 2 years. Note: In children and adolescents, mood can be irritable and duration must be at least 1 year

    2. Presence while depressed of 2 or more of the following:

      a. Poor appetite or overeating

      b. Insomnia or hypersomnia

      c. Low energy or fatigue

      d. Low self-esteem

      e. Poor concentration or difficulty making decisions

      f. Feelings of hopelessness

    3. During the 2-year period (1 year for children or adolescents) of the disturbance, the person has never been without the symptoms in Criteria 1 and 2 for more than 2 months at a time

    4. No Major Depressive Episode has been present during the first 2 years of the disturbance (1 year for children and adolescents); i.e., the disturbance is not better accounted for by chronic Major Depressive Disorder or Major Depressive Disorder in partial remission

    5. There has never been a Manic Episode, a Mixed Episode, or a Hypomanic Episode, and criteria have never been met for Cyclothymic Disorder

    6. The disturbance does not occur exclusively during the course of a chronic Psychotic Disorder, such as Schizophrenia or Delusional Disorder

    7. The symptoms are not due to the direct physiological effects of a substance (e.g., a drug of abuse, a medication) or a general medical condition (e.g., hypohydroidism)

    8. The symptoms cause clinically significant distress or impairment in social, occupational, or other important areas of functioning

  D. The Primary Care Evaluation of Mental Disorders (PRIME-MD) is a brief diagnostic assessment procedure that has been shown to be accurate in diagnosing mental disorders in the primary care setting

IV. MEDICAL CAUSES OF DEPRESSION

It is important to perform a thorough physical examination prior to initiating therapy to rule out medically related causes that require specific treatments

  A. Endocrine: Hypo- or hyperthyroidism, hyperparathyroidism, Cushing's disease, diabetes, Addison's disease, or menopause

  B. Infectious: AIDS, tertiary syphilis, tuberculosis, mononucleosis, or hepatitis

  C. Inflammatory: Systemic lupus erythematosus (SLE), rheumatoid arthritis and other connective tissue diseases

  D. Neurologic: Multiple sclerosis (MS), Parkinson's disease, complex partial seizures, CNS tumors, dementia, or stroke

  E. Nutritional: Vitamin deficiencies (B_{12}, folate, niacin, thiamine, or C)

  F. Pharmacologic: ß-blockers, corticosteroids, contraceptives, Cimetidine (Tagamet), Phenothiazines, α-methyldopa, or anticholinesterases

V. TREATMENT

  • The first consideration with a depressed patient is candidacy for either inpatient or outpatient psychotherapy

  • Factors that should initiate inpatient therapy include suicidality (ideation, plan), lethality, and psychosis

  • Patient education is important to increase compliance

PSY

Three-Phase Approach to Drug Treatment of Depression

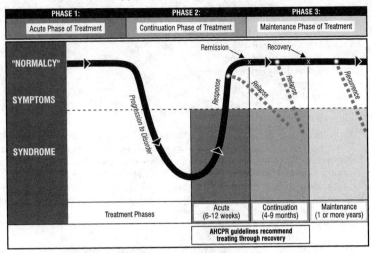

A. Selective serotonin reuptake inhibitors (SSRIs)

1. Act by increasing concentration of serotonin by blocking its reuptake
2. First line therapy in treatment of depression secondary to their favorable side effect profile
   a. **Sertraline (Zoloft):** 50mg PO QAM (may increase to 200mg/day)
   b. **Fluoxetine (Prozac):** 20mg PO QAM (may increase to 80mg/day), tends to be more "activating"
   c. **Paroxetine (Paxil):** 20mg PO QAM (may increase to 50mg/day), tends to be more "calming"
   d. **Citalopram (Celexa):** 20mg PO QD, may increase to 40mg/day
3. Side effects: Anxiety, insomnia, tremor, dizziness, somnolence, diaphoresis, impotence, sexual dysfunction, anorexia, nausea, and diarrhea
4. The side effect of sexual dysfunction may respond to dosage reduction or drug holidays. Also, the use of Viagra, Bupropion, Buspirone or Cyproheptadine (in doses of 4–12mg taken 1–2hrs before coitus) may be helpful
5. The GI side effects may be reduced by smaller increments of dosage during the early phase of treatment and administration with food. The GI side effects are often transitory and may improve after a week of treatment

B. Atypical

1. **Venlafaxine (Effexor XL):** 75mg PO QD (may increase to 225mg/day)—SSRI and norepinephrine uptake inhibitor. This mediation can cause a sustained elevation of supine diastolic BP that is dosage-related
2. **Nefazodone (Serzone):** 100mg BID (may increase to 600mg/day). Side effects: orthostatic hypotension, nausea and diarrhea. Advantage: no weight gain, sexual dysfunction or agitation
3. **Bupropion Hydrochloride (Wellbutrin)**
   a. **Wellbutrin:** Dosage should begin at 200mg/day, given as 100mg BID. May increase to 300mg/day, given as 100mg TID (no closer together than 6hrs apart), no sooner than 3 days after beginning therapy. Extreme caution should be used when prescribing Wellbutrin to patients with a history of seizure, head injury, or other predisposing factors toward seizure (long acting form likely reduces seizure risk)
   b. **Wellbutrin SR** May reduce seizure risk. Begin with 150mg PO QD and may increase to 300mg QD
4. **Mirtazapine (Remeron):** 15mg HS, may increase to 45mg/day. Presynaptic and 2 antagonists plus 5 HT_2 and 5 HT_3 antagonists with antihistamine activity. Side effects include somnolence, weight gain, dizziness, and dry mouth

C. Tricyclic Antidepressants (TCA)

1. Act by increasing the amount of **norepinephrine** and **serotonin** in the body. May also involve downregulation of receptors of these neurotransmitters

a. **Amitriptyline (Elavil):** 25mg PO TID or 50–100mg PO QHS (may increase to 150mg/day). Avoid in elderly patients

b. **Imipramine (Tofranil):** 75–150mg PO QHS or in divided doses

c. **Doxepin (Sinequan):** 25mg PO TID or 75mg PO QHS (may increase to 150mg/day). Caution with elderly patients

d. **Nortriptyline (Pamelor):** 25mg PO TID–QID (may increase to 150mg/day)

2. Side effects: Dry mouth, constipation, blurred vision, urinary hesitancy, orthostatic hypotension, potentiates heart block with EKG changes (e.g., prolonged PR and QRS intervals), tremor or sedation (especially with Amitriptyline) (See Chapter 104, Medication Use in the Elderly)

D. Monoamine oxidase inhibitors (MAOIs)

1. Act by inhibiting the enzyme monoamine oxidase which oxidizes norepinephrine, serotonin, dopamine, and tyramine

2. Have become third line agents in treating depression and should be prescribed by a psychiatrist

a. **Phenelzine (Nardil)**

b. **Tranylcypromine (Parnate)**

3. Side effects: Dry mouth, sexual dysfunction, orthostatic hypotension or acute hypertension (rapid progression to hypertensive crisis and death have occurred)

4. **Warnings for MAOIs**

a. No additional drugs (including nonprescription drugs) should be administered without consultation with the physician prescribing the MAOI

b. Drugs to avoid:Meperidine (Demerol), cough medications with Dextromethorphan, nasal decongestants, appetite suppressants, and asthma inhalers

c. A low tyramine diet must be followed. Foods to avoid: cheese, red wine, beer, liqueurs, yeast or protein extracts, fava beans, or pickled or smoked fish

d. Contraindicated: Concomitant treatment with SSRIs or tricyclic antidepressants

E. Electroconvulsive therapy

1. Useful for refractory depression

2. Works well in the elderly population (especially when antidepressant side effects are not tolerated)

3. Contraindications: intracranial mass, recent MI, recent CVA

CLINICAL PEARLS

• Once the diagnosis of depression is made, it is important to assess whether the depression is unipolar (depression only) or bipolar (severe mood swings between depression and elation). This is a critical distinction because of the different treatment regimens of these 2 conditions

• Approximately 65–70% of patients respond to antidepressant drug therapy and can enjoy a complete recovery from their depression. ECT, when indicated, will work in 10–15% of the remaining patients, which leaves 20% of depressed patients resistant to standard therapy

• Reviewing the side effect profile of antidepressant medications is important for the physician who infrequently prescribes them. Side effect profiles should be discussed with patients and their families

• Patients who have suffered from major depression are at risk for relapse and recurrence. Is this episode of depression an initial episode or a recurrence?

• Following full symptom remission after the first episode of depression, a minimum of 6–9 months of maintenance antidepressant therapy is recommended. Treatment should continue for at least 1 year after remission of a second episode. Indefinite antidepressant maintenance therapy may be necessary after a third episode of major depression

• Recurrence risk after the first, second and third episodes of major depression is 50%, 70% and 90% respectively

PSY

References

Epperson C. Postpartum major depression: detection and treatment. Am Fam Phys 1999;59:2247.

Gallo JJ. Depression without sadness: alternative presentations of depression in late life. Am Fam Phys 1999;60:820–6.

Michelson D, et al. Changes in weight during a 1-year trial of fluoxetine. Am J Psychiatry Aug 1999;156:1170–6.

Reynolds CF, et al. Nortriptyline and interpersonal psychotherapy as maintenance therapies for recurrent major depression: a randomized controlled trial in patients older than 59 years. JAMA 1999;282:39–45.

Judd LL. Therapeutic use of psychotropic medications. In HPIM-12 2139.

American Psychiatric Association. Task Force on DSM-IV. Diagnostic and statistical manual of mental disorders. 4th ed. rev. Washington, D.C.: American Psychiatric Association, 1994.

Spitzer RL, et al. Utility of a new procedure for diagnosing mental disorders in primary care. The PRIME-MD 1000 study. JAMA 1994; 272(22):1749–56.

Douglas Knutson, MD
Daniel M. Neides, MD

101. ALCOHOL AND OTHER DRUGS OF ABUSE

I. SCREENING
A. Eliciting an alcohol and drug history
1. Ask patients: "Have you ever had a health, legal, or personal problem as a result of alcohol or drugs?" and "When was your last drink or use of drugs?"
2. Answering "yes" to the first question and "within the last 24 hours" to the second question is almost 95% sensitive for diagnosing alcoholism
3. Asking a patient "How much do you drink?" or "Do you use drugs?" often results in dishonest answers

B. CAGE Questions: 2 out of 4 positive answers to the CAGE questions is also fairly sensitive and specific for alcoholism
1. Have you ever tried to **C**ut down?
2. Do you get **A**nnoyed when people question your drinking?
3. Do you feel **G**uilty about drinking?
4. Have you ever needed an **E**ye opener?

II. ALCOHOL
A. Definitions
1. **Abuse:** A pathological pattern of use involving social, occupational, or functional impairment
2. **Dependence:** Abuse plus evidence of tolerance

B. Clues that your patient is an alcoholic
1. Laboratory tests
   a. Elevated GGT (> 35 units)
   b. High or high-normal MCV (> 95)
   c. AST/ALT>2 (suggests alcohol induced liver disease)
   d. Serum uric acid > 7mg/dL
   e. Serum triglycerides >180mg/dL
2. Other clues: Inconsistent mild HTN, insomnia or anxiety, unexplained hepatitis or cirrhosis, history of pancreatitis without stones

C. Signs and symptoms of withdrawal: Symptoms begin 5–10hrs after the last drink and peak at 2–3 days; usually improve by 4–5 days
1. Withdrawal: Tremor, increased pulse, blood pressure, or temperature, insomnia, or anxiety
2. Delirium tremens (DTs): Can occur in 5% of alcoholic withdrawals. Entails confusion, hallucinations, delusions, and/or grand mal seizures

D. Prophylaxis for withdrawal (Inpatient management)
1. **Phenobarbital:** 30–60mg PO or IV scheduled Q6hrs to alternate with **Valium** 10–20mg PO or IV Q6hrs. Alternate these medications so that the patient will receive 1 of them every 3hrs. Wean them over 3–5 days by decreasing amounts and then frequency of medications as symptoms tolerate
2. **Thiamine:** 100mg IM QD for 3 days to avoid Wernicke's encephalopathy
3. **Folate:** 1mg PO QD

E. Treatment for delerium tremens (DTs): Benzodiazepines remain first line. However, symptoms may persist despite very large doses
1. **Chlordiazepoxide (Librium):** 100mg IV or PO Q2–6hrs PRN (with a maximum dose of 500mg/24hrs) *—or—*
2. **Valium:** 5–20mg IV or PO Q2–6hrs PRN may be used
3. The object of treatment is to avoid seizures and keep patient from self-harm

4. **Dilantin** is rarely necessary, and anti-psychotics should be avoided as they can lower the seizure threshold

III. BENZODIAZEPINES

A. Signs and symptoms of withdrawal are similar to those of alcohol, but they can persist for a longer period of time

B. Prophylaxis

1. **Clonazepam** (or another long-acting benzodiazepine) at an equivalent dose to the total daily use of the abuser
2. If inpatient: Decrease dosage by 10% of the original dose every day
3. If outpatient: Decrease dosage by 15% every week

IV. OPIATES

A. Withdrawal: Called "Jonesing"; symptoms include HTN, nausea, sweating, abdominal cramping, diarrhea, insomnia, and pain

B. Prophylaxis: 2 methods

1. **Methadone** taper (Methadone detox clinic): Methadone is an alternative opiate used to avoid symptoms. Determine amount of opiate used by the addict and give equivalent Methadone:
   1mg **Methadone** = 3mg **Morphine** = 1mg **Heroin** = 20mg **Demerol**
   Most start with 10–25mg **Methadone** twice every day
   Wean 10–20% of original dosage every day
2. **Clonidine:** Decreases sympathetic over-activity and treats the symptoms without using alternative opiates
   a. Two #2 **Clonidine (Catapres)** patches if < 150 lb —*or*— three #2 **Clonidine** patches if > 150 lb —*plus*— 0.2mg **Clonidine** PO Q6hrs for 48hrs
   i. Patches should be removed after 1 week
   ii. Measure *supine* and *upright* blood pressures prior to PO doses and hold if upright systolic pressure is < 90
   b. For relief of other symptoms:
   i. **Bentyl:** 20mg PO Q6hrs (for abdominal cramping)
   ii. **Motrin:** 800mg PO Q6hrs (for pain relief)
   iii. **Kaopectate:** 30cc PO Q6hrs (for diarrhea)
   iv. **Benadryl:** 25–50mg PO QPM PRN for 2 days (for insomnia)

V. COCAINE

A. Has no withdrawal syndrome, but does have intense cravings

B. Desipramine 200mg PO QHS may decrease cravings in some cases (for 4–6 weeks)

CLINICAL PEARLS

- Denial is an integral part of alcohol or drug abuse—family denial may be as strong as patient denial
- For every abuser there is an enabler—*both* need rehabilitation
- Once the patient has been successfully detoxified, a referral must be made to the appropriate program or agency (e.g., Alcoholics Anonymous) to help the patient remain sober

References

Burge SK, Schneider FD. Alcohol-related problems: recognition and intervention. Am Fam Phys 1999;59:361.

Prater CD, Miller K, et al. Outpatient detoxification of the addicted or alcoholic patient. Am Fam Phys 1999;60:1175–83.

Swift RM. Drug therapy for alcohol dependence. N Engl J Med May 13, 1999;340:1482–90.

O'Connor PG, Schottenfeld RS. Patients with alcohol problems. N Engl J Med 1998;338:592–602.

Adams WL, Barry KL, Fleming MF. Screening for problem drinking in older primary care patients. JAMA 1996;276:1964–7.

Eighth special report to the U.S. Congress on alcohol and health from the Secretary of Health and Human Services. Rockville, Md.: U.S. Dept. of Health and Human Services, Public Health Service, National Institutes of Health, National Institute on Alcohol Abuse and Alcoholism, 1994; DHHS publication no. 94–3699.

US Public Health Service. Alcohol and other drugs of abuse in adolescents. Am Fam Phys 1994;50:1737–40.

PSY

Lahmeyer HW, et al. Psychoactive substance abuse. In: Flaherty JA, et al. Psychiatry diagnosis and therapy. Norwalk, CT: Appleton & Lange, 1993:266–83.
Morse RM, et al. The definition of alcoholism. JAMA 1992;268:1012.

Daniel M. Neides, MD

102. ATTENTION DEFICIT HYPERACTIVITY DISORDER

DEFINITION: A behavior problem that is characterized by a short attention span, impulsivity, a low frustration tolerance, distractibility, and hyperactivity

I. INTRODUCTION
  A. Prevalence of 2–6% of school-aged children
  B. Male to female ratio: 3–8:1
  C. Onset is usually before age 4
  D. Etiology is unknown but a there is a strong genetic component
  E. Increased risk for ADHD with fetal alcohol syndrome, fetal exposure to drugs of abuse, past brain injury, and AIDS

II. HISTORY AND PHYSICAL EXAM
  A. History
    1. Specific description of behaviors. The parent is a biased source and may have inppropriate expectations for their child's developmental level
    2. Emotional history: Irritability, temper tantrums, sleep problems, or history of colic
    3. Parent and teacher input: Essential in making the diagnosis
    4. Conner's Parent Rating Scale and Comprehensive Teacher Rating Scale will assess for conduct problems, learning problems, psychosomatic problems, hyperactivity, and anxiety
  B. Physical: Thorough physical exam including neurologic exam
  C. Lab: Generally lab studies are *not indicated* unless directed by the history or physical exam
    1. Complete blood count, iron studies, lead level, thyroid tests
    2. Consider chromosomal studies if mental retardation or fragile X (etc.) are suspected
    3. EEG if seizures (absence seizures) are suspected

III. DIAGNOSIS: DSM-IV CRITERIA FOR ADHD
  A. Either 1 or 2:
    1. **Inattention:** At least 6 of the following symptoms of inattention have persisted for at least 6 months to a degree that is maladaptive and inconsistent with developmental level
      a. Often fails to give close attention to details or makes careless mistakes in schoolwork, work, or other activities
      b. Often has difficulty sustaining attention in tasks or play activities
      c. Often does not seem to listen to what is being said
      d. Often does not follow through on instructions and fails to finish schoolwork, chores, or duties in the workplace
      e. Often has difficulties organizing tasks and activities
      f. Often avoids or strongly dislikes tasks that require sustained mental effort
      g. Often loses things necessary for tasks or activities
      h. Often distracted by extraneous stimuli
      i. Often forgetful in daily activities
    2. **Hyperactivity—Impulsivity:** At least 4 of the following symptoms of hyperactivity have persisted for at least 6 months to a degree that is maladaptive and inconsistent with developmental level
      a. Hyperactivity
        i. Often fidgets with hands or feet or squirms in seat
        ii. Leaves seat in classroom
        iii. Often runs about or climbs excessively in situations where it is inappropriate
        iv. Often has difficulty quietly playing or engaging in leisure activity

       b. Impulsivity
         i. Often blurts out answers before the questions have been completed
         ii. Often has difficulty waiting in lines or awaiting turns in games
  B. Onset no later than 7 years of age
  C. Symptoms must be present in 2 or more situations (e.g., school, work, home)
  D. The disturbance causes clinically significant distress or impairment in social, academic, or occupational functioning
  E. Does not occur exclusively during the course of a pervasive developmental disorder, schizophrenia, or other psychotic disorder and is not better accounted for by a mood disorder, anxiety disorder, dissociative disorder, or personality disorder

IV. DIFFERENTIAL DIAGNOSIS OF ADHD

  A. Dysfunctional family
    1. Acute family stressors: E.g., divorce, death
    2. Poor parenting: Lack of limit setting, teen parents, parental depression, mental illness in parents
  B. Learning disability: Performance several grade levels below expectations for age
  C. Mental retardation or lower IQ
  D. Hearing or visual disorder
  E. Oppositional defiant disorder
  F. Conduct disorder
  G. Cognitive impairment from other disorders
    1. Lead poisoning
    2. Medication reaction (Theophylline, Phenobarbital, antihistamines)
    3. Hyperthyroidism
  H. Childhood depression
  I. Inappropriate parental expectations for normal developmental maturity
  J. Tourette's syndrome
  K. Absence seizures

V. TREATMENT

  A. Parental interventions
    1. Rules and limits: must be *consistent* and *firm* in enforcing them; consequences should be *predictable*
    2. Environmental structure: routines at home will help the child accept consistency
    3. Reinforce positive behavior: One method involves a "token economy system" where the child earns tokens for good behavior, doing homework, finishing tasks, etc. and then trades in the tokens for rewards
    4. Set aside time each day where all of the attention is on the child (reading or playing age appropriate games)
    5. Provide a special place for doing homework that is quiet and free of distractions
  B. Teacher interventions
    1. Seat the child in the front of the classroom
    2. Allow the child to move around occasionally by having him/her hand out papers or erase the chalkboard
    3. Keep instructions brief and clear
    4. Give the student positive reinforcement whenever possible
    5. A weekly report will allow parents to monitor behavior
    6. Supervise the child closely in the cafeteria or the playground (fighting or acting up)
  C. Medications
    • 80% of ADHD patients who take psychostimulants (Ritalin, Cylert, and Dexedrine) show an improved response
    • Adverse effects of the drugs include anorexia, sleep disturbances, irritability, dysphoria, headache, abdominal pain, and growth delay
    • Do NOT start a medication at the beginning of the school year—verify that the child does indeed require therapy
    • "Drug holidays" over weekends or school holidays are not recommended (especially if the child wants to participate in weekend activities). This area is controversial. Therapy should be individualized for child. Some may do fine on a drug holiday during play time (summer vacation), while others may need continuous therapy

PSY

• Repeat the behavior rating scale 2–4 weeks after initiating therapy to monitor efficacy
• Monitor for side effects at 2 month intervals initially. May decrease frequency of visits if child is stable (e.g., every 6 months)

1. **Methylphenidate (Ritalin):** 0.3–0.5mg/kg/dose
   a. Initially 5mg QD–BID. If started QD the first dose is usually in the morning. If BID add the second dose at lunch. Should be taken 30–45 minutes before meals
   b. May titrate in increments of 2.5–5.0mg. Keep on lowest dose to effect appropriate response while monitoring side effects. (Available 5, 10, 20mg scored tablets)
   c. Average dose is 20–30mg/day. Max. dose 60mg/day
   d. Peak effect 2hrs after ingestion, most effects gone after 6hrs
   e. Some children may need a mid-afternoon dose to concentrate on homework or extra-curricular activities. If there is a difficulty with sleeping, the last dose should not be taken after 6 PM
   f. Side effects: Weight loss, elevated blood pressure, difficulty with sleep
   g. **Methylphenidate sustained release (Ritalin-SR):** Available 20mg tablets
      i. Sustained release with 8hr duration of action
      ii. Dose is the same as for immediate release preparation
      iii. May be combined with immediate release
      iv. Must be swallowed whole
      v. Less potential for abuse (street value)

2. **Amphetamine mixtures (Adderall)**
   i. 5mg QD or BID, may increase by 5mg, every week up to 40mg/day
   ii. In children 3–5 years of age, the initial dosage is 2.5mg QD, may increase by 2.5 mg Q week till optimium response is attained

3. **Pemoline (Cylert)** 0.5–3.0mg/kg/day (available 18.75, 37.5, 75mg tablets)
   a. May be administered in a single morning dose usually starting with 37.5mg
   b. May increase by increments of 18.75mg
   c. Must monitor liver function tests closely secondary to potential liver toxicity
   d. Side effects: Weight loss, difficulty with sleep, hepatic dysfunction, abuse potential

4. **Dextroamphetamine Sulfate (Dexedrine):** 0.2–0.4mg/kg/dose
   a. Alternative drug when Ritalin is not effective or side effects occur
   b. Usually given in the morning only but may be dosed BID
   c. High potential for *abuse*
   d. Side effects: Weight loss, HTN, difficulty with sleep

5. **Tricyclic Antidepressants (Imipramine** or **Desipramine)**
   a. May be a third line of therapy if psychostimulants fail or produce undersirable side effects
   b. Both may be dosed 1–4mg/kg/day usually divided BID (may be given QD)
   c. More appropriate for older adolescents or adults secondary to potential cardiovascular side effects
   d. Consider psychiatry referral

PSY

CLINICAL PEARLS
• The normal attention span is approximately 3–5 minutes per year of age
• Controlled studies have NOT shown that children with ADHD benefit from dietary control of sugar and other additives
• ADHD is a *clinical diagnosis* that requires integration of many factors. Medications should not be started simply to pacify the parents
• Recognizing and treating ADHD is extremely important for the patient's long-term prognosis. Recent studies have shown that untreated hyperactive boys showed a significantly higher rate of adult psychiatric problems including antisocial and drug abuse disorders

References
Goldman LS, et al. Diagnosis and treatment of attention-deficit/hyperactivity disorder in children and adolescents. JAMA 1998;279:1100–7.
Sheflin AJ. Attention deficit disorders: a family physician perspective. Family Practice Recertification 1994; 16(8):21–32.
Pliszka SR. Attention-deficit hyperactivity disorder: a clinical review. Am Fam Phys 1991;43:1267.
The NIH consensus statement on attention-deficit/hyperactivity disorder: http://odp.od.nih.gov/consensus/

XI. Care of the Geriatric Patient

GERI

Edward T. Bope, MD

103. PERIODIC HEALTH SCREENING IN THE ELDERLY

I. HISTORY—ANNUAL
A. Updated medical and family history
B. Review of systems: Symptoms of transient ischemic attack (TIA), chest pain, shortness of breath/dyspnea on exertion, orthopnea, weight loss, symptoms of peripheral arterial disease
C. Dietary intake: Malnutrition, calcium supplementation
D. Physical activity/regular exercise
E. Tobacco, alcohol, and drug use
F. Functional status at home
G. Mental status changes: Screen for dementia even in asymptomatic patients
H. Depression and suicide attempts
I. Sexual health and satisfaction

II. PHYSICAL—ANNUAL
A. Height and weight
B. Blood pressure
C. Visual acuity and funduscopic exam (Glaucoma—increased cup to disc ratio, increased intraocular pressure, loss of temporal vision)
D. Hearing test and otoscopic exam
E. Breast exam
F. Pelvic exam (and Pap smear): Every 1–3 years until age 65. May discontinue after 65 if previous Pap tests have been within normal limits. Screening elderly asymptomatic women without risk factors is not recommended
G. Skin exam
H. Consider digital rectal exam
I. Palpation of thyroid

III. LABORATORY—ANNUAL
A. Dipstick urinalysis with complete urinalysis if positive
B. TSH for women or symptomatic men
C. Consider fasting cholesterol profile (If normal at age 65, may discontinue monitoring)
D. Fecal occult blood test every year or yearly flexible sigmoidoscopy or both (Not recommended for or against by USPSTF due to lack of evidence)
E. Consider yearly serum PSA for all men age > 50 (Not recommended by USPSTF)
F. Serum glucose: Obese patients, family history of DM, history of gestational diabetes
G. PPD for high risk patients with booster test 1 week after first negative PPD (chronic care facilities) (See Chapter 34, Tuberculosis Screening)

IV. OTHER TESTS
A. Flexible sigmoidoscopy plus barium enema or colonoscopy every 3–5 years for patients with familial polyposis coli or cancer family syndrome
B. ECG: 2 or more cardiac risk factors (high cholesterol, HTN, DM, smoking, family history of CAD), patients who could endanger public safety (e.g., pilots), or sedentary patients starting an exercise program (may consider stress testing—See Chapter 43, Cardiac Stress Testing). Not recommended in asymptomatic patients without risk factors
C. Mammogram (every 2 years until age 50, then every year). May be stopped after age 70 unless pathology is detected during clinical exam

V. PREVENTIVE MEDICINE
A. Immunizations
   1. dT (every 10 years)
   2. Influenza vaccine (every year)

GERI

3. Pneumococcal vaccine (given once, if patient has not already received it)
4. Hepatitis B vaccine for high risk patients

B. Hypertension: Mortality due to stroke or cardiovascular disease is decreased with treatment of diastolic *or* systolic hypertension. Treatment of patients older than age 60 with isolated systolic hypertension resulted in 36% fewer strokes, 32% fewer nonfatal and fatal cardiovascular events, 27% fewer nonfatal MI's and a decrease in the death rate of 13%. Medications used were **Chlorthalidone** 12.5–25mg and **Atenolol** 25–50mg per day. There was not an increase in depression or dementia at these doses (See 1991 JAMA reference below: SHEP Cooperative Research Group)

C. Assessment for risk of falling: (See Chapter 105, Falls in the Elderly)

D. Exercise: Beneficial effects on blood pressure, cardiovascular conditioning, bone density, mood, and prevention of insomnia. Helpful with constipation and prevention of falls

E. Mental health: Screening for depression. (See Chapter 100, Depression and Dysthymia)

F. Substance abuse: Counseling on alcohol and tobacco abuse

G. Medication toxicity and interactions: (See Chapter 104, Medication Use in the Elderly, and Chapter 77, Drug Interactions)

H. Consider estrogen replacement therapy: (See Chapter 25, Menopause and Hormone Replacement Therapy)

I. Nutrition
1. Malnutrition: Consider home health/Meals On Wheels, etc.
2. Calcium 1000–1500mg QD and Vitamin D$_3$ 800 IU QD
3. Obesity: Counseling on diet and exercise/lifestyle changes

J. Dental health

K. Safety: Seatbelts, helmets, hot water, fire detectors

CLINICAL PEARLS
- Approximately 25% of men and 38% of women between ages 65 and 75 are overweight
- The annual incidence of falls in people in the community between ages 70 and 75 is 25–35%. 5–10% of all falls result in serious injury
- Cerebrovascular disease is the third leading cause of death in the US
- Screening for lung cancer in asymptomatic patients is not recommended
- The American College of Physicians (ACP), the Canadian Task Force (CTF), and the US Preventive Services Task Force (USPSTF) have all *recommended against* screening asymptomatic patients without risk factors with resting ECGs or exercise stress tests
- Consider chemoprophylaxis with Aspirin if greater than age 40 with risk factors for MI

References

Frame PS, et al. U.S. Preventive Services Task Force: highlights of the 1996 report. Am Fam Phys 1997;55(2):567–76.

U.S. Preventive Services Task Force. Guide to clinical preventive services. 2d ed. Baltimore: Williams & Wilkins, 1996.

Krumholz HM, Seeman TE. Lack of association between cholesterol and CAD mortality and morbidity and all-cause mortality in persons older than 70 years. JAMA 1994;272:1335–40.

Amery A, Schaepdryver AD. Introduction: The European working party on high blood pressure in the elderly (EWPHE). Am J Med 1991; 90(Suppl 3A):3.

SHEP Cooperative Research Group: prevention of stroke by antihypertensive drug treatment in older persons with isolated systolic hypertension. Final results of the Systolic Hypertension in the Elderly Program (SHEP). JAMA 1991;265:3255.

Miriam M. Chan, PharmD

104. MEDICATION USE IN THE ELDERLY

I. GERIATRIC DRUG USE ISSUES

   A. The elderly use more medications than any other age group because they often have multiple diseases that require treatment

   B. The average home-dwelling elderly uses 4.5 different prescription drugs at the same time, while nursing home resident receives an average of 7 drugs

   C. Polypharmacy and age-related physiological changes contribute to the increased incidence of adverse drug events and noncompliance in the elderly population

   D. An estimated 3 to 10% of all hospital admissions for elderly patients are caused by iatrogenic complication of medication use. Subtle but important side effects such as sedation or cognitive impairment resulting in falls may go unrecognized

   E. Elderly patients experience a large proportion of adverse drug effects as a result of drug interactions

II. EFFECTS OF AGING ON PHARMACOTHERAPY

   A. Altered absorption: Drug absorption may decrease as a result of low acid production (e.g., Ketoconazole). The significance of changes in the GI tract during aging is not clear

   B. Changes in drug distribution

   1. Elderly persons have more body fat, less total body water and lean body mass than younger adults. Therefore, lipid-soluble drugs (e.g., Diazepam) will have increased body store and hence prolonged effects. On the other hand, water-soluble drugs (e.g., Cimetidine and Lithium) and drugs bound to muscle (e.g., Digoxin) will have higher serum concentrations and hence increased toxicity

   2. Serum albumin concentration often declines, especially in frail elderly. Drugs that are highly protein bound (e.g., Phenytoin, Warfarin) will have increased pharmacologic action because there will be more drug available in free (active) form

   C. Drug clearance and aging

   1. Hepatic metabolism of certain drugs may diminish with age. Drugs that undergo Phase I metabolism (e.g., Diazepam, Alprazolam) will have a prolonged activity

   2. Renal elimination of drugs is affected as renal function declines by approximately 10% each decade after the age of 40 years. Serum creatinine may overestimate renal function in the elderly because of decreased muscle mass. Creatinine clearance (CrCl) is a more useful measurement of renal function (See Chapter 115, Formulas, for estimation of CrCl). Drugs that depend on renal elimination (e.g., aminoglycosides, Digoxin, H_2 blockers) will require dosage adjustment according to CrCl

   D. Pharmacodynamics: Older patients appear to be more sensitive to Benzodiazepines, Opiates, Warfarin, and agents with anticholinergic side effects. The apparent increase in receptor sensitivity can result in greater therapeutic effect as well as an increased potential for toxicity

III. RECOGNIZING AND PREVENTING ADVERSE DRUG REACTIONS

   A. Adverse drug reactions may mimic the characteristics of disease states. Drug induced cognitive impairment may be mistaken for senile dementia. Drugs with strong anticholinergic properties can cause many somatic symptoms such as dry mouth, constipation, confusion, and urinary retention

   B. The susceptibility of older persons to adverse drug reactions can be assessed by determining the risk associated with specific drugs

   C. See Clinical Pearls below for "MASTER"—A guide for rational drug therapy in the elderly

GERI

IV. COMMONLY PRESCRIBED DRUGS REQUIRING SPECIAL CONSIDERATIONS

DRUGS	ADVERSE EFFECTS	SPECIAL CONSIDERATIONS
Antiarrhythmics, e.g. Lidocaine, Procainamide, Quinidine, Disopyramide (Norpace)	↑ half-life and thus ↑ frequency of adverse events. Disopyramide also has anticholinergic side effects.	Reduce dose and use with close monitoring Procainamide and Disopyramide will need dosage adjustment according to CrCl.
Antihypertensive, α-blockers: Doxazosin (Cardura), Prazosin (Minipress), Terazosin (Hytrin)	Postural hypotension especially during initial therapy. Other common adverse effects are dizziness, headache and syncope	Give low dose at bedtime and titrated slowly. Monitor orthostatic blood pressure. Doxazosin and Terazosin may improve the symptoms of BPH in elderly hypertensive men
Antihypertensive, centrally acting agents: Clonidine (Catapress), Guanabenz (Wytensin), Methyldopa (Aldomet)	Adverse CNS effects (i.e. fatigue, sedation, dry mouth)	Prescribe with caution in the elderly. Use lowest possible dose and monitor carefully. Rebound hypertension may occur with abrupt cessation
Antimicrobials, renally excreted: e.g. Acyclovir, aminoglycosides,	↓ clearance, ↑ serum concentration and ↑ toxicity	Adjust dose according to creatinine clearance. Measure serum concentration if possible.
Antipsychotic agents	All cause sedation, hypotension, anticholinergic and extrapyramidal symptoms. Tardive dyskinesia can develop even with short-term, low-dose use.	Start with a low dose and titrate slowly. Close follow-up is important. Low-potency drugs (Chlorpromazine, Thioridazine) are very sedating, hypotensive and anticholinergic, but produce less extrapyramidal symptoms. High-potency drugs (Haloperidol) have more prominent extrapyramidal symptoms but are less anticholinergic, sedating and hypotensive
Barbiturates, e.g. Phenobarbital, Secobarbital	Are fat soluble and thus have prolonged duration. Are enzyme inducers and may cause drug interactions with other concomitant medications	Use safer alternatives.
Benzodiazepines, long-acting: e.g. Chlordiazepoxide (Librium), Clonazepam (Klonopin), Diazepam, (Valium), Flurazepam (Dalmane)	Are lipid soluble and have active metabolites. ↑ half-life, leading to excess CNS effects (e.g. confusion, oversedation, falls and fractures)	Evaluate the need for a benzodiazepine (BDZ). When it is used, select a short or intermediate acting agent. Start with lowest possible dose and limit use to short term. Monitor closely. Short-acting BDZ: Triazolam (Halcion). Intermediate-acting BDZ: Alprazolam (Xanax), Lorazepam (Ativan), Oxazepam (Serax), Temazepam (Restoril)
Beta-blockers	↑ CNS adverse reactions (e.g. depression, fatigue), especially with more lipophilic agents (e.g. Propranolol, Metoprolol). Worsening diseases that are common in elderly, such as asthma, and PVD. May mask symptoms of hypoglycemia	Agents with less lipid solubility (e.g. Atenolol) have less CNS side effects. Cardio-selective agents (e.g. Atenolol, Metoprolol) in small doses cause less bronchoconstriction and less disturbance of glucose and lipid metabolism. Agents with intrinsic sympathomimetic activity (e.g. Pindolol) produce less peripheral vasoconstriction.
Beta-blockers, Ophthalmic: Timolol (Timoptic), Betaxolol (Betoptic), Carteolol (Ocupress), Levobunolol (Betagan), Metipranolol (OptiPranolol)	Systemic absorption may occur from topical administration and can cause exacerbations of asthma and bronchospasm, confusion and heart block	Be cautious when using in elderly person who has other concomitant illness
Digoxin	↑ toxicity caused by ↓ clearance and ↓ muscle mass. In addition, elderly are more sensitive to Digoxin. Toxicity may be subtle and can occur even at normal serum concentrations	Evaluate the need for Digoxin. Reduce both loading and maintenance doses. Watch for drug interactions especially with antiarrhythmics and diuretics. Monitor closely with serum concentrations and signs of toxicity (e.g. GI upset, CNS disturbances, arrhythmias)
Diphenhydramine (Benadryl)	Confusion, fall and urinary retention	Commonly used as a hypnotic, but its strong anticholinergic effects make it undesirable for use in the elderly
H₂ blockers Note: OTC products are now available	Adverse CNS effects (e.g. confusion, psychosis, hallucinations), especially with Cimetidine. ↑ risk of drug interaction	Adjust dose according to creatinine clearance. Monitor closely for drug interactions. Cimetidine inhibits the hepatic metabolism of drugs such as benzodiazepines, Carbamazepine, Quinidine, Theophylline, Terfenadine, and Warfarin. Ranitidine has less drug interactions than Cimetidine

GERI

DRUGS	ADVERSE EFFECTS	SPECIAL CONSIDERATIONS
Narcotics	↑ sensitivity to analgesic effects, respiratory depression, and CNS effects (e.g. confusion, somnolence). ↑ incidence of nausea and constipation	Start with smaller doses or longer dosing interval. Use bowel stimulants (e.g. Pericolace) as soon as narcotic therapy is begun. Meperidine and propoxyphene have active metabolites which can accumulate in patients with decreased renal function and cause seizures.
NSAIDs Note OTC drug use	↑ gastric ulceration and hemorrhage. ↑ renal toxicity. ↑ CNS effects (e.g. dizziness, confusion). ↑ risk of drug interaction.	Recognize high-risk patient for gastropathy and acute renal failure. Reduce dosage/duration of therapy if feasible. Monitor closely for adverse reactions, drug interactions and compliance. Administer prophylactic therapy when appropriate.
Over-the-counter cold remedies: Most contain decongestants (sympathomimetics) and/or antihistamines	Decongestants may effect blood pressure control. Antihistamines are sedating and can produce anticholinergic side effects	Limit use to short term. Be aware of the alcohol content in some of the products.
SSRIs: fluoxetine (Prozac), paroxetine (Paxil), sertraline (Zoloft), citalopram (Celexa)	Agitation and insomnia, nausea and GI discomfort, headache and weight loss. ↑ risk of drug interaction	Give dose in the morning to avoid sleep interruption. Fluoxetine has a long half-life and active metabolites. Both fluoxetine and paroxetine are potent enzyme inhibitors and are more likely to cause drug interactions with other concomitant medications
Sulfonylureas	Prone to hypoglycemia. Because the elderly often have a blunted metabolic response, hypoglycemia is more subtle in presentation	Start with a low dose and increase slowly. Use a second generation agent, i.e. glipizide (Glucotrol), glyburide (DiaBeta, Glynase), glimepiride (Amaryl). Glipizide is metabolized to inactive metabolites and is preferable for patients with decreased renal function
Theophylline	↑ clearance, ↑ serum concentrations and ↑ toxicity	Reduce dose and monitor serum concentration and signs of toxicity. Watch for drug-drug interactions
Thiazide diuretics	Susceptible to fluid and electrolyte disturbances (↓K⁺, ↓Na⁺, ↑ uric acid, volume depletion) and glucose intolerance	Use HCTZ at doses of 6.25 to 12.5 mg/day. Higher doses have more side effects without any significant increase in efficacy
Tricyclic antidepressants (TCAs)	Susceptible to adverse effects including anticholinergic effects, cardiac toxicity, cognitive decline, orthostatic hypotension, and sedation. This is particularly problematic in the very old and the more frail elderly patients.	Reduce dose and titrate slowly. Of the TCAs, desipramine (Norpramin) and nortriptyline (Pamelor) are preferred agents because they have lower rate of side effects. Avoid amitriptyline and imipramine which are highly anticholinergic, doxepin (Sinequan) which is very sedating, and protriptyline (Vivactil) which has a long half-life
Warfarin	Enhanced activity and prolonged duration	Start with a low dose and increase slowly. Monitor frequently. Watch for drug-drug interactions. Be aware of increased risk of falls and head trauma in the elderly

CLINICAL PEARLS

Use the acronym **MASTER** developed by Garnett and Barr as a guide for rational drug therapy in the elderly:

- **M**inimize number of drugs used and simplify medication schedules. Discontinue drug whenever possible
- **A**lternatives should be considered. Avoid drugs that pose high risk to older persons. Select the most cost-effective alternative
- **S**tart low, go slow. Start at the lowest possible dosage and increase slowly
- **T**itrate the dose according to response. Monitor plasma levels if applicable. Monitor patients for adverse reactions
- **E**ducate patients about their drug therapy and their potential side effects. Be aware of visual, hearing and memory impairment and adjust instruction accordingly. Encourage and routinely check for compliance
- **R**eview regularly patient's medications, including OTC products and home remedies. Assess for drug-disease and drug-drug interactions

GERI

References

McEvoy GK, ed. The American hospital formulary service. Bethesda, MD: American Society of Health-System Pharmacists, 1996.

Abrams WB, Beers MH, Berkow R, ed. The Merck manual of geriatrics. 2nd ed. Merck & Co., Inc. 1995;255–76.

Chutka DS, Evans JM, Fleming KC, et al. Drug prescribing for elderly patients. Mayo Clin Proc 1995;70:685–93.

Willcox SM, Himmelstein DU, Woolhandler S. Inappropriate drug prescribing for the community dwelling elderly. JAMA 1994;272:292–6.

Chrischilles EA, Segar ET, Wallace RB. Self-reported adverse drug reactions and related resource use: a study of community-dwelling persons 65 years of age and older. Ann Intern Med 1992;117:634–40.

Beers MH, Ouslander JG. Risk factors in geriatric drug prescribing a practical guide to avoiding problems. Drugs 1989;37:105–12.

Michael B. Weinstock, MD

105. FALLS IN THE ELDERLY

I. BACKGROUND

A. Falls in the elderly are a common problem which can often be avoided by taking a careful history, performing a complete physical examination and searching for factors contributing to falls (medications, alcohol, dehydration, environmental factors)

B. Fractures commonly sustained as a result of falls include fractures of the wrist, hip and vertebrae. Injuries are the sixth leading cause of death for elderly people and most are due to falls. 55% of the elderly who fall do so repeatedly. The annual incidence of falls of elderly persons in the community ages 70–75 is 25–35%

II. USE OF MEDICATIONS

A. Frequently assess meds for risks and benefits

B. Try to reduce number/dosage of meds being taken

C. Change meds to those that are less centrally acting, shortest duration of action, have less effect on postural hypotension

III. OTHER RISK FACTORS/INTERVENTIONS

A. **Reduced vision:** Refraction, cataract extraction

B. **Reduced hearing:** Removal of cerumen; hearing aid

C. **Vestibular dysfunction:** Refer for neurologic or ENT evaluation

D. **Poor balance or gait:** Check for vitamin deficiency; cervical spondylosis, treatment of foot disorders (calluses, bunions); appropriate footwear; balance and gait training

E. **Dementia:** Increased supervision

F. **Postural hypotension:** Rehydration, dorsiflexion exercise, elevate head of bed, counsel on getting up slowly

G. **Musculoskeletal disorder:** Diagnostic evaluation; muscular strengthening exercises; walking aid

IV. ENVIRONMENTAL MODIFICATIONS

A. **Lighting:** Reduce glare, shadows; install night lights

B. **Floors:** Remove loose rugs; remove obstructions

C. **Stairs:** Secure handrails; contrasting tape on steps

D. **Bathroom:** Grab bars; nonskid bathtub; raised toilet seat

CLINICAL PEARLS

- In elderly women with hip fractures, the mortality is approximately 20% in the first year
- Confusion may be a reason for a fall or a result of a fall. Subdural hematoma is a treatable and often overlooked sequelae of falling
- 5 to 10% of falls result in a serious injury
- Elderly patients on Benzodiazepines have a 29 times increased risk of falling

GERI

References

Lawson J. et al. Diagnosis of geriatric patients with severe dizziness. J Am Geriatr Soc Jan 1999;47:12–7.

Lord SR, et al. Effects of shoe collar height and sole hardness on balance in older women. J Am Geriatr Soc Jun 1999;47:681–4.

Lazarou J, et al. Incidence of adverse drug reactions in hospitalized patients. A meta-analysis of prospective studies. JAMA 1998;276:1200–5.

Grisso JA, et al. Risk factors for falls as a cause of hip fractures in women. N Engl J Med 1991;324:1326.

Rubenstein LZ, et al. The value of assessing falls in an elderly population. Ann Intern Med 1990;113:308.

Tinetti ME, Speechley M. Prevention of falls among the elderly. N Engl J Med 1989;320:1055.

Charles Levy, MD
Marc Duerden, MD
Michael B. Weinstock, MD

106. COMPRESSION FRACTURES

I. HISTORY—See also Chapter 68, Osteoprosis

    A. Patient typically complains of low thoracic pain which began suddenly following activity involving flexion of the thoracic spine (bending, lifting) or simply after coughing or laughing

    B. High risk groups include thin, caucasian, post-menopausal women. Other risk factors include smoking, chronic alcoholism, treatment with steroids, vitamin D or calcium deficiency, osteoporosis, advanced age, anticonvulsant medications, renal or hepatic insufficiency, hyperthyroidism, hyperparathyroidism, and cancer

II. PHYSICAL EXAMINATION

    A. Exam is often normal

    B. Examine for focal neurologic deficits (strength, sensation)

    C. Observe posture and gait, height, and spine

    D. Palpate for point tenderness over painful area

III. LABORATORY

    A. Consider serum calcium, phosphorus, alkaline phosphatase, thyroid studies, serum protein electrophoresis and erythrocyte sedimentation rate

    B. These studies are normal in primary osteoporosis

IV. RADIOLOGY

    A normal x-ray of the thoracic and lumbar spine helps to rule out a compression fracture. If a compression fracture is present, it is often difficult to determine acute vs. chronic

V. TREATMENT—Back pain secondary to compression fractures is self limited and usually resolves in 4–6 weeks. Uncomplicated fractures are stable and do not need surgical intervention

    A. Pain relief

        1. **Analgesics**

            a. NSAIDs

                i. **Naprosyn:** 375mg PO TID on the first day, then 375mg PO BID with meals

                ii. Use caution in the geriatric patient. Side effects include GI toxicity, confusion, renal failure, constipation

            b. **Acetaminophen (Tylenol):** 650mg PO Q4–6hrs PRN pain. May use concurrently with NSAIDs

            c. Opiate pain medications

            d. **Calcitonin:** 100 units SQ 3 ×/week

                i. Provides effective *analgesia* and inhibits osteoclastic activity

                ii. Duration of therapy can be for the symptomatic course (4–6 weeks) or as long as 12–18 months to treat the underlying disease process

        2. **Heat** (heating pad) and massage

        3. **Braces:** Hyperextension thoracolumbosacral orthoses (TLSO)

GERI

a. Start with a **"Warm N Form"** TLSO individually form fitted (usually by a physical therapist). It is cheaper and well tolerated

b. More restriction may be obtained with **Jewett** and **CASH** braces, and, for even more restriction, a molded plastic TLSO (fitted by an orthotist)

c. Prolonged use may contribute to disuse atrophy of erector spinal muscles

B. Rehabilitation/maintenance of conditioning

1. Begin with isometric exercises and advance to exercises involving active lumbothoracic extension (walking, swimming). Avoid exercises in flexion, as they increase the incidence of new compression fractures

2. Consider physical and occupational therapy

C. Treatment of chronic pain

1. Chronic pain may develop secondary to postural changes, especially with the accumulation of compression fractures. As kyphosis develops, spinal ligaments may be placed in unaccustomed stretch. In advanced cases the lower rib cage may abut the iliac crests

2. Physical and occupational therapy will strengthen thoracolumbar extensors and minimize flexion

3. Assistive devices such as long-handled "reachers" and shoehorns can decrease risky postures and minimize flexion

4. Gait training with a cane can improve stability and decrease the risk of hip fractures

5. Braces (TLSO) as previously mentioned. Tolerance may be limited by COPD, hernia, obesity, short stature

VI. PREVENTION

A. Adequate calcium intake

1. Especially important from adolescence to age 30 when peak skeletal mass is being determined

2. Recommend 1000–1500mg/day. This is equivalent to three 8 oz glasses of milk and 2 slices of calcium enriched bread per day. If this is not possible then stress calcium replacement (vitamins)

B. Weight bearing exercises: Walking, running, etc.

C. Estrogen replacement therapy—See Chapter 25, Menopause and Hormone Replacement Therapy

D. Osteoporosis: See Chapter 68, Osteoporosis

CLINICAL PEARLS

• Persistence of pain raises the suspicion of underlying malignancy, especially multiple myeloma

References

Goldberg L, Elliot DL. Exercise for prevention and treatment of illness. Philadelphia: F. A. Davis, 1994.

Delias JA. Rehabilitation medicine: principles and practice. 2nd ed. Philadelphia: J. B. Lippincott, 1993.

Kottke FJ. Krusen's handbook of physical medicine and rehabilitation. 4th ed. Philadelphia:W.B. Saunders, 1990.

GERI

107. URINARY INCONTINENCE IN THE ELDERLY

I. ANATOMY AND PHYSIOLOGY OF MICTURITION
A. Two muscle groups
1. Detrusor (smooth muscle surrounding bladder)
2. Sphincter (pelvic floor and bladder neck muscles plus the bladder-urethral angle)
B. Innervation
1. Voiding is a reflex: When the bladder fills to a certain stretch point, voiding occurs unless inhibited by higher function centers in the cerebral cortex
2. Cholinergic to detrusor causes contraction (and voiding)
3. Cholinergic to sphincter causes relaxation (and voiding)
4. Adrenergic (alpha) to sphincter provides increased tone and continued continence
C. Pharmacology
1. Anticholinergics (antihistamines, tricyclics, antipsychotics) prevent both detrusor contraction and sphincter relaxation and thereby cause urinary retention
2. Adrenergics (decongestants) cause persistent sphincter tone and retention
3. α-adrenergic blockers (Prazosin, Terazosin, Cardura) decrease sphincter tone

II. DIAGNOSIS
A. Types of incontinence, mechanisms, history and possible physical findings. A combination of types is often present:

TYPE	MECHANISMS	HISTORY	POSSIBLE FINDINGS
Urge	Detrusor instability. Unstable spastic bladder: CNS lesions (stroke), demyelinating diseases, infection, tumors	Intense urgency followed by incontinence, nocturnal wetting. May be triggered by running water	Normal PVR*
Stress	Inadequate sphincter tone, atrophic urethra (estrogen deficiency), altered bladder neck angle, perineal trauma	Incontinence associated with increased intra-abdominal pressure (transferred to the bladder) (e.g., cough, sneeze, laugh, lifting)	Normal PVR, reproducible incontinence with Valsalva maneuver (with full bladder), atrophic urethritis/vaginitis
Overflow	Detrusor hypotonia. Impaired sensation from CVA or neuropathy (diabetes, B12 deficiency, herniated disc), or outflow tract obstruction (BPH, mass, urethral stricture).	Frequent leaking of small amounts, dribbling, urgency, (prostatism), nocturnal wetting. Occurs secondary to bladder overdistention.	Large PVR, palpable bladder, cystocele, enlarged prostate, neuropathy (diabetes, injury), fecal impaction, hydronephrosis
Functional	Normal urinary system, but unable to reach toilet in time. Infection.	Functionally impaired patient (demented, sedated, arthritic, CVA, bed-ridden, restrained, acutely ill)	Impaired mobility
Iatrogenic	Medication effects (see section I.C.), cause incontinence through various mechanisms	Use of diuretics, anticholinergics (antihistamines, tricyclics), adrenergic agonists and antagonists, sedatives, CCB†	Resolution of incontinence when medication is stopped

* PVR: post-void residual urine volume measured by catheterization or ultrasound; † CCB: calcium channel blocker
Adapted from Rosenthal AJ, McMurtry CT. Urinary incontinence in the elderly. Postgrad Med 1995;97(5):110.

B. Physical examination
1. Mental status
2. Mobility and dexterity
3. Neuro (herniated disc, tumor, MS, B_{12} deficiency)
4. Abdominal exam (distended bladder, mass)
5. Rectal (tone, prostate exam, mass, presence of stool)
6. Pelvic (cystocele, atrophy)
C. Laboratory and other evaluation
1. Urinalysis (+/- culture if dysuria is present)
2. BUN, creatinine, glucose (consider electrolytes and calcium)
3. Post-void residual (PVR) volume measurement (normal is < 50mL)
4. Incontinence diary of voids and incontinent episodes (include triggers and volume)

GERI

III. MANGEMENT

A. Mixed types are common; various permutations are acceptable

TYPE	NON-PHARMACOLOGIC	PHARMACOLOGIC
Urge	Timed-voiding bladder training (see III. B.), dietary modifications*	**Oxybutynin (Ditropan)** 2.5-5.0mg TID **Flavoxate (Urispas)** 100-200mg TID-QID **Tolterodine (Detrol)** 2mg BID, may be decreased to 1mg BID according to individual response and tolerance **Imipramine (Tofranil)** 10-25mg QD to TID **Estrogen replacement therapy** (oral or topical)
Stress	Pelvic floor exercises (Kegel) (see III. C.), keep bladder volumes down, tampon trial‡	**Premarin** 0.625mg QD or intravaginal estrogen cream 1g TIW† **Phenylpropanolamine** 25mg QD-BID **Pseudoephedrine (Sudafed)** 60mg Q6-8hrs **Imipramine (Tofranil)** 10-25mg QD to TID
Overflow	Relieve the obstruction (e.g. TURP) timed-voiding Q4-6hr schedule, intermittent catheterization	**Terazosin (Hytrin)** 1mg QHS (may titrate to max of 10mg/d) **Doxazosin (Cardura)** 1mg QD (may titrate to max of 8mg/d) **Finasteride(Proscar)** 5mg QD for at least 6 months§ **Bethanechol (Urecholine)** 5-25mg BID to QID
Functional	Improve environment (bedside commode, voiding reminder)	Not applicable
Iatrogenic	Discontinue suspected medications	Continually reevaluate all medication use in the elderly.

*Caffeine may increase detrusor spacitiy as wll as cause diuresis; alcohol causes diuresis and decreased mobility.
†For use in women with evidence of atrophic urethritis (ie postmenopausal);
‡Inserting a tampon (changed at least once a day) into the vagina may help support the urethral-bladder junction;
§For use in men with BPH

B. Timed-voiding bladder training schedule (patient instructions)
1. Void every 2hrs while awake and every 2–4hrs during the night (individualize)
2. Increase voiding schedule by 30 minutes each week until reasonable (Q4hr void)
3. Even if the patient feels the need to void, have him or her make every effort to wait until the scheduled time before voiding
4. Have the patient make every effort to void on schedule, even if there is no urge to void at that time

C. Pelvic floor strengthening exercises (Kegel), (patient instructions)
1. Identify pelvic floor muscles by practicing voiding teaspoon-like amounts. The muscles used to start and stop flow are the pelvic floor muscles
2. 5 times a day (or with each void), practice contracting and holding these muscles tight for 5 seconds, 10 repetitions (total of 50 repetitions per day)
3. Regular daily repetitions (weeks to months) are necessary for this technique to work

D. Additional patient information
1. *Understanding Incontinence—A Patient's Guide* (AHCPR #96-0684) from U.S. Public Health Service, Agency for Health Care Research Clearing House: Call (800) 358-9295
2. National Association for Continence Resource Guide and Newsletter: 800-BLADDER; 864-579-7900; www.nafc.org

E. When to refer
1. An elevated PVR (>150–200) may indicate a significant underlying obstruction and further evaluation is warranted
2. Hematuria (gross or microscopic) needs to be evaluated for neoplasms or stones
3. If surgical intervention is likely (suspicion of prostate cancer, high grade cystocele, severe stress incontinence)
4. Unclear diagnosis or unsuccessful management

IV. CAUSES OF TRANSIENT INCONTINENCE (DIAPPERS)

D	Delerium or confusion
I	Infection
A	Atrophy (urethritis or vaginitis)
P	Pharmacologic: Sedatives or hypnotics, anticholinergic drugs, α-adrenoceptor agonists and antagonists, calcium channel blockers
P	Psychologic (Depression)
E	Endocrine disorder (Hypercalcemia or hyperglycemia)
R	Restricted mobility
S	Stool impaction

GERI

CLINICAL PEARLS
- Urge incontinence is the most common type of incontinence in the elderly, accounting for up to 70% of cases
- Approximately 8–12 million Americans have incontinence
- Many of the medications used to treat incontinence in the elderly have potential adverse effects. Start low and titrate upward. Evaluate for adverse effects at each visit

References

Bo K, et al. Single blind, randomized controlled trial of pelvic floor exercises, electrical stimulation, vaginal cones, and no treatment in management of genuine stress incontinence in women. BMJ Feb 20, 1999;318:487–93.

Burgio KL, et al. Behavioral vs. drug treatment for urge urinary incontinence in older women. A randomized controlled trial. JAMA Dec 16, 1998;280:1995–2000, and Resnick NM. Improving treatment of urinary incontinence [Editorial]. JAMA Dec 16, 1998;280:2034–5.

Fantl JA, Newman DK, Colling J, et al. Urinary Incontinence in Adults: Acute and Chronic Management. Clinical Practice Guideline No. 2, 1996 Update. Rockville, MD: U.S. Department of Health and Human Services. Public Health Service, Agency for Health Care Policy and Research. AHCPR Publication No. 96–0682, Mar 1996.

Mold JW. Pharmacotherapy of urinary incontinence. Am Fam Phys 1996;54:673.

Goodson JD. Approach to incontinence and other forms of lower urinary tract dysfunction. From: Primary care medicine: office evaluation and management of the adult patient. 3rd ed. Philadelphia:J. B. Lippincott, 1995.

Rosenthal AJ, McMurtry CT. Urinary incontinence in the elderly. Postgrad Med 1995;97(5):109–21.

Weiss BD. Nonpharmacologic treatment of urinary incontinence. Am Fam Phys 1991;44:579–86.

Michael B. Weinstock, MD
Edward T. Bope, MD

108. EVALUATION OF MENTAL STATUS CHANGES

DEFINITION
A. **Delirium:** A disturbance of consciousness marked by agitation and confusion, delusion, and occasional hallucinations—duration hours to weeks
B. **Dementia:** Organic loss of mental function—duration months to years

I. DIFFERENTIAL DIAGNOSIS OF DELIRIUM
A. **Drugs:** Anticholinergics, Narcotics and Benzodiazepines, H_2 receptor blockers, β-blockers, steroids and NSAIDs, ethanol (intoxication or withdrawal), Digoxin, Phenytoin
B. **Fluids and Electrolytes:** Sodium, calcium or magnesium disorders, hyper/hypovolemia
C. **CNS:** Alzheimer's disease, CVA/Multi-infarct dementia, subdural/epidural hematoma/subarachnoid hemorrhage, hypertension, seizure, unmasked dementia (Question family on patient's previous level of functioning. E.g., "When did they stop driving and shopping independently?")
D. **Infectious:** HIV/AIDS dementia, syphilis, meningitis/encephalitis/brain abscess, Lyme disease, measles (subacute sclerosing panencephalitis). Note: In the elderly almost any infection (pneumonia, urosepsis, sepsis, etc.) can cause acute reversible mental status changes
E. **Metabolic:** Renal or hepatic failure, anemia, hyper/hypoglycemia, Wernicke's encephalopathy, hypoxemia/hypercapnia
F. **Endocrine:** Thyroid disorders, adrenal dysfunction
G. **Psychiatric:** Depression, psychosis, mania
H. **Miscellaneous:** Vitamin deficiency (B_{12}, folate, thiamine), hypo/hyperthermia, myocardial infarction, pulmonary embolus, change in environment, sundowner's, pain, sleep loss, depression

II. HISTORY: Obtain from the patient and 1 or more family members
A. Medications
B. Mode of onset (abrupt versus gradual), progression of symptoms
C. Duration of symptoms

GERI

    D. Mental status history: Is patient confused or agitated, somnolent or unresponsive?
    E. Sleep history
    F. Previous head trauma (causing loss of consciousness)
    G. Alcohol use, tranquilizers, medications (including OTC meds), drugs of abuse, dietary habits
    H. Psychiatric and/or suicidal symptoms
    I. Non-Alzheimer's causes (i.e., infectious, metabolic, mass, vascular, etc.)—see Differential Diagnosis above
    J. Family history: Alzheimer's disease, Huntington's disease

III. PHYSICAL EXAM
    A. General: Vital signs and temperature
        1. Hypoventilation: Oxygen induced respiratory suppression with COPD or narcotics
        2. Hyperventilation (MI, PE, COPD, asthma)
    B. Ophthalmologic exam: Papilledema—(space occupying lesion or HTN encephalopathy), meiotic pupils (opiates), blown pupil (herniation), Kayser-Fleischer rings (Wilson's disease)
    C. Neck: Carotid bruits, JVD, nuchal rigidity, C-spine tenderness in trauma
    D. Pulmonary: Rales, decreased breath sounds, etc.
    E. Cardiovascular: Afib (embolic CVA), murmur (AS, AR), distant heart sounds (effusion)
    F. Abdomen: Acute abdomen, hepatomegaly
    G. Skin: Temperature, tenting (dehydration), rash (petechiae)
    H. Neuro: Check cranial nerve exam and for focal neurological, muscle strength, cerebellar function, mental status exam

IV. LABS (when indicated)
    A. CBC, electrolytes, glucose, BUN/creatinine, calcium and magnesium, liver function tests
    B. ABG's/oxygen saturation
    C. Blood alcohol level and toxicology screen
    D. HIV (selected patients)
    E. Syphilis serology
    F. Thyroid studies (TSH and T4)
    G. Vitamin B_{12}, folate
    H. Ceruloplasmin (Wilson's disease), lead level
    I. TB skin test

V. OTHER TESTS
    A. Head CT or MRI (CVA, multi-infarct dementia, atrophy, mass, hydrocephalus)
    B. Lumbar puncture (Meningitis—bacterial, viral, fungal, TB)
    C. Carotid dopplers
    D. Cardiac ECHO
    E. Functional Activities Questionnaire (FAQ): The best standardized test for early onset dementia
    F. Mini-Mental State Examination (MMSE): To establish a baseline for future evaluations

VI. REVERSIBLE CAUSES OF DEMENTIA (a mnemonic)

D	**Drugs:**	Prescription, alcohol, BDZ, OTC, Benadryl, anticholinergic
E	**Emotion:**	Depression, psychosis
M	**Metabolic:**	Thyroid, electrolytes
E	**Eyes and ears:**	Deafness, blindness
N	**Nutritional:**	B_{12} deficiency
T	**Tumor, trauma:**	Subdural hematoma
I	**Infectious:**	Syphilis, HIV dementia, cerebral toxoplasmosis, cryptococcus
A	**Autoimmune/cerebritis, arteriosclerosis:**	Multi-infarct dementia

GERI

VII. MANAGEMENT OF DELIRIUM WITH AGITATION
A. Avoid the precipitating factors, correct the medical problem
B. Support the patient with proper intake, light and pain control
C. Control behavior with minimal chemical or physical restraint
    1. **Neuroleptics**: **Haloperidol (Haldol):** 0.5–1.0mg PO or IM—slow onset
    2. **Benzodiazepines:** E.g., **Lorazepam (Ativan)** 0.05–1.0mg PO—rapid onset

VIII. THE MINI-MENTAL STATUS EXAM
A. Instructions for Administration of Mini-Mental State Examination

Orientation	1. Ask for the date. Then ask specifically for parts omitted, e.g. "Can you also tell us what season it is?" Score one point for each correct answer. 2. Ask in turn, "Can you tell me the name of this hospital?" (town, county, etc.). Score one point for each correct answer.
Registration	Ask the patient if you may test his/her memory. Then say the names of 3 unrelated objects, clearly and slowly, about one second for each. After you have said all 3, ask the patient to repeat them. This first repetition determines his/her score (0–3) but keep saying them until he/she can repeat all 3, up to 6 trials. If 3 are not eventually learned, recall cannot be meaningfully tested.
Attention and Calculation	Ask the patient to spell out the word "world" backwards. The score is the number of letters in correct order (e.g. DLROW=5; DLRW=4; DLORW, DLW=3; OW=2; DRLWO=1).
Recall	Ask the patient if he/she can recall the 3 words you previously asked him/her to remember. Score 0–3.
Language	*Naming:* Show the patient a wristwatch and ask him/her what IT is. Repeat for pencil. Score 0–2.
	Repetition: Ask the patient to repeat the sentence after you. Allow only one trial. Score 0 or 1.
	3-stage command: Give the patient a piece of blank paper and repeat the command. Score 1 point for each part correctly executed.
	Reading: On a blank piece of paper print the sentence, "Close your eyes." in letters large enough for the patient to see clearly. Ask him/her to read it and do what it says. Score 1 point only if he actually closes his eyes.
	Writing: Give the patient a blank piece of paper and ask him/her to write a sentence for you. Do not dictate a sentence; it is to be written spontaneously. It must contain a subject and verb and be sensible. Correct grammar and punctuation are not necessary.
	Copying: On a clean piece of paper, draw intersecting pentagons, each side about 1 in., and ask him/her to copy it exactly as it is. All 10 angles must be present and 2 must intersect to score 1 point. Tremor and rotation are ignored.

GERI

B. Mini-Mental State Examination (MMSE):

Maximum Score	Score	
5	( )	**ORIENTATION** What is the (year) (season) (date) (day) (month) ?
5	( )	Where are we: (state) (county) (town or city) (hospital) (floor).
3	( )	**REGISTRATION** Name 3 common objects (e.g. "apple," "table," "penny"):] Take 1 second to say each. Then ask the patient to repeat all 3 after you have said them. Give 1 point for each correct answer. Then repeat them until he/she learns all three. Count trials and record. Trials:
5	( )	**ATTENTION AND CALCULATION** Spell "world" backwards. The score is the number of letters in correct order (D___ L___ R___ O___ W___).
3	( )	**RECALL** Ask for the 3 objects repeated above. Give 1 point for each correct answer. [Note: recall cannot be tested if all 3 objects were not remembered during registration.]
		LANGUAGE
2	( )	Name a "pencil," and "watch." (2 points)
1	( )	Repeat the following. "No ifs, ands, or buts." (1 point)
3	( )	Follow a 3-stage command: "Take a paper in your right hand, fold it in half, and put it on the floor." (3 points)
		Read and obey the following:
1	( )	Close your eyes. (1 point)
1	( )	Write a sentence. (1 point)
1	( )	Copy the following design (1 point)

Total score:_____

Adapted from Folucin MF, Folmein SE. Mini-Mental State. J Psychiatric Rev 1975; 12:196–8; and Coclurell JR and
  Folucin MF Mini-Mental State Examination (MMSE). Psychopharm Bull 1988; 24(4):689–92.

CLINICAL PEARLS
- Hypertension should not be corrected too rapidly as this could lead to cerebral hypoperfusion, especially during an acute CVA
- Hypoglycemia from insulin overdose may outlast the effects of one amp of D50
- The effect of opiates may outlast one amp of Narcan
- A seizure or postictal state in a child may be only a symptom of underlying meningitis

PATIENT RESOURCES FOR DEMENTIA
- Memory and aging: Alzheimer's disease and related disorders, and many other materials. Alzheimer's Association, 919 N. Michigan Av., Suite 1100, Chicago, IL, 60611; telephone (800) 272–3900
- Memory loss: What's normal, what's not. American Academy of Family Physicians, 11400 Tomahawk Creek Parkway, Leawood, KS 66211-2672; telephone (800) 944–0000

References

Geerlings MI, et al. Association between memory complaints and incident Alzheimer's disease in elderly people with normal baseline cognition. Am J Psychiatry Apr 1999;156:531–7.

Vedhara K, et al. Chronic stress in elderly carers of demented patients and antibody response to influenza vaccination. Lancet Feb 20, 1999;353:627–31.

Clinical Practice Guideline. Recognition and initial assessment of Alzheimer's disease and related dementias. AHCPR Publication No. 97-R123, Sep 1996.

Consensus conference. Differential diagnosis of dementing diseases. JAMA 1987; 258;3411–6.

GERI

Siu AL. Screening for dementia and investigating its causes. Ann Intern Med 1991;115:122–32.
US Public Health Service. Cognitive and functional impairment. Am Fam Phys 1995;51:633.
Evans DA et al. Prevalence of Alzheimer's disease in a community population of older persons. Higher than previously reported. JAMA 1989;262:2551–6.
Early identification of Alzheimer's disease and related dementias. Am Fam Phys 1997;55:1303.
Stewart JT. Managing behavior problems in the demented patient. Am Fam Phys 1995;52:2311.

Michael B. Weinstock, MD

109. ADDRESSING CODE STATUS

Code status will need to be addressed with critically ill patients, patients with terminal conditions (such as cancer or end-stage AIDS) and will need to be addressed with family members or a power of attorney when a patient is unresponsive. If there is a disagreement between a patient and the family, the patient's wishes always come first!

I. IN THE AMBULATORY SETTING
A. Encourage all patients to have a living will
B. Discuss with the patients (or the family, if the patient has granted them power of attorney) several options for intervention:
1. Full code: Doing "everything" including chest compressions, intubation, and using vasopressors (ACLS medications)
2. No code (Do not resuscitate—DNR). This includes providing continuing medical management, but no chest compressions or intubation
3. Comfort care only

II. WHILE ON CALL
A. Code status is preferably addressed by someone who knows the patient and will provide the patient with continuity of care. As a resident, code status is often addressed on a new patient who is "crashing"
B. First, introduce yourself. State your position at the hospital and your association with the patient
C. Explain the patient's condition, and that you are currently "doing everything that can be done," but need to confirm *the patient's wishes*, in case "their heart and lungs stop working"
D. A good way to phrase the question when discussing code status with a family member is to ask what *the patient's wishes* would be. This helps alleviate guilt on the part of the family members making the decision
E. Ask if there are any questions. Stress your availability to answer questions, should any arise

CLINICAL PEARLS
- It is impractical to perform chest compressions on a patient who is not receiving adequate ventilation, or to intubate a pulseless patient without performing chest compressions
- Consider involving other physicians or other health care professionals
- Hospital ethics committees are often available for consultation for the most difficult situations
- $1/2$ of all patients survive the initial resuscitation, $1/3$ survive for 24hrs, and $1/8$ survive to leave the hospital

GERI

References
Ebell MH. Practical guidelines for do-not-resuscitate orders. Am Fam Phys 1994; 50:1293–9.
Jayes RL, et al. Do-not-resuscitate orders in intensive care units: current practices and recent changes. JAMA 1993;270:2213–7.

XII. HIV and AIDS

HIV

Michael B. Weinstock, MD

110. AMBULATORY HIV/AIDS MANAGEMENT

The optimal management of patients with HIV/AIDS is a constantly evolving process. These recommendations are intended for physicians with experience in treating patients with HIV/AIDS who have a baseline level of knowledge. Prescribing antiretroviral medications should only be done by, or in conjunction with, physicians who have experience with these medications. These recommendations are for management of *adults* with HIV and AIDS. For diagnosis and management of symptoms, see Chapters 110 through 114.

These recommendations are current as of July, 2000

I. HISTORY

A. History of present illness: In addition to standard history, ask specifically about: Fatigue, weight loss, weakness, fever, chills, night sweats, lymphadenopathy, rash or skin changes, oral lesions, dysphagia/odynophagia, change in vision, cough, dyspnea, easy bruising, diarrhea, nausea/vomiting, abdominal pain, dysuria, vaginal/penile discharge, yeast infections, anal pain, headaches, confusion/seizures

B. Past medical history: Inquire about hospitalizations/operations, drug allergies (sulfa), immunizations, medications (potential interactions), history of infectious diseases (varicella/zoster, TB or positive skin tests, HSV, hepatitis, STD's), recent blood donation (notify collector)

C. Social history: Possible mode of infection, current sexual practices, drug use, smoking and alcohol, diet, stressors, support systems.

II. PHYSICAL EXAMINATION

A. General exam (cachexia)
B. Ophthalmic exam (visual field defects, fundi)
C. Dermatologic exam (seborrheic dermatitis, Kaposi's sarcoma, tinea, varicella, HSV, etc.)
D. Oral and dental exam (candidiasis, oral hairy leukoplakia, HSV, KS)
E. Pulmonary
F. Cardiovascular
G. Abdominal exam
H. Neurologic exam (baseline)
I. Consider rectal exam (condyloma, perirectal HSV)
J. Genital exam (candida, HSV, chancre, HPV, etc.)

III. LABORATORY AND OTHER DIAGNOSTIC EVALUATIONS

TESTING AND IMMUNIZATIONS DURING THE INITIAL EVALUATION

Laboratory	Other tests	Immunizations
CBC with differential and platelets	Chest radiograph	Pneumococcal vaccine
Chemistry panel	PPD skin testing (no anergy screen necessary)	Hepatitis B vaccine (if seronegative)
Liver enzymes	PAP smear	Hepatitis A vaccine
Syphilis serology		Influenza vaccine
Hepatitis A, B, C screen		
Toxoplasma titer (IgG)		(Varicella vaccine *for household contacts* with no history of chickenpox)
CD4 count (cells/mm^3)		
Viral load (copies/cc)		

HIV

A. Laboratory and other tests
    1. CD4 count: See below under section V—Antiretroviral therapy
    2. Viral load testing: See below under section V—Antiretroviral therapy

3. Hepatitis B serology—HBsAb, HBsAg, HbcAb: See Chapter 55, Diagnosis and Management of Hepatitis B
4. Hepatitis A serology
   a. If IgG positive, then they are immune
   b. If IgG negative, then vaccinate
5. Hepatitis C serology
6. PPD skin testing: Anergy testing is not recommended as it is not reproducible. See Chapter 34, Tuberculosis Screening for TB prophylaxis recommendations
7. PAP smear: Cervical dysplasia is increased 8–11 times

B. Immunizations

1. Pneumococcal vaccine (cost ~$10): Strongly recommended
   a. Recommended for all patients with HIV with CD4 counts over 200. Optional for patients with CD4 counts less than 200 as the response to vaccination is poor. A one time follow up vaccination is recommended at 5 years
   b. Impact on viral load: May transiently increase the viral load. Viral load testing should be delayed for 4 weeks after the immunization
   c. General: Incidence of pneumococcal pneumonia is increased over 20 times in patients with HIV and the risk of pneumococcal bacteremia is increased 150–300 fold higher than age matched controls without HIV. Pneumococcal vaccine should be given at the earliest opportunity and repeated once at 5 years. One study showed that 88% of asymptomatic HIV infected patients responded to at least 1 component of the 23-valent vaccines
2. Influenza vaccine (cost ~ $5): Generally recommended
   a. Recommended by the centers for disease control (CDC)
   b. Impact on viral load: May raise the viral load, therefore, viral load testing should be delayed for 4 weeks after the immunization
   c. General: Patients with HIV do not have worse infections with influenza than non-infected patients, however, the advantage of preventing influenza is that the symptoms will not be confused with symptoms of an opportunistic infection and unnecessary evaluations will be avoided. Other advantages include the increased risk of persons with HIV for bacterial infections that commonly complicate influenza. Protective antibody titers develop in 52–89% of patients with asymptomatic disease and 13–58% of patients with AIDS
3. Hepatitis B vaccine: Generally recommended
   a. Recommended for individuals who continue to engage in high risk behaviors and who do not have serologic evidence of past infection with hepatitis B. See above
   b. General: Patients with HIV and hepatitis B have a 19–37% risk of becoming chronic carriers (3–6 times higher risk than patients without HIV). Response rate to the vaccine is 25–60%
4. Hepatitis A vaccine: Generally recommended for those who engage in anal intercourse and for travelers
5. Hemophilis Influenzae type B: Same as for non-infected patients
6. Diphtheria/tetanus: Same as for non-infected patients
7. MMR: Same as for non-infected patients
8. Travel vaccines: Same as for non-infected patients, but no live vaccines
9. Varicella
   a. Vaccine: Not recommended for persons infected with HIV secondary to the risk of disseminated viral infection. It is recommended for household contacts of persons with HIV if they have not had chickenpox
   b. Immune globulin: With significant exposure to chicken pox or shingles in patients without history of either condition (or negative antibody titer) give Varicella Zoster Immune Globulin (VZIG) 5 vials (1.25mL each) IM if < 96hrs post exposure (preferable within 48hrs)
10. Vaccines not to give
    a. Oral polio vaccine (OPV)
    b. Varicella vaccine (Household contacts who have not had chickenpox should receive the vaccine)
    c. Other live vaccines

HIV

C. Prevention of infection
1. Pets: Should not empty litter boxes or bird cages
2. Exposure to water: Water should be boiled with outbreaks of cryptosporidia, etc.
3. Exposure to feces

D. Other information: See end of chapter for important phone numbers for patients and physicians. Provide patient with written information on HIV/AIDS, support groups, unsafe and safe sexual and IV drug use practices. Certain sexual practices are safe for patient to continue to engage in (activities which do not exchange body fluids) and should be discussed explicitly with the patient. Past contacts should be notified, but this can be deferred until the doctor patient relationship has been better established. Explain to patient the need for frequent visits and blood tests. Stress your availability to answer medical and psychosocial questions

IV. PROPHYLAXIS
A. PCP prophylaxis
1. Pneumocystis is (probably) a protozoa which is common in the environment. Most children have antibodies by age 2–3 years. Most common site is pulmonary, but infection may occur in extra-pulmonary sites as well (e.g., skin, lymph nodes, spleen, brain)
2. **Trimethoprim/Sulfamethoxazole (TMP/SMX)** is first line for prophylaxis. It is low cost, effective, and it has activity against toxoplasmosis and many bacterial infections in addition to *Pneumocystis carinii*. If it is not tolerated due to rash, GI upset, or fever, a desensitization protocol may be attempted
3. Indications for PCP prophylaxis
   a. Prior PCP
   b. CD4 < 200 cells/mm³
   c. HIV associated thrush
   d. Unexplained fevers > 100°F for greater than 2 weeks
4. **TMP/SMX** initiation protocol: Tolerated better if started as a low dose (½ DS tab QOD) and gradually increased
5. If an allergic rash develops, then treat symptoms with sedating antihistamines (**Diphenhydramine** or **Hydroxyzine**)
6. **TMP/SMX** desensitization: Very slow initiation may be attempted for patients who had previous non-anaphylactic reactions to TMP/SMX
7. Patients who have CD4 count increase to > 200 for 3–6 months may discontinue *primary* PCP prophylaxis

MEDICATIONS USED FOR PNEUMOCYSTIS (PCP) PROPHYLAXIS
PROPHYLAXIS OF PNEUMOCYSTIS PNEUMONIA (PCP)

MEDICATION	DOSE	COST/MO. (AWP 7/00)	RELAPSE RATE	SIDE EFFECTS
Trimethoprim-sulfamethoxazole DS	One PO QD (preferred) or One PO TIW or One SS PO QD	$10	<5%/yr	Rash, nausea/vomiting, fever, anemia neutropenia, Stevens-Johnson
Dapsone	100mg PO QD (preferred) or 50mg PO QD	$6	5–20%/yr	Rash, agranulocytosis, aplastic anemia, hemolytic anemia in G6PD deficiency
Aerolized pentamidine	300mg per month administered over 30–45 minutes per Respirgard II nebulizer	$95 plus cost of administration	15–25%/yr	Bronchospasm (consider pre-treat with albuterol MDI), increased incidence of upper lobe disease and extra-pulmonary PCP
Atovaquone(Mepron)	750mg PO BID with meal	$910		Rash, diarrhea, nausea

B. Mycobacterium avium complex (MAC) prophylaxis
1. Common in food and water. Causes disease in up to 40% of late stage patients with HIV infection who do not take MAC prophylaxis
2. Symptoms include fever and night sweats, weight loss, abdominal pain, increased alkaline phosphatase and anemia
3. Indications: CD4 < 50 cells/mm³
4. If Clarithromycin or Azithromycin are used, then screen for MAC first by obtaining a MAC culture. (To treat MAC, you must use a macrolide in combination therapy. If a macrolide is started on a patient who already has MAC disease, they would essentially have macrolide

HIV

MAC monotherapy). There is about a 27% incidence of resistance to macrolides in patients who develop MAC while on prophylaxis with macrolides)
5. Preferred agents are Clarithromycin and Azithromycin
6. Patients who have CD4 count increase to > 100 for 3–6 months may discontinue primary prophylaxis

PROPHYLAXIS OF MYCROBACTERIUM AVIUM COMPLEX (MAC)

Medication	Dose	Cost/yr. (AWP 7/00)	Side effects and precautions
Clarithromycin (Biaxin)	500mg BID	$2347	GI disturbances
Azithromycin (Zithromax)	1200mg per week (Two 600mg tabs with or without food)	$1635	GI disturbances
Rifabutin (Mycobutin)	300mg QD	$3743	Neutropenia, thrombocytopenia, rash and GI, uveitis, drug-drug interactions with protease inhibitors

C. **Tuberculosis** (See Chapter 34, Tuberculosis Screening)
D. **Cryptococcus**
  1. Cryptococcus is a fungus, acquired by inhalation
  2. Indications
    a. Primary prophylaxis not recommended because there is no reduction in mortality and cryptococcal meningitis is easily diagnosed with serum cryptococcal antigen (95% sensitive) and is treatable
    b. Secondary prophylaxis recommended
      i. **Fluconazole (Diflucan):** 200–400mg QD
      ii. Alternative medication—**Amphotericin B:** 0.5–1 mg/kg IV 1–2 ×/week
E. **CMV disease (retinitis)**
  1. CMV is a viral infection often causing blindness as a result of retinitis
  2. Indications: Ophthalmologist exams every 6 months with CD4 counts less than 50 cells/mm^3 or visual symptoms
  3. Medications: A decreased incidence of CMV retinitis has been shown with oral **Ganciclovir** used as prophylaxis, however it is not recommended due to the high toxicity, high number of pills and high cost
F. **Toxoplasmosis**
  1. Primary prophylaxis: Indications—CD4 < 100 and positive IgG
  2. Medications are basically the same as for PCP (same doses, see chart above for PCP)
    a. First line: **TMP/SMX**
    b. Second line: **Dapsone**

V. ANTIRETROVIRAL THERAPY
  Currently, two HIV enzymes can be inhibited with medications: reverse transcriptase and HIV protease. Nucleoside analogs and nonnucleoside analogs both work to inhibit reverse transcriptase. Protease inhibitors work to inhibit HIV protease. See following table on antiretroviral medications
  1. Pathogenesis of HIV
    a. HIV is a retrovirus. It is incorporated into CD4 cells by the binding of the HIV envelope protein gp120 to the CD4 receptor and a second receptor (possibly a chemokine receptor). Once inside the cell the HIV RNA is converted into DNA by the enzyme *reverse transcriptase* and then incorporated into the host cell's DNA. Next, messenger RNA (mRNA) is made which is then translated to make the proteins that will eventually form into the virus. These proteins are cleaved into the active form of HIV by the enzyme *HIV protease*. These active viral components are then packaged and put into circulation as infectious virions
    b. Nucleoside and nonnucleoside analogs both work by inhibiting reverse transcriptase. Protease inhibitors block HIV protease which results in noninfectious viral particles which have reduced reverse transcriptase activity

HIV

    c. HIV pathogenesis is a very active process. Even during early, asymptomatic disease there are approximately 10 billion HIV viral particles produced and destroyed each day. The half life of plasma virus is about 6hrs

    d. In addition to active viral replication in the blood, there is viral replication in the lymphoid system, CSF and other sites

    e. Decreases in plasma viral load are not always paralleled by decreases in these other locations or in genital secretions. A patient with a non-detectable plasma viral load should not be considered to be noninfectious

2. Viral load testing (the level of HIV RNA in the plasma)

    a. The viral load measures the amount of virus in 1 cc of plasma. It ranges from "non-detectable" (<25 to <400 copies/cc (depending on the lab) to >750,000 copies/cc (the upper limit of the test). The viral load count *routinely varies by a factor of 3 (0.5 log).* This variability may be decreased by multiple measurements

    b. Alpha and beta slope

        i. Alpha slope (the first decline): Upon initiating an effective antiretroviral regimen there is a rapid fall in HIV in plasma and in acutely infected CD4 cells which can account for 99% of HIV in blood. This change can be seen by 2–4 weeks

        ii. Beta slope (the second decline): Reflects a decline in HIV infected macrophages, latently infected CD4 cells and HIV released from other compartments (HIV trapped in follicular dendritic cells of lymph follicles). Change generally occurs at 10–12 weeks

    c. Uses

        i. Viral load is the strongest predictor of progression (should still be correlated with the CD4 count and the clinical picture)

        ii. Useful for therapeutic monitoring: Decreases in viral load during therapy are strongly associated with a decrease in risk of subsequent disease progression

    d. Limitations: Viral load testing does not test:

        i. Immune function

        ii. CD4 regenerative reserve

        iii. Susceptibility to antiretroviral agents

        iv. Infectivity

        v. Viral phenotype (syncytium vs. non-syncytium inducing forms)

        vi. Virus in lymph nodes, CNS, genital secretions

    e. Cost: ~$80–292 per test

    f. Method

        i. 2 baseline assays should be done 2–4 weeks apart

        ii. Viral load should be checked 2–4 weeks after starting or changing therapy (alpha slope) and then at 10–12 weeks (beta slope)

        iii. Testing should be done by the same laboratory using the same test (the HIV PCR test may give values twice that of the bDNA test)

        iv. Viral load may be increased by vaccinations and active infections (TB increases viral load 5–160 fold and pneumococcal pneumonia increases viral load by 3–5 fold). Wait 4 weeks after vaccinations to perform viral load testing

3. CD4 count

    a. CD4 count = WBC × percent lymphocytes × lymphocytes that are CD4 cells. Therefore, anything which affects the WBC count may influence the CD4 count (infection, drugs, steroids). CD4 count normally *varies by 30%,* but this variation can be accounted for by multiple measurements of the CD4 count. Should be checked 2 weeks apart, by the same laboratory to reduce variation. The "% CD4" count stays fairly constant and should be looked at in conjunction with the CD4 count

    b. Should be used in conjunction with the viral load and the clinical picture to make decisions about antiretroviral therapy

    c. Is an independent risk factor for opportunistic infections

    d. Cost: ~$100 per test

4. General considerations with antiretroviral therapy

    a. Never use monotherapy

    b. Don't add a protease inhibitor to a failing regimen (same as using monotherapy because

HIV

the virus is likely resistant to the current agents)

c. At least 2 agents should be changed at once (add 2 agents, change 1 and add 1, etc.)

d. Use full dose therapy (to prevent resistance)

e. Emphasize adherence at every visit

f. Think about drug interactions (more of a concern with the protease inhibitors)

g. Monitor viral load (see above)

h. Think ahead about what you can change if resistance develops

5. Initiation of therapy

CONSIDERATIONS FOR INITIATION OF ANTIRETROVIRAL THERAPY
1. Viral load (PCR) > 10,000 - 20,000 copies/ml
2. Symptomatic HIV disease*
3. CD4 count less then 500/mm³ (or CD4% <25)
4. Progressive decline in CD4 cells
5. Progressive rise in viral load
6. Persons with primary infection (should receive therapy as part of a clinical trial if available)
*Symptomatic disease includes symptoms such as recurrent mucosal candidiasis, oral hairy leukoplakia (OHL), chronic and unexplained fever, night sweats, and weight loss

a. Consideration of initiation of therapy should be a lifelong commitment by the patient and the physician. The goal of treatment is to change HIV from a chronic disease that is always fatal into a chronic disease (similar to diabetes) where the virus is suppressed through the duration of a patient's life by the continual use of medications

b. 100% compliance should be repeatedly stressed. If this is not possible at the present time, then antiretroviral therapy should be delayed until this is possible

c. Decisions on the initiation of therapy should take into account the whole clinical picture including history and exam, CD4 count and viral load. If a patient has had HIV for 10 years and their CD4 count has been stable at 400–500 and the viral load is above 5–10,000, there is not a clear recommendation of initiating therapy

d. As always, doctors can make a recommendation of initiating therapy. But the final decision is left up to the patients

6. Goal: To decrease viral load to non-detectable

7. Choices for initial therapy

a. Strong consideration should be given to dosing frequency and side effects of the regimen, as these medications may be taken for the duration of the patient's life, and compliance issues are important

b. Consideration for cost, side effects and drug interactions (see table at IX. below)

c. See below for choices for alternative antiretroviral regimens

HIV

8. Correlation between virologic response at 6 months and adherence

Adherence to HAART	VL < 500 copies/ml
>95% adherence	81%
90-95% adherence	64%
80-90% adherence	50%
70-80% adherence	24%
<70% adherence	6%

9. Choices for initial antiretroviral therapy for patients who are antiretroviral naïve—There are 3 main choices for therapy:
   a. 3 nucleosides (AZT + 3TC + Abacavir)
   b. 2 nucs and a non-nuc
   c. 2 nucs and 1 (or 2) PI's

DHHS RECOMMENDATIONS FOR INITIAL THERAPY

Column A	Column B
Indinavir	AZT + ddI
Nelfinavir	d4T + ddI
Ritonavir	AZT + ddC
Saquinavir — SGC	AZT + 3TC**
Ritonavir + Saquinavir — SGC	d4T + 3TC**
Efavirenz	ddI + 3TC**

Pick one from column A and one from column B
**High level resistance to 3TC develops within 2–4 weeks in partially suppressive regimens
Not recommended:
All monotherapy
AZT/d4T, ddC/ddI, d4T/ddC, 3TC/ddC

VI. CHANGING THERAPY—Indications for changing therapy:
A. Treatment failure
   1. Clinically significant increase in viral load
   2. Failure to achieve desired reduction in viral load after initiation of therapy
   3. Declining CD4 count (Caution: CD4 counts may take 3–6 months or longer to increase after potent suppression of the viral load)
   4. Possible indications
      a. Discordance: Fall in viral load and continued fall in CD4 counts
      b. Clinical disease progression despite obtaining target viral burden
B. Unacceptable toxicity of regimen
C. Noncompliance due to difficulty of regimen (if there is noncompliance because a patient is unwilling to take the meds, then consider deferral of antiretroviral therapy until patient can make an absolute commitment)
D. Current use of a suboptimal regimen (monotherapy) with detectable or rising viral load (if patient has been on monotherapy for a long time with potent suppression, then consider continuing therapy)
E. If medications are held for toxicity, it is best to stop all medications at once and not just 1 medication (to decrease chance of resistance)
F. Goal: The goal is to decrease viral load to non-detectable (ranges from less than 400 copies/mL to < 20 copies/mL depending on the assay used)

HIV

G. Empiric selection for changing antiretroviral regimens

Prior Regimen	New Regimen
2 NRTIs + PI	2 new NRTIs plus NNRTI or Dual PIs (RTV + SQV, RTV +IDV, NFV + SQV)
2 NRTIs + NNRTI	2 new NRTIs + PI or SQV + RTV
ABC + AZT + 3TC	2 new NRTIs (ddI + d4T) + either PI or NNRTI
2 NRTIs	2 new NRTIs + PI or NNRTI

VII. RESISTANCE TESTING

A. Advantages
1. Virologic outcome is superior (early data)
2. Number of drugs changed is reduced

B. General
1. Must be done while a patient is taking medications
2. Results are limited to the dominant strains (>20% of the total population). This means that a result of resistant is probably accurate, while a result of sensitive may or may not be accurate (if there is resistance, but < 20% of the viral population)
3. A viral load of > 1,000 is required
4. Interpretation is complex and there are a multiplicity of mutations and differing levels of resistance

VIII. INTENSIFICATION

A. The addition of 1 or 2 agents to an existing regimen that has resulted in suppression that is incomplete

B. Indications
1. Failure to reach targeted threshold
2. Confirmed rebound in a patient with previously undetectable virus

C. Possibilities
1. Addition of HU to a ddI containing regimen
2. Addition of a second PI to a PI containing regimen
3. Addition of third NRTI (ABC or 3TC)

IX. CONTRAINDICATIONS AND DRUG INTERACTIONS

Medication	Adult Dose	Monitoring	Side Effects	AWP-3/00	Available
-- Nucleoside analog reverse transcriptase inhibitors (NRTIs) --					
Zidovudine (Retrovir) AZT	200mg TID or 300mg BID	CBC every 2-4 weeks for 3 months, then every 3 months	Anemia - Hb < 8.0 (1.8%), neutropenia - ANC < 750 (5.4%), headache (27%), fatigue (23%), nausea (29%), myalgia (6%)	$3822	caps: 100mg tabs: 300mg
Didanosine (Videx) ddI	If > 60kg: 400mg QD -or- 200mg BID If < 60kg: 250mg QD -or- 125mg BID if -empty stomach	Intermittent CBC and LFT's	Acute pancreatitis (5-9%), painful peripheral neuropathy (5-12%), nausea/vomiting, hepatic failure	$2717 $1698	Sachets: 100, 167, 250mg Tabs: 25, 50, 100, 150, 200
Zalcitabine (HIVID) ddC	If > 45kg: 0.75mg Q 8 hours If < 45kg: 0.375mg Q 8 hours	Intermittent CBC and LFT's	Peripheral neuropathy (17-31%), rash, stomatitis, esophageal irritation, pancreatitis (1%)	$2437 $2092	Tabs: 0.75, 0.375mg
Stavudine (Zerit) d4T	40mg BID if > 60kg 30mg BID if < 60kg	Intermittent creatinine and LFT's	Peripheral neuropathy, elevated liver enzymes	$3408 $3296	Caps: 15, 20, 30, 40mg
Lamivudine (Epivir) 3TC	150mg BID	CBC every 2-4 weeks for 3 months, then every 3 months	3TC plus AZT: Anemia - Hb < 8.0 (2.9%), neutropenia - ANC < 750 (7.2%), headache (35%), fatigue (27%), nausea (33%), myalgia (8%)	$3271	Tabs: 150mg
Abacavir (Ziagen) ABC	300mg BID	Intermittent	Hypersensitivity (2-5%), n/v, malaise, morbilliform rash. DO NOT RECHALLENGE!	$4396	Tabs: 300mg
Combivir	One pill BID (AZT 300mg and 3TC 150mg)	Same as AZT and 3TC	Same as AZT plus 3TC	$7093	tabs
-- Nonnucleoside reverse transcriptase inhibitors (NNRTIs) --					
Nevirapine (Viramune) NVP	200mg QD X 14 d. then 200mg BID	Intermittent LFT's	Rash (17%), increased GGT > 450 U/L (2.4%)	$3343	tabs: 200mg
Delavirdine (Rescriptor) DLV	400mg TID	Intermittent CBC and LFT's	Rash (30%), increased LFT's, HA, nausea, diarrhea, fatigue, anemia, neutropenia	$3395	tabs: 100, 200mg
Efavirenz (Sustiva) EFV	600mg QHS	Intermittent	Dizziness, disconnectedness, somnolence, insomnia, bad dreams, confusion, amnesia, agitation, poor concentration, rash (5%).	$4730	Caps: 50, 100, 200mg
-- Protease inhibitors (PIs) --					
Saquinavir (Fortovase) FTV	1200mg TID with food (400mg BID with RIT)	Intermittent glucose, cholesterol, triglycerides, LFT's	Diarrhea (19%), nausea (11%), fatigue (5%), headaches (5%)	$7476	Soft gel caps: 200mg
Ritonavir (Norvir) RIT	600mg BID (400mg BID with FTV)	Same	Monotherapy: Nausea/vomiting (13-26%), abd. pain (3-7%), circumoral paresthesias (3-6%), increased LFT's, increased chol.	$8013	caps: 100mg
Indinavir (Crixivan) IDV	800mg Q8 hours -empty stomach or light foods	Same	Monotherapy: Nausea (12%), vomiting (4%), increased bilirubin (8%), abdominal pain (9%), nephrolithiasis (3%)	$5562	Caps: 200, 333 400mg
Nelfinavir (Viracept) NFV	1250 BID -or- 750mg TID	Same	Mild GI: Diarrhea (15-20%), flatulence (4-7%)	$8121	tabs: 250mg
Amprenavir (Agenerase) AMP	1200mg BID	Same	GI (10-30%), rash (20-25%), Stevens-Johnson syndrome (1%), paresthesias-perioral or peripheral (10-30%)	$7613	caps: 50, 150mg + 15mg/ml

HIV

DRUGS THAT SHOULD NOT BE USED WITH PROTEASE INHIBITORS OR NNRTIs*

Drug Category	Indinavir	Ritonavir	Saquinavir	Nelfinavir	Delavirdine	Efavirenz	Amprenavir
Analgesics	(none)	meperidine, piroxicam, propoxyphene	(none)	(none)	(none)	(none)	(none)
Cardiac	(none)	amiodarone, encainide, flecainide, proprafenone, quinidine	(none)	(none)	(none)	(none)	amiodarone, quinidine
Lipid lowering agents	simvastatin, lovastatin	simvastatin, lovastatin	simvastatin, lovastatin	simvastatin, lovastatin	simvastatin, lovastatin	(none)	simvastatin, lovastatin, provastatin, atorvastatin, cerivastatin
Anti-Mycobacterial	rifampin	rifampin	rifampin, rifabutin	rifampin	rifampin, rifabutin	rifampin	rifampin
Ca++ channel blocker	(none)	bepridil	(none)	(none)	(none)	(none)	bepridil
Antihistamine	astemizole, terfenadine	astemizole, terfenadine	astemizole, terfenadine	astemizole, terfenadine	astemizole, terfenadine	astemizole, terfenadine	astemizole
GI	cisapride	cisapride	cisapride	cisapride	cisapride, blockers	cisapride	cisapride
Antidepressant	(none)	bupropion	(none)	(none)	(none)	(none)	(none)
Neuroleptic	(none)	clozapine, pimozide	(none)	(none)	(none)	(none)	(none)
Psychotropic	midazolam, triazolam	clorazepate, diazepam, estazolam, flurazepam, midazolam, triazolam, zolpidem	midazolam, triazolam	midazolam, triazolam	midazolam, triazolam	midazolam, triazolam	midazolam, triazolam, tricyclics
Ergot Alkaloid (vasoconstrictor)	dihydroergotamine, ergotamine (various forms)	dihydroergotamine, ergotamine (various forms)	dihydroergotamine, ergotamine (various forms)	dihydroergotamine, ergotamine (various forms)	dihydroergotamine (DHE 45), ergotamine (various forms)	dihydroergotamine (DHE 45), ergotamine (various forms)	dihydroergotamine, ergotamine (various forms)

*Alternatives: Analgesics — ASA, oxycodone, acetaminophen; Rifabutin (MAC) — clarithromycin, ethambutol, azithromycin; Antihistamine — loratadine; Antidepressant — fluoxetine, desipramine; Psychotrophic — temazepam, forazepam; Lipid-lowering — atorvastatin, pravastatin, fluvastatin, cerivastatin

DRUGS INTERACTIONS: PROTEASE INHIBITORS AND NON-NUCLEOSIDE REVERSE TRANSCRIPTASE INHIBITORS
Effect of Drug on Levels (AUCs)/Dose

Drug Affected	Ritonavir	Saquinavir	Nelfinavir	Amprenavir	Nevirapine	Delavirdine	Efavirenz
Indinavir (IDV)	Levels: IDV ↑ 2-5x Dose: Limited data for IDV 400mg bid + RTV 400mg bid, or IDV 800mg bid + RTV 100-200 mg bid	Levels: IDV no effect SQV ↑ 4-7x** Dose: Insufficient data	Levels: IDV ↑ 50% NFV ↑ 80% Dose: Limited data for IDV 1200mg bid + NFV 1250mg bid	Levels: IDV ↓ 38% APV ↑ 53% Dose: IDV 800mg tid, APV 800mg tid	Levels: IDV ↓ 28% NVP no effect Dose: Standard	Levels: IDV ↑ 40% Dose: IDV 600mg q 8h	Levels: IDV ↓ 31% Dose: IDV 1000mg q 8h
Ritonavir (RTV)		Levels: RTV no effect SQV ↑ 20x* ** Dose: Invirase or Fortovase 400mg bid + RTV 400mg bid	Levels: RTV no effect NFV ↑ 1.5x Dose: Limited data for RTV 400mg bid + NFV 500-750mg bid	Levels: No data	Levels: RTV ↓ 11% NVP no effect Dose: Standard	Levels: RTV ↑ 70% Dose: No data	Levels: RTV ↑ 18% EFV ↑ 21% Dose: RTV 600mg bid (500mg bid for intolerance)
Saquinavir (SQV)			Levels: SQV ↑ 3-5x NFV ↑ 20%** Dose: Standard NFV Fortovase 800mg tid (or 1200 bid)	Levels: APV ↓ 32% SQV** ↓ 19% Dose: SQV 800mg tid, APV 800mg tid	Levels: SQV ↓ 25% NVP no effect Dose: No Data	Levels: SQV ↑ 5x** DLV no effect Dose: Fortovase 800 mg tid, DLV standard (monitor transaminase levels)	Levels: SQV ↓ 62% EFV ↓ 12% Co-administration not recommended
Nelfinavir (NFV)				Levels: NFV ↑ 15% APV ↑ 9% Dose: NFV 750mg tid, APV 800mg tid	Levels: NFV ↑ 10% NVP no effect Dose: Standard	Levels: NFV ↑ 2x DLV ↓ 50% Dose: No data (monitor for neutropenic complications)	Levels: NFV ↑ 20% Dose: Standard
Nevirapine						No Data	No Data
Delavirdine					No Data		No Data
Efavirenz (EFV)				Levels: EFV ↑ 15% APV ↓ 36% Dose: Standard doses	No Data	No Data	

*Conducted with Invirase   **Conducted with Fortovase

CLINICAL PEARLS
- Using AZT during pregnancy can significantly decrease maternal transmission of HIV to the fetus. The reduction in transmission with AZT monotherapy is ~ $2/3$ (~25% with placebo and ~8% with AZT). Most clinicians now recommend 3 drug antiretroviral therapy (which contains AZT—even if AZT experienced) for all pregnant women
- The average fall in CD4 counts without therapy is about 50–80/year
- CD4 counts and viral load both independently predict risk for HIV disease progression. Using both together can provide even more diagnostic information

HIV

• Openness and honesty are paramount. Most AIDS patients will also be getting information from sources other than their physician, including the internet and friends infected with HIV. Desperation makes a believer out of a cynic. Ask your patients what other interventions they are trying

• See Chapter 114, Post-exposure Prophylaxis of HIV, for risk of transmission with various exposures (e.g., needle sharing, anal sex, etc.) to an HIV infected source

NATIONAL RESOURCES:

1. National AIDS Hotline .... 800-342-2437(AIDS)
2. National Sexually Transmitted Disease Hotline 800-227-8922
3. Experimental Drug Trial Information .... 800-874-2572 (TRIALS-A)
4. American Foundation for AIDS Research (AMFAR) .... 800-392-6327; 212-806-1600; www.amfar.org
5. National Assoc. of People With AIDS (NAPWA) 202-898-0414;www.napwa.org
6. Body Positive (Support for people HIV+) 212-566-7333;www.thebody.com

LOCAL / STATE RESOURCES: (To be filled in)

1. (Local/State) _____ AIDS Hotline ...._____
2. (Local/State) _____ HIV Support groups ...._____
3. (Local/State) _____ AIDS Task Force ...._____
4. Other local/state resources _____ ...._____

References

Gallant JE. Strategies for long-term success in the treatment of HIV infection. JAMA 2000;283:1329–34.

Carpenter CC, et al. Antiretroviral therapy in adults: updated recommendations of the International AIDS Society—USA Panel. JAMA 2000;283:381–90.

Bartlett JG. 1999 Medical management of HIV infection. Johns Hopkins Univ, Dept of infectious diseases. Baltimore, MD, 1999. Note: Available at http://www.hopkins-aids.edu/publication/book/book_toc.html

Dornadula G, Zhang H, VanUitert B, et al. Residual HIV-1 RNA in blood plasma of patients taking suppressive highly active antiretroviral therapy. JAMA 1999;282:1627–32.

Ledergerber B, Matthias Egger M, et al. AIDS-related opportunistic illnesses occurring after initiation of potent antiretroviral therapy. JAMA 1999;282:2220–6.

Martinez MA, Cabana M, Ibanez A, Clotet B, Arno A, Ruiz L.Human immunodeficiency virus type 1 genetic evolution in patients with prolonged suppression of plasma viremia. Virology1999;256:180–7.

Natarajan V, Bosche M, Metcalf JA, et al.HIV-1 replication in patients with undetectable plasma virus receiving HAART. Lancet 1999;353:119–20.

U.S. Public Health Service (USPHS) and Infectious Diseases Society of America (IDSA). 1999 USPHS/IDSA guidelines for the prevention of opportunistic infections in persons infected with human immunodeficiency virus. MMWR Aug 20 1999; 48(RR-10):1–59, 61–6.

Guidelines for the use of antiretroviral agents in HIV-infected adults and adolescents. Department of Health and Human Services and Henry J. Kaiser Family Foundation. MMWR Morb Mortal Wkly Rep. 1998 Apr 24;47(RR-5):43–82.

Vergeront JM, et al. Meeting the challenge of early identification of HIV infection in primary care. WMJ (United States), Dec 1998;97(11):52–61.

Hirsch MS, et al. Antiretroviral drug resistance testing in adults with HIV infection: implications for clinical management. International AIDS Society—USA Panel. JAMA Jun 1998;279(24):1984–91.

Mellors JW et al. Plasma viral load and CD4+ lymphocytes as prognostic markers of HIV-1 infection. Ann Intern Med J Jun 15, 1997;126:946–54.

HIV

111. AIDS-DEFINING CONDITIONS

INDICATOR CONDITIONS IN CASE DEFINITION OF AIDS (ADULTS)
  Candidiasis of esophagus, trachea, bronchi or lungs
  Cervical cancer, invasive*†
  Coccidioidomycosis, extrapulmonary*
  Cryptococcosis, extrapulmonary
  Cryptosporidiosis with diarrhea >1 month
  Cytomegalovirus of any organ other than liver, spleen or lymph nodes
  Herpes simplex with mucocutaneous ulcer >1 month or bronchitis, pneumonitis, esophagitis
  Histoplasmosis, extrapulmonary*
  HIV-associated dementia*: Disabling cognitive and/or motor dysfunction interfering with occupation or activities of daily living
  HIV-associated wasting*: Involuntary weight loss >10% of baseline plus chronic diarrhea (≥2 loose stools/day ≥30 days) or chronic weakness and documented enigmatic fever ≥30 days
  Isosporiasis with diarrhea >1 mo*
  Kaposi's sarcoma in patient under 60 yrs (or over 60 yrs*)
  Lymphoma of brain in patient under 60 yrs (or over 60 yrs*)
  Lymphoma, non-Hodgkins of B-cell or unknown immunologic phenotype and histology showing small, noncleaved lymphoma or immunoblastic sarcoma
  Mycobacterium avium or *M. kansasii*, disseminated
  Mycobacterium tuberculosis, disseminated*
  Mycobacterium tuberculosis, pulmonary*†
  *Nocardiosis**
  Pneumocystis carinii pneumonia
  Pneumonia, recurrent-bacterial (≥2 episodes in 12 months)*†
  Progressive multifocal leukoencephalopathy
  Salmonella septicemia (non-typhoid), recurrent*
  Strongyloidosis, extraintestinal
  Toxoplasmosis of internal organ
  Wasting syndrome due to HIV (as defined above—HIV-associated wasting)

*Requires positive HIV serology
†Added in the revised case definition 1993

All patients with CD4 < 200 are considered to have AIDS based on the 1993 revised case definition

HIV

112. CD4 CELL COUNTS AND ASSOCIATED CLINICAL MANIFESTATIONS

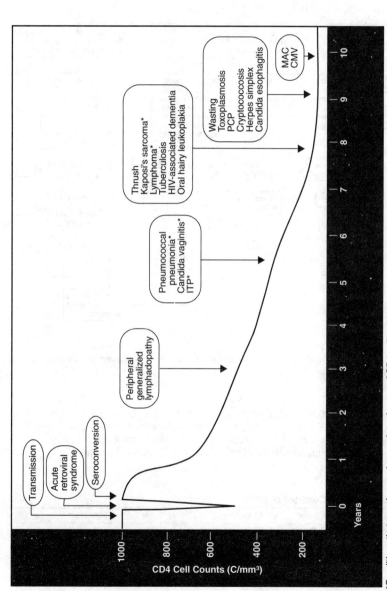

*Conditions that are observed over a broad range of CD4 cell counts

Source: Adapted from American Medical Association. HIV early intervention. Physician guidelines. 2nd ed. Chicago: American Medical Association, copyright © 1994 and Bartlett J. The Johns Hopkins hospital guide to medical care of patients with HIV infection. 4th ed. Baltimore: Williams & Wilkins, 1994. © John G. Bartlett, M.D., 1994. Used with permission.

HIV

113. WORK-UP IN PATIENTS WITH HIV/AIDS

I. HEADACHE

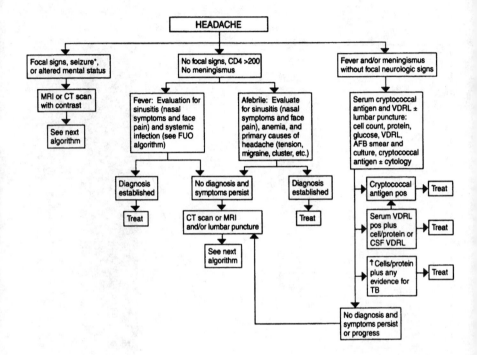

* Causes of seizures: HIV encephalitis (50%), toxoplasmosis (25%), cryptococcal meningitis (15%), lymphoma (5%), metabolic (5%)

Source: Bartlett JG. 1999 medical management of HIV infection. Baltimore, MD. Copyright © 1997, 1998, 1999, 2000 The Johns Hopkins University on behalf of its Division of Infectious Diseases and AIDS Service. All rights reserved. Used with permission.
http://hopkins-aids.edu/publications/book/ch7_1nerve_head.html

Head Scan (CT With Contrast or MRI)

Disorder	Number	Pattern	Enhancement	Location
Toxoplasmosis	1–many	Ring mass	+ +	Basal ganglia
Lymphoma	1–several	Solid mass	+ + +	Periventricular
PML	1–several	No mass	0	Subcortical white
Cryptococcosis	0–many	Punctate	0	Basal ganglia
CMV	1–several	Confluent	+ +	Periventricular
HIV encephalitis	1–several	Confluent	0	Deep white

II. ACUTE DIARRHEA

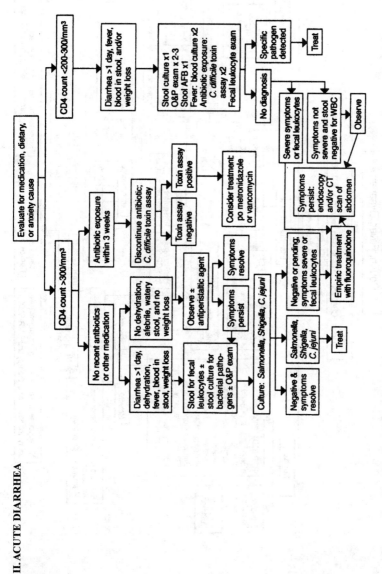

Source: Bartlett JG. 1999 medical management of HIV infection. Baltimore, MD. Copyright © 1997, 1998, 1999, 2000 The Johns Hopkins University on behalf of its Division of Infectious Diseases and AIDS Service. All rights reserved. Used with permission.
http://hopkins-aids.edu/publications/book/Chart269.html

III. PULMONARY COMPLICATIONS

HIV

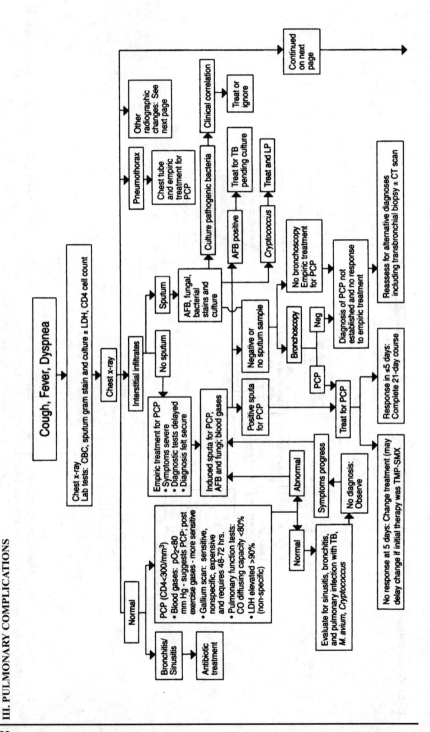

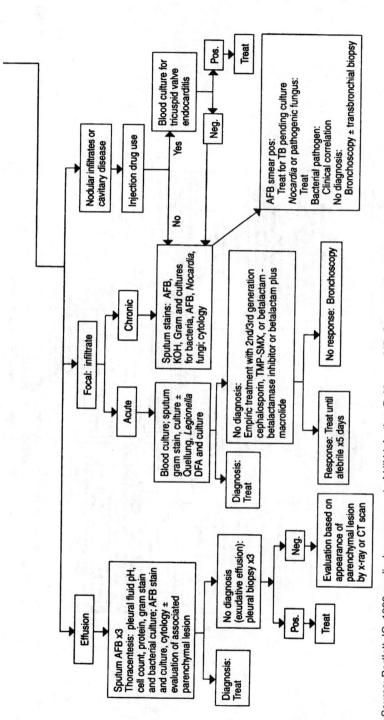

http://hopkins-aids.edu/publications/book/ch7_1pul.html#cou

HIV

IV. FEVER OF UNKNOWN ORIGIN *(FUO)*

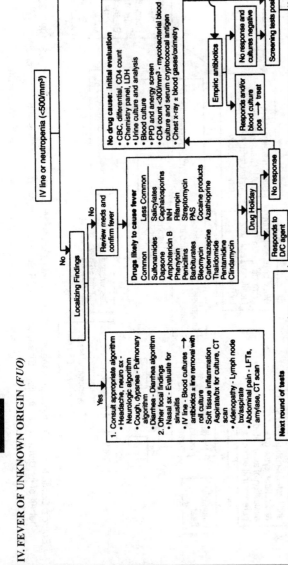

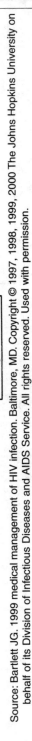

HIV

114. POST-EXPOSURE PROPHYLAXIS OF HIV

I. TRANSMISSION: HIV is transmitted by transfer of blood or body fluids
   A. Body fluids that are documented to carry sufficient virus include blood, semen, vaginal secretions, cerebrospinal fluid (CSF), synovial fluid, pleural fluid, peritoneal fluid, pericardial fluid and amniotic fluid
   B. Body fluids *not considered* to be at risk include feces, nasal secretions, sputum, saliva, sweat, tears, urine and vomitus. The safest policy for health care workers is to use universal precautions with all body fluids

II. PREVALENCE/EPIDEMIOLOGY
   A. The three groups with the highest prevalence of HIV are gay men, IV drug abusers and hemophiliacs. Wives of hemophiliac men have a rate of 20–25%. The rate in prostitutes varies with location and with concomitant IV drug use. Other routes of infection include heterosexual transmission, blood transfusions, pregnancy, breast milk
   B. As of December, 1995, all blood is screened for both HIV antibody and antigen. The use of this new technique has decreased the risk of HIV infected blood to less than one in 500,000 units of blood. Non-intimate contact and household exposure does not increase risk of transmission of HIV

III. RISK OF TRANSMISSION
   A. **Occupational exposure:** Pooled data from 23 prospective studies showed that risk after occupational exposure to needles and other contaminated devices was 0.33 percent (20 infections after 6,135 exposures). Risk is increased with
      1. Deep injury
      2. Visible blood on the injuring device
      3. Injection directly in to blood vessel
      4. Source patient with high viral titer (high viral load, end-stage AIDS, etc.)
   B. **Needle stick:** Risk of transmission varies by type of needle (hollow vs. solid), depth of penetration, amount of blood transferred, use of gloves, and the amount of virus in infected blood (asymptomatic vs. symptomatic patients)
   C. **Risk with mucocutaneous exposures:** 1 infection in 1,443 mucosal exposures (0.09%)
   D. **Risk with exposure to intact skin:** No conversions have been documented (no infections after 2,712 instances of exposure)
   E. **Risk after exposure:**

RISK OF HIV TRANSMISSION WITH SINGLE EXPOSURE FROM AN HIV-INFECTED SOURCE

Exposure	Probability / 10,000 exposures
Needle sharing	67
Percutaneous (occupational exposure)	30
Receptive anal intercourse	10-30
Receptive vaginal intercourse	8-20
Insertive vaginal sex	3-9
Insertive anal sex	3

HIV

IV. MANAGEMENT

A. Public health service statement on management of occupational exposures to HIV and recommendations for postexposure prophylaxis (MMWR, 47:RR-7)

B. Recommendations: Evaluate risk including exposure code (EC) and HIV status of body fluid/blood. Recommendations below are for a positive HIV status of body fluid/blood

  1. EC 1: Small volume exposure (few drops, limited time) to compromised skin (chapped skin, abrasion) or mucous membrane
    ➤ Offer, but toxicity of PEP may outweigh benefit

  2. EC 2: Larger volume exposure to compromised skin/mucous membranes OR less severe percutaneous exposure (superficial scratch, solid needle)
    ➤ Consider AZT/3TC without protease inhibitor (see below for doses)

  3. EC 3: Severe percutaneous exposure (large bore hollow needle, deep puncture, etc.)
    ➤ Three drug regimen (see below for dosing)

C. Timing: Initiate as soon as possible, preferably within 1–2hrs postexposure. Therapy after 72hrs is probably not effective

D. Testing: Immediately after exposure, then at 6 weeks, 3 months and 6 months. Testing at 1 year is optional (4% may seroconvert after 6 months). The antiretroviral syndrome (acute febrile illness) occurs 50–70% of the time and occurs within 2–4 weeks after exposure. Also need testing for HCV, HBV, GC, *chlamydia*. Pregnancy test if appropriate

E. Treatment regimen: AZT/3TC (may be given as **Combivir** one pill BID) +/- **Indinavir** (800mg TID) or **Nelfinavir** (1250mg BID)—see above. See Chapter 110 for table on antiretroviral therapy, drug monitoring, side effects, and cost. Note: **d4T** may be substituted for AZT if necessary

F. Duration: The optimal duration is unknown. Recommendations are 4 weeks

CLINICAL PEARLS

- The CDC does not recommend postexposure prophylaxis after exposure to urine
- The risk of sexual exposure to a person with *N. Gonorrhea* is 20–25% per contact
- The prevalence of AIDS in US prisons is 14 times that in the general population. Prison rape may represent a high risk exposure

References

Bamberger JD, et al. Postexposure prophylaxis for human immunodeficiency virus (HIV) infection following sexual assault. Am J Med March 1999;106:323–6.

Henderson DK. Postexposure chemoprophylaxis for occupational exposures to the human immunodeficiency virus. JAMA March 1999;281:931–6.

1999 Medical management of HIV infection. John G. Bartlett, MD. Johns Hopkins University, Dept. of infectious diseases. Baltimore, MD, 1999 Note: Available at http://www.hopkins-aids.edu/publication/book/book_toc.html.

Kats MH and Gerberding JL. Postexposure treatment of people exposed to the human immunodeficiency virus through sexual contact or injection drug use. N Engl J Med 1997; 336:1097–1100.

HIV

XIII. Appendix

APPX

115. FORMULAS

A. Anion gap:

$$AG = Na^+ - (Cl^- + HCO_3)$$

$$Normal = 8\text{--}16 \ mEq / L$$

B. Creatinine clearance (CrCl):

1. $CrCl \ (male) = \dfrac{(140 - age) \times weight \ (kg)}{Serum \ creatinine \times 72}$

2. $CrCl \ (female) = 0.85 \times CrCl \ (male)$

C. Fractional excretion of sodium:

$$Fe_{Na} = \frac{U_{Na} / P_{Na}}{U_{Cr} / P_{Cr}} \times 100$$

D. Serum osmolality:

$$Osm = 2(Na^+ + K^+) + (Glucose / 18) + (BUN / 2.8)$$

E. A–a Gradient:

$$= (713 \times F_1O_2) - (PaCO_2 \times 1.2) - PaO_2$$

Note: Pressures are at sea level
F_1O_2 at room air is 0.21
(Normal A–a Gradient = 5–15)

F. Corrected sodium with hyperglycemia:

$$Corrected \ Na^+ = Na^+ + [1.6 \times (Glucose - 140) / 100]$$

G. LDL Cholesterol:

$$LDL \ cholesterol = Total \ cholesterol - HDL \ cholesterol - \left(\frac{triglycerides}{5} \right)$$

APPX

Michael B. Weinstock, MD

116. SYMPTOMATIC MEDICATIONS: COLDS AND FLU, SINUSITIS, BRONCHITIS, ETC.

DRUG	COMPONENTS	ADULT DOSE	PEDIATRIC DOSE	OTC/Rx
		ANTITUSSIVES		
Hycodan	Hydrocodone bitartrate 5mg, Homatropine methylbromide 1.5mg, per tab or per 5mL	5mL or 1 tab PO Q4–6hrs PRN	Under 6 y/o: Not rec. 6–12 y/o: 2.5mL or 1 tab PO Q4–6hrs PRN — max dose 15mL/day	Rx (Class III)
Robitussin Pediatric	Dextromethorphan 7.5mg per 5mL	—	Under 2y/o: Not rec. 2–6 y/o: 5mL PO Q6–8hrs 6–12 y/o: 10mL PO Q6–8hrs	OTC
Tessalon	Benzonatate 100mg	100mg PO TID — max dose 600mg/day	Under 10 y/o: Not rec. Over 10 y/o: Same as adult	Rx
		ANTITUSSIVES, EXPECTORANTS		
Humibid DM	Dextromethorphan 30mg, Guaifenesin 600mg per tab, sustained release	1–2 tabs PO Q12hrs	Under 2 y/o: Not rec. 2–6 y/o: ½ tab PO Q12hrs 6–12 y/o: 1 tab PO Q12hrs	Rx
Hycotuss, Vicodin Tuss	Hydrocodone bitartrate 5mg, Guaifenesin 100mg per 5mL	5mL PO after meals and QHS, at least 4 hours apart — max dose 30mL/day	Under 6 y/o: Not rec. 6–12 y/o: 2.5–5mL PO Q4–6	Rx (Class III)
Tussi-Organidin	Codeine phosphate 10mg, Iodinated glycerol 30mg per 5mL	5–10mL PO Q4hrs	Under 6 y/o: Not rec. 6–12 y/o: 5mL PO Q4–6hrs	Rx (Class V)
Robitussin DM	Dextromethorphan 10mg, Guaifenesin 100mg per 5mL	10mL PO Q4hrs	Under 2 y/o: Not rec. 2–6 y/o: 2.5mL PO Q4hrs 6–12 y/o: 5mL PO Q4hrs	OTC
Robitussin A–C	Codeine phosphate 10mg, Guaifenesin 100mg per 5mL	10mL PO Q4hrs	Under 6 y/o: Not rec. 6–12 y/o: 5mL PO Q4hrs	Rx (Class V)
		ANTITUSSIVE, EXPECTORANTS, SYMPATHOMIMETICS		
Duratuss HD	Hydrocodone bitartrate 5mg, Guaifenesin 100mg, Pseudoephedrine 30mg per 5mL	10mL PO Q4–6hrs	Under 6 y/o: Not rec. 6–12 y/o: 5mL PO Q4–6hrs	Rx (Class III)
Naldecon CX	Codeine phosphate 10mg, Guaifenesin 200mg, Phenylpropanolamine 12.5mg per 5mL	10mL PO Q4hrs	Not recommended	Rx (Class V)
Naldecon DX, Robitussin CF	Dextromethorphan 10mg, Guaifenesin (Naldecon DX: 200mg; Robitussin CF: 100mg), Phenylpropano-amine 12.5mg per 5 mL	10mL PO Q4hrs	Under 2 y/o: Not rec. 2–6 y/o: 2.5mL PO Q4hrs 6–12 y/o: 5–10mL PO Q4hrs	OTC
Robitussin DAC	Codeine phosphate 10mg, Guaifenesin 100mg, Pseudoephedrine 30mg per 5mL	5–10mL PO Q4hrs — max dose 40mL/day	Under 6 y/o: Not rec. 6–12 y/o: 5mL PO Q4–6hrs — max dose 20mL/day	Rx (Class V)
		ANTITUSSIVES, ANTIHISTAMINES, SYMPATHOMIMETICS		
Actifed with codeine	Codeine phosphate 10mg, Triprolidine 1.25mg, Pseudoephedrine 30mg per 5mL	10mL PO TID–QID	Under 2 y/o: Not rec. 2–6 y/o: 2.5mL PO TID–QID 6–12 y/o: 5–10mL PO TID–QID	Rx (Class V)
Bromfed-DM, Dimetane-DX	Dextromethorphan 10mg, Brompheniramine 2mg, Pseudoephedrine 30mg per 5mL	10mL PO Q4hrs	Under 2 y/o: Not rec. 2–6 y/o: 2.5mL PO Q4hrs 6–12 y/o: 5mL PO Q4hrs	Rx
Rondec-DM	Dextromethorphan 15mg, Carbinoxamine 4mg, Pseudoephedrine 60mg per 5mL	5mL PO QID	Under 18 months: Use Rondec-DM drops 18 mo.–6 y/o: 2.5mL PO QID Over 6 y/o: Same as adults	Rx

DRUG	COMPONENTS	ADULT DOSE	PEDIATRIC DOSE	OTC/Rx
Triaminic Nite Light	Dextromethorphan7.5mg, Chlorpheniramine 1mg, Pseudoephedrine 15mg per 5mL	20mL PO Q6hrs	Under 3 months: Not rec. 3–12 mo. (12–17 lbs): 1.25mL PO Q6hrs 1–2 y/o (18–23 lbs): 2.5mL PO Q6hrs 2–6 y/o: 5mL PO Q6hrs 6–12 y/o: 10mL PO Q6hrs	OTC
Dimetapp DM	Dextromethorphan 10mg, Brompheniramine 2mg, Phenylpropanolamine 12.5mg per 5mL	10mL PO Q4hrs	Under 2 y/o: Not rec. 2–6 y/o: 2.5mL PO Q4hrs 6–12 y/o: 5mL PO Q4hrs	OTC
SYMPATHOMIMETICS				
Afrin	Pseudoephedrine 120mg SR	1 tab PO Q12hrs	Not recommended	OTC
Sudafed Sudafed 12 HR Sudafed Liquid	Pseudoephedrine 30, 60mg; 120mg (Sudafed 12HR); 30mg/5mL (liquid)	60mg PO Q4–6hrs or 1 12-hour tab Q12hrs — max dose 240mg/day	Under 2 y/o: Not rec. 2–6 y/o: 2.5mL PO Q4–6hrs 6–12 y/o: 5mL PO Q4–6hrs	OTC
SYMPATHOMIMETICS, EXPECTORANTS				
Entex	Phenylephrine 5mg, Phenylpropanolamine 45mg, Guaifenesin 200mg	1 cap PO QID with food or liquid	Use liquid	Rx
Entex LA	Phenylpropanolamine 75mg, Guaifenesin 400mg, sustained release	1 tab PO Q12hrs	Under 6 y/o: Not rec. 6–12 y/o: ½ tab PO Q12hrs	Rx
Entex PSE	Phenylpropanolamine 120mg, Guaifenesin 600mg, sustained release	1 tab PO Q12hrs	Under 6 y/o: Not rec. 6–12 y/o: ½ tab PO Q12hrs	Rx
Entex LIQ	Phenylephrine 5mg, Phenylpropanolamine 20mg, Guaifenesin 100mg per 5mL	10mL PO QID	Under 2 y/o: Not rec. 2–4 y/o: 2.5mL PO QID 4–6 y/o: 5mL PO QID 6–12 y/o: 7.5mL PO Q4hrs	Rx
Naldecon EX Child	Phenylpropanolamine 6.25mg, Guaifenesin 100mg per 5mL	not applicable	Under 2 y/o: Not rec. 2–6 y/o: 5mL PO Q4hrs 6–12 y/o: 10mL PO QID	OTC
Naldecon EX Ped drops	Phenylpropanolamine 6.25mg, Guaifenesin 100mg per 5mL	not applicable	Under 2 y/o: Not rec. 1–3 mo.: 0.25mL PO Q4hrs 4–6 mo.: 0.5mL PO Q4hrs 7–9 mo.: 0.75mL PO Q4hrs 10 mo.–2 y/o: 1mL PO Q4hrs	OTC
Robitussin PE	Pseudoephedrine 30mg, Guaifenesin 100mg per 5mL	10mL PO Q4hrs	Under 2 y/o: Not rec. 2–6 y/o: 2.5mL PO Q4hrs 6–12 y/o: 5mL PO Q4hrs	OTC
Triaminic expectorant	Phenylpropanolamine 6.25mg, Guaifenesin 50mg per 5mL	20mL PO Q4hrs	Under 3 mo.: Not rec. 3 mo.–1 y/o: 1.25mL PO Q4hrs 1–2 y/o: 2.5mL PO Q4hrs 2–6 y/o: 5mL PO Q4hrs 6–12 y/o: 10mL PO Q4hrs	OTC
EXPECTORANTS				
Organidin	Iodinated glycerol 30mg	2 tabs QID with liquid	Up to half adult dose	Rx
Robitussin	Guaifenesin 100mg per 5mL	10–20mL PO Q4hrs	Under 2 y/o: Not rec. 2–6 y/o: 2.5–5mL PO Q4hrs 6–12 y/o: 5–10mL PO Q4hrs	OTC
Humibid LA	Guaifenesin 600mg, sustained release, scored tabs	1–2 tabs PO Q12hrs	Under 2 y/o: Not rec. 2–6 y/o: ½ tab PO Q12hrs 6–12 y/o: 1 tab PO Q12hrs	Rx
Naldecon Senior EX	Guaifenesin 100mg per 5mL	10mL PO Q4hrs	Not recommended	OTC
ANTIHISTAMINES				
Atarax	Hydroxyzine 10mg/tab Hydroxyzine 10mg/5mL	25mg PO TID–QID	Under 6 y/o: 50mg PO daily Over 6 y/o: 50–100mg PO QD	Rx
Benadryl	Diphenhydramine 25, 50mg Diphenhydramine 12.5mg/5mL	25–50mg PO TID–QID	Over 20 lbs: 5–10mL PO TID–QID — max dose 5mg/kg/day	OTC
Chlor-trimeton	Chlorpheniramine 4mg tabs Chlorpheniramine 2mg/5mL	4mg PO Q4–6hrs	Under 2 y/o: Not rec. 2–5 y/o: 2.5mL PO Q4–6hrs 6–11 y/o: 5mL PO Q4–6hrs	OTC
Claritin	Loratadine 10 mg tabs	1 PO QD on empty stomach	Under 12 y/o: Not rec.	Rx
Seldane	Terfenadine 60mg tabs	1 PO BID	Under 12 y/o: Not rec.	Rx
Hismanal	Astemizole 10mg tabs	1 PO QD on empty stomach	Under 12 y/o: Not rec.	Rx

— *See Chapter 59, Allergic Rhinitis/Seasonal Allergies, for information on nasal inhalers and ophthalmic solutions.*

APPX

DRUG	COMPONENTS	ADULT DOSE	PEDIATRIC DOSE	OTC/Rx
		ANTIHISTAMINES, SYMPATHOMIMETICS		
Actifed **Actifed syrup**	Triprolidine 2.5mg, Pseudoephedrine 60mg Note: Syrup contains ½ amount per 5mL	1 tab or 10mL PO, Q4–6hrs PRN	Under 6 y/o: Not rec. Over 6 y/o: ½ tab or 5mL, Q4–6hrs PRN max. 4 doses/day	OTC
Dimetapp	Brompheniramine 2 mg, Phenylpropanolamine 12.5mg per 5mL	10mL PO Q4hrs	Under 2 y/o: Not rec. 2–6 y/o: 2.5–5mL PO Q4hrs 6–12 y/o: 5–10mL PO Q4hrs	OTC
Dimetapp **extentabs**	Brompheniramine 12mg, Phenylpropanolamine 75mg	1 tab PO Q12hrs	Not recommended	OTC
Rondec	Carbinoxamine 4mg, Pseudoephedrine 60mg per tab or by 5mL	1 tab or 5mL PO QID	Under 18 mo.: Not rec. 18 mo.–6 y/o: 2.5mL PO QID	Rx
Rondec TR	Carbinoxamine 4mg, Pseudoephedrine 120mg per sustained release tab	1 tab PO Q12hrs	Not recommended	Rx
Seldane-D (non-sedating)	Terfenadine 60mg Pseudoephedrine 120mg per sustained release tab	1 tab PO BID	Not recommended	Rx

APPX

117. ADULT ADVANCED CARDIAC LIFE SUPPORT (ACLS) PROTOCOLS

Source: Emergency Cardiac Care Committee and Subcommittees, American Heart Association. Guidelines for cardiopulmonary resuscitation and emergency cardiac care, III: adult advanced cardiac life support. JAMA 1992; 268:2199-2241. Copyright 1992, American Medical Association. Used with permission.

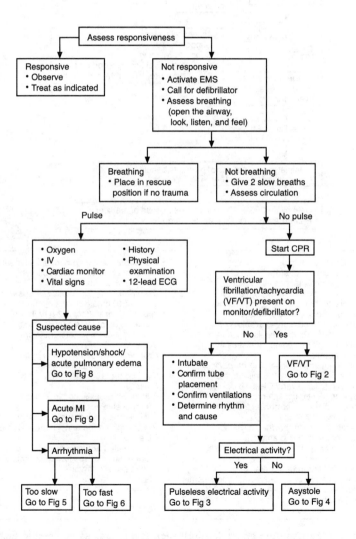

Figure 1. Universal algorithm for adult emergency cardiac care (ECC).

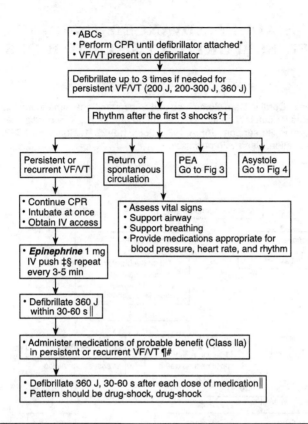

- ABCs
- Perform CPR until defibrillator attached*
- VF/VT present on defibrillator

Defibrillate up to 3 times if needed for persistent VF/VT (200 J, 200-300 J, 360 J)

Rhythm after the first 3 shocks?†

| Persistent or recurrent VF/VT | Return of spontaneous circulation | PEA Go to Fig 3 | Asystole Go to Fig 4 |

- Continue CPR
- Intubate at once
- Obtain IV access

- Assess vital signs
- Support airway
- Support breathing
- Provide medications appropriate for blood pressure, heart rate, and rhythm

- *Epinephrine* 1 mg IV push ‡§ repeat every 3-5 min

- Defibrillate 360 J within 30-60 s ‖

- Administer medications of probable benefit (Class IIa) in persistent or recurrent VF/VT ¶#

- Defibrillate 360 J, 30-60 s after each dose of medication‖
- Pattern should be drug-shock, drug-shock

Class I: definitely helpful
Class IIa: acceptable, probably helpful
Class IIb: acceptable, possibly helpful
Class III: not indicated, may be harmful
*Precordial thump is a Class IIb action in witnessed arrest, no pulse, and no defibrillator immediately available.
†Hypothermic cardiac arrest is treated differently after this point. See section on hypothermia.
‡The recommended dose of *epinephrine* is 1 mg IV push every 3-5 min. If this approach fails, several Class IIb dosing regimens can be considered:
- Intermediate: *epinephrine* 2-5 mg IV push, every 3-5 min
- Escalating: *epinephrine* 1mg-3mg-5 mg IV push (3 min apart)
- High: *epinephrine* 0.1 mg/kg IV push, every 3-5 min
§*Sodium bicarbonate* (1mEq/kg) is Class I if patient has known preexisting hyperkalemia
‖Multiple sequenced shocks (200 J, 200-300 J, 360 J) are acceptable here (Class I), especially when medications are delayed

¶ • *Lidocaine* 1.5 mg/kg IV push. Repeat in 3-5 min to total loading dose of 3 mg/kg; then use
- *Bretylium* 5 mg/kg IV push. Repeat in 5 min at 10 mg/kg
- *Magnesium sulfate* 1-2 g IV in torsades de pointes or suspected hypomagnesemic state or severe refractory VF
- *Procainamide* 30 mg/min in refractory VF (maximum total 17 mg/kg)
• *Sodium bicarbonate* (1mEq/kg IV):
  Class IIa
  - if known preexisting bicarbonate-responsive acidosis
  - if overdose with tricyclic antidepressants
  - to alkalinize the urine in drug overdoses
  Class IIb
  - if intubated and continued long arrest interval
  - upon return of spontaneous circulation after long arrest interval
  Class III
  - hypoxic lactic acidosis

Figure 2. Algorithm for ventricular fibrillation and pulseless ventricular tachycardia (VF/VT)

PEA includes
- Electromechanical dissociation (EMD)
- Pseudo-EMD
- Idioventricular rhythms
- Ventricular escape rhythms
- Bradyasystolic rhythms
- Postdefibrillation idioventricular rhythms

- Continue CPR
- Intubate at once
- Obtain IV access
- Assess blood flow using Doppler ultrasound

↓

Consider possible causes
(Parentheses = possible therapies and treatments)
- Hypovolemia (volume infusion)
- Hypoxia (ventilation)
- Cardiac tamponade (pericardiocentesis)
- Tension pneumothorax (needle decompression)
- Hypothermia (see hypothermia algorithm, Section IV)
- Massive pulmonary embolism (surgery, ***thrombolytics***)
- Drug overdoses such as tricyclics, digitalis, β-blockers, calcium channel blockers
- Hyperkalemia*
- Acidosis†
- Massive acute myocardial infarction (go to Fig 9)

↓

- ***Epinephrine*** 1 mg IV push, *‡ repeat every 3-5 min

↓

- If absolute bradycardia (<60 beats/min) or relative bradycardia, give ***atropine*** 1mg IV
- Repeat every 3-5 min up to a total of 0.04 mg/kg§

Class I: definitely helpful
Class IIa: acceptable, probably helpful
Class IIb: acceptable, possibly helpful
Class III: not indicated, may be harmful
****Sodium bicarbonate*** 1mEq/kg is Class I if patient has known preexisting hyperkalemia.
†***Sodium bicarbonate*** 1mEq/kg:
   Class IIa
- if known preexisting bicarbonate-responsive acidosis
- if overdose with tricyclic antidepressants
- to alkalinize the urine in drug overdoses
   Class IIb
- if intubated and continued long arrest interval
- upon return of spontaneous circulation after long arrest interval
   Class III
- hypoxic lactic acidosis
‡The recommended dose of ***epinephrine*** is 1 mg IV push every 3-5 min.
   If this approach fails, several Class IIb dosing regimens can be considered.
- Intermediate:***epinephrine*** 2-5 mg IV push, every 3-5 min
- Escalating:***epinephrine*** 1mg-3mg-5 mg IV push (3 min apart)
- High:***epinephrine*** 0.1 mg/kg IV push, every 3-5 min
§Shorter ***atropine*** dosing intervals are possibly helpful in cardiac arrest (Class IIb).

Figure 3. Algorithm for pulseless electrical activity (PEA) (electromechanical dissociation [EMD]).

APPX

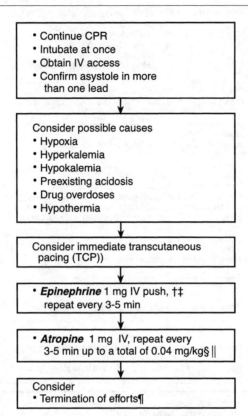

- Continue CPR
- Intubate at once
- Obtain IV access
- Confirm asystole in more than one lead

Consider possible causes
- Hypoxia
- Hyperkalemia
- Hypokalemia
- Preexisting acidosis
- Drug overdoses
- Hypothermia

Consider immediate transcutaneous pacing (TCP))

- *Epinephrine* 1 mg IV push, †‡ repeat every 3-5 min

- *Atropine* 1 mg IV, repeat every 3-5 min up to a total of 0.04 mg/kg§ ||

Consider
- Termination of efforts¶

Class I: definitely helpful
Class IIa: acceptable, probably helpful
Class IIb: acceptable, possibly helpful
Class III: not indicated, may be harmful
*TCP is a Class IIb intervention. Lack of success may be due to delays in pacing. To be effective TCP must be performed early, simultaneously with drugs. Evidence does not support routine use of TCP for asystole.
†The recommended dose of *epinephrine* is 1 mg IV push every 3-5 min. If this approach fails, several Class IIb dosing regimens can be considered:
- Intermediate: *epinephrine* 2-5 mg IV push, every 3-5 min
- Escalating: *epinephrine* 1mg-3mg-5 mg IV push (3 min apart)
- High: *epinephrine* 0.1 mg/kg IV push, every 3-5 min
‡*Sodium bicarbonate* 1mEq/kg is Class I if patient has known preexisting hyperkalemia.

§Shorter *atropine* dosing intervals are Class IIb in asystolic arrest .
|| *Sodium bicarbonate* 1mEq/kg:
Class IIa
- if known preexisting bicarbonate-responsive acidosis
- if overdose with tricyclic antidepressants
- to alkalinize the urine in drug overdoses
Class IIb
- if intubated and continued long arrest interval
- upon return of spontaneous circulation after long arrest interval
Class III
- hypoxic lactic acidosis
¶If patient remains in asystole or other agonal rhythms after successful intubation and initial medications and no reversible causes are identified, consider termination of resuscitative efforts by a physician. Consider interval since arrest.

Figure 4. Asystole treatment algorithm.

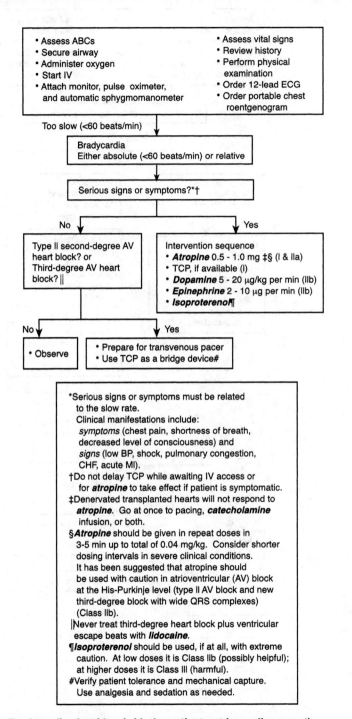

Figure 5. Bradycardia algorithm (with the patient not in cardiac arrest).

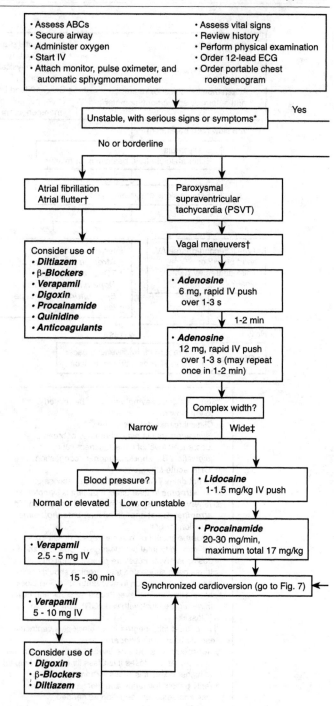

Figure 6. Tachycardia algorithm.

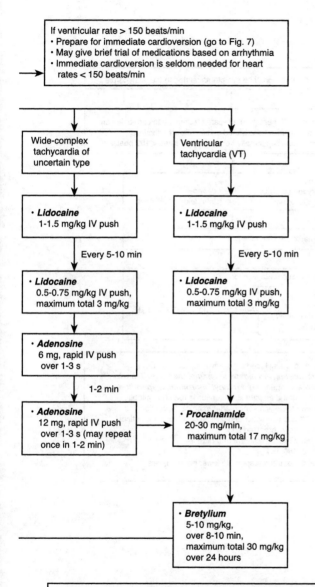

If ventricular rate > 150 beats/min
- Prepare for immediate cardioversion (go to Fig. 7)
- May give brief trial of medications based on arrhythmia
- Immediate cardioversion is seldom needed for heart rates < 150 beats/min

Wide-complex tachycardia of uncertain type

Ventricular tachycardia (VT)

- *Lidocaine* 1-1.5 mg/kg IV push

- *Lidocaine* 1-1.5 mg/kg IV push

Every 5-10 min

Every 5-10 min

- *Lidocaine* 0.5-0.75 mg/kg IV push, maximum total 3 mg/kg

- *Lidocaine* 0.5-0.75 mg/kg IV push, maximum total 3 mg/kg

- *Adenosine* 6 mg, rapid IV push over 1-3 s

1-2 min

- *Adenosine* 12 mg, rapid IV push over 1-3 s (may repeat once in 1-2 min)

- *Procainamide* 20-30 mg/min, maximum total 17 mg/kg

- *Bretylium* 5-10 mg/kg, over 8-10 min, maximum total 30 mg/kg over 24 hours

*Unstable condition must be related to the tachycardia. Signs and symptoms may include chest pain, shortness of breath, decreased level of consciousness, low blood pressure (BP), shock, pulmonary congestion, congestive heart failure, acute myocardial infarction.
†Carotid sinus pressure is contraindicated in patients with carotid bruits; avoid ice water immersion in patients with ischemic heart disease.
‡If the wide-complex tachycardia is known with certainty to be PSVT and BP is normal/elevated, sequence can include *verapamil*.

Figure 6. Tachycardia algorithm (continued).

APPX

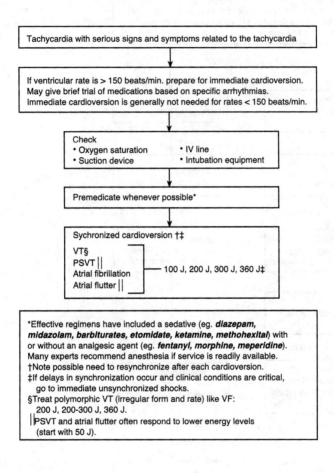

Figure 7. Electrical cardioversion algorithm (with the patient not in cardiac arrest).

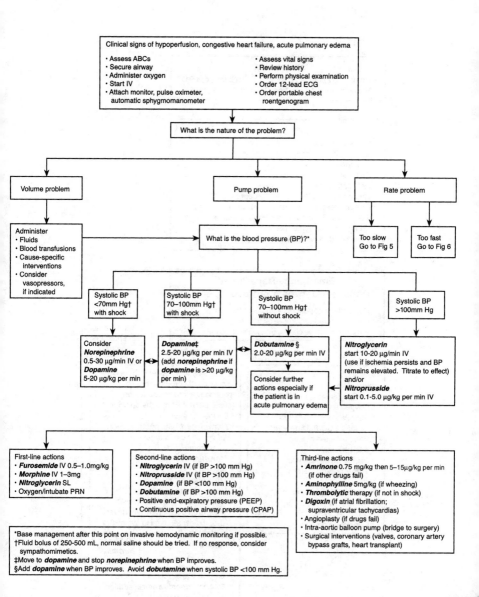

Figure 8. Algorithm for hypotension, shock, and acute pulmonary edema.

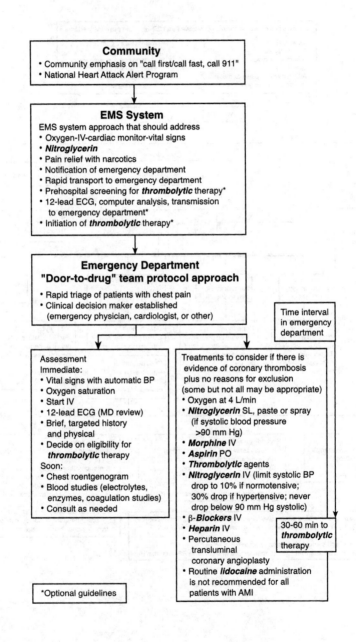

Community
- Community emphasis on "call first/call fast, call 911"
- National Heart Attack Alert Program

EMS System
EMS system approach that should address
- Oxygen-IV-cardiac monitor-vital signs
- *Nitroglycerin*
- Pain relief with narcotics
- Notification of emergency department
- Rapid transport to emergency department
- Prehospital screening for *thrombolytic* therapy*
- 12-lead ECG, computer analysis, transmission to emergency department*
- Initiation of *thrombolytic* therapy*

Emergency Department
"Door-to-drug" team protocol approach
- Rapid triage of patients with chest pain
- Clinical decision maker established (emergency physician, cardiologist, or other)

Time interval in emergency department

Assessment
Immediate:
- Vital signs with automatic BP
- Oxygen saturation
- Start IV
- 12-lead ECG (MD review)
- Brief, targeted history and physical
- Decide on eligibility for *thrombolytic* therapy
Soon:
- Chest roentgenogram
- Blood studies (electrolytes, enzymes, coagulation studies)
- Consult as needed

Treatments to consider if there is evidence of coronary thrombosis plus no reasons for exclusion (some but not all may be appropriate)
- Oxygen at 4 L/min
- *Nitroglycerin* SL, paste or spray (if systolic blood pressure >90 mm Hg)
- *Morphine* IV
- *Aspirin* PO
- *Thrombolytic* agents
- *Nitroglycerin* IV (limit systolic BP drop to 10% if normotensive; 30% drop if hypertensive; never drop below 90 mm Hg systolic)
- β-*Blockers* IV
- *Heparin* IV
- Percutaneous transluminal coronary angioplasty
- Routine *lidocaine* administration is not recommended for all patients with AMI

30-60 min to *thrombolytic* therapy

*Optional guidelines

APPX

Figure 9. Acute myocardial infarction (AMI) algorithm. Recommendations for early treatment of patients with chest pain and possible AMI.

Miriam Chan, PharmD

118. COMMON ADULT EMERGENCY DRUG DOSAGE[1]

Drug	Indications	Dosage	Comments
Adenosine	1. PSVT 2. Wide QRS-complex tachy-cardia of uncertain type	6mg rapid IVP over 1–3 sec; if no response in 1–2 min, repeat 6 or 12mg rapid IVP over 1–3 sec.	Common side effects: transient chest pain, flushing and dyspnea
Atropine	1. Symptomatic bradycardia 2. AV block at the nodal level 3. Asystole Note: Will not work with cardiac transplant patients	0.5–1.0mg IVP Q3–5 min 1mg IVP Q 3–5 min	Maximum dose: 3mg (0.04mg/kg)
Bretylium	1. Refractory VF/pulseless VT 2. Resistant VT, wide-complex tachycardia of uncertain type	5mg/kg IVP, then 10mg/kg Q5 min 5–10mg/kg IVPB over 8–10 min	1. Maximum dose: 30–35mg/kg 2. Maintenance drip: 1–2mg/min (Conc: 2g in 500mL D_5W or NS)
Epinephrine	1. Cardiac arrest 2. As a vasopressor in sympto-matic bradycardia	Recommended dose: 1mg (1:10,000) IVP Q3–5 min If this fails, may use: 2–5mg IVP Q3–5 min or 1mg-3mg-5mg IVP 3 min apart or 0.1mg/kg IVP Q3–5 min 2–10mcg/min IV infusion. titrate to effect	May use continuous infusion via central line: 30mg/250mL at 100mL/hr (comparable to 1mg Q5 min)
Isoproterenol	1. Refractory torsades de pointes 2. Symptomatic bradycardia	Use low doses: 2–10mcg/min IV infusion, titrate to effect	At high doses, it can exacerbate ischemia and arrhythmia
Lidocaine	1. VF/pulseless VT 2. PVCs, VT, wide-complex tachycardia of uncertain type, wide complex PSVT	1.5mg/kg IVP, repeat in 3–5 min 1.0–1.5mg/kg IVP, repeat with 0.5–0.75mg/kg IVP Q 5–10 min	1. Maximum dose: 3mg/kg 2. Maintenance drip: 2–4mg/min (Conc: 2g in 500mL D_5W or NS)
Magnesium Sulfate	1. Torsades de pointes 2. Suspected hypomagnesemia 3. Severe refractory VF/pulseless VT	1–2g/100mL infuse over 1–2 min during cardiac arrest	In acute MI patient with docu-mented Mg deficiency, $MgSO_4$ may be given as 1–2g / 50–100mL over 5–60 min, followed by an infusion of 0.5–1g/hr × 24 hr
Procainamide	1. PVCs, recurrent VT, wide-complex tachycardia of uncertain type 2. Refractory VF / pulseless VT	20–30mg/min IV infusion until effect, maximum dose = 17mg/kg. S/E Hypotension, or QRS > 50% its orignal width (May give as 1g in 50mL D_5W or NS)	1. Maintenance drip: 1–4mg/min (Conc: 2g in 500mL D_5W or NS) 2. Avoid use in patients with prolonged QT interval or torsades de pointes
Sodium Bicarbonate	1. Hyperkalemia 2. Not recommended for routine use during arrest (use appropri-ately according to clinical situation)	Use ABG to guide therapy. If ABG unavailable, 1mEq/kg IVP then ½ dose Q 10 min	Adequate ventilation and restoration of tissue perfusion are essential
Verapamil	1. To control ventricular rate in atrial fibrillation and atrial flutter 2. Narrow-complex PSVT	2.5–5mg IVP over 2 min, repeat PRN. 5–10mg Q 15–30 min to a maximum of 20mg	1. In elderly, give 2–4mg over 3–4 min 2. S/E — Hypotension

APPX

---

[1] This table is a summary of ACLS drug dosage recommendations (JAMA, 1992;268:2199–2241). It is intended to serve only as a quick reference. One should refer to appropriate references for detailed information.

Miriam Chan, PharmD

119. PREPARATION OF INFUSION FOR ADULT EMERGENCY DRUGS

Drug	Dosage Range	Infusion Concentration	Drip Rate (mL/hr) (assume a 70kg patient)
Bretylium	1–2mg/min	2g/500mL	1mg/min = 15mL/hr
Dobutamine	2.0–20mcg/kg/min	500mg/250mL	2mcg/kg/min = 4mL/hr
Dopamine	2.0–20mcg/kg/min	400mg/250mL	5mcg/kg/min = 13mL/hr
Epinephrine	2–10mcg/min	2mg/250mL	2mcg/min = 15mL/hr
Isoproterenol	2–10mcg/min	2mg/250mL	2mcg/min = 15mL/hr
Lidocaine	2–4mg/min	2g/500mL	2mg/mL = 30mL/hr
Nitroglycerin (IV)	start 10–20mcg/min	50mg/250mL	10mcg/min = 3mL/hr
Nitroprusside	0.1–5.0mcg/kg/min	50mg/250mL	0.1mcg/kg/min = 2mL/hr
Norepinephrine	0.5–30mcg/min	8mg/250mL	0.5mcg/min = 1mL/hr
Phenylephrine	start 25–40mcg/min	50mg/250mL	50mcg/min = 15mL/hr
Procainamide	1–4mg/min	2g/500mL	1mg/min = 15mL/hr

INDEX

Note: Chapter titles are in all capitals

INDEX

INDEX

INDEX

INDEX

INDEX

INDEX

INDEX

INDEX

INDEX

Frequently Called Consultants

Allergy Name _____
Office _____
Beeper _____

Cardiology Name _____
Office _____
Beeper _____

Dentistry Name _____
Office _____
Beeper _____

Dermatology Name _____
Office _____
Beeper _____

Endocrinology Name _____
Office _____
Beeper _____

GI Name _____
Office _____
Beeper _____

Heme/Onc Name _____
Office _____
Beeper _____

Infectious Disease Name _____
Office _____
Beeper _____

Nephrology Name _____
Office _____
Beeper _____

Neurology Name _____
Office _____
Beeper _____

OB/GYN Name _____
Office _____
Beeper _____

Ophthalmology   Name _____
                    Office _____
                    Beeper _____

Podiatry   Name _____
                    Office _____
                    Beeper _____

Psychiatry   Name _____
                    Office _____
                    Beeper _____

Rheumatology   Name _____
                    Office _____
                    Beeper _____

SURGERY

General   Name _____
                    Office _____
                    Beeper _____

Neurologic   Name _____
                    Office _____
                    Beeper _____

Orthopedic   Name _____
                    Office _____
                    Beeper _____

Plastic   Name _____
                    Office _____
                    Beeper _____

Urologic   Name _____
                    Office _____
                    Beeper _____

Vascular/Thoracic Name _____
                       Office _____
                       Beeper _____

Notes

FREQUENTLY USED PHONE NUMBERS

Admitting .... _____

CT Scan .... _____

Diabetes Education .... _____

ECG .... _____

EEG .... _____

Emergency Room .... _____

Lab .... _____

Labor & Delivery .... _____

MRI .... _____

Medical Records .... _____

Newborn Nursery .... _____

Pathology .... _____

Peripheral Vascular Lab .... _____

PFT Lab .... _____

Pharmacy .... _____

Physical Therapy .... _____

Protective Services .... _____

X-ray .... _____

_____   .... _____

_____   .... _____

_____   .... _____